Research Methods in Athletic Training

Research Methods in Athletic Training

Brent L. Arnold, PhD, ATC
Virginia Commonwealth University
Richmond, VA

Bruce M. Gansneder, PhD
University of Virginia
Charlottesville, VA

David H. Perrin, PhD, ATC, FACSM
University of North Carolina–Greensboro
Greensboro, NC

F.A. Davis Company • Philadelphia

F. A. Davis Company
1915 Arch Street
Philadelphia, PA 19103
www.fadavis.com

Copyright © 2005 by F. A. Davis Company

Printed in the United States of America

Last digit indicates print number: 10 9 8 7 6 5 4 3 2 1

Acquisitions Editor: Christa Fratantoro
Design and Illustration Manager: Joan Wendt
Developmental Editors: Laura Horowitz and Melissa Reed

Library of Congress Cataloging-in-Publication Data

Arnold, Brent L.
  Research methods in athletic training / Brent L. Arnold, Bruce Gansneder, David Perrin.
    p. ; cm.
  Includes bibliographical references and index.
  ISBN 0-8036-0778-4 (softcover : alk. paper)
  1. Sports medicine—Research—Methodology. 2. Physical education and training—Research—Methodology.
[DNLM: 1. Sports—education. 2. Athletic Injuries—prevention & control. 3. Research—methods. 4. Research Design. 5. Writing. QT 260 A7522r 2005] I. Gansneder, Bruce Michael, 1941- II. Perrin, David H., 1954- III. Title.
  RC1210.A755 2005
  617.1'027'072—dc22

                                                                                    2004014305

Acknowledgments

Many people deserve recognition and thanks for their support of this book. At F.A. Davis Company, Jean Francois lit the fire, and Acquisitions Editor Christa Fratantoro carried the torch to the book's completion. Thanks are also extended to Laura Horowitz and Melissa Reed, Developmental Editors; Susan Rhyner, Head of Creative Development; Bob Butler, Production Manager; Jonel Sofian, Designer; and Joan Wendt, Design and Illustrations Manager.

For their careful review of the manuscript, we would like to thank the following athletic training educators:

- Scott Doberstein, MS, LATC, CSCS, University of Wisconsin-La Crosse, La Crosse, Wisconsin;
- William Holcomb, PhD, ATC/L, CSCS, University of Las Vegas, Las Vegas, Nevada;
- Daniel R. Sedory, MS, ATC, NHLAT, University of New Hampshire, Durham, New Hampshire; and
- Stacy Walker, PhD, ATC, LAT, Ball State University, Muncie, Indiana.

Special thanks to Chad Starkey, PhD, ATC, Northeastern University, Boston, Massachusetts, for his reviews and for writing the Foreword. His excitement for the book kept us moving in the right direction.

We thank Sandra Shultz, PhD, ATC, CSCS, for sharing her gift for grant writing as author of Chapter 19, "Introduction to Grant Writing and Research Funding Sources." Also, thanks to Sandy, Kevin Guskiewicz, PhD, ATC, and Carl Mattacola, PhD, ATC, for their "real" fictional boxes.

Finally, we thank the many master's degree students in athletic training and doctoral students in sports medicine who attended the University of Virginia from 1986 to 2001. Your enthusiasm for conducting research in athletic training provided the impetus to write this book.

Contributor

Sandra Shultz, PhD, ATC, CSCS
University of North Carolina–Greensboro
Greensboro, NC

Preface

We have written *Research Methods in Athletic Training* after guiding several hundred athletic training master's degree students through the process of conducting a research project over the past 20 years. We have also directed nearly 50 sports medicine doctoral student dissertations along the way. Many of these doctoral students participated in the mentoring of the master's degree student research projects.

Our target audience for this text is entry level and post-certification graduate students in athletic training, and certified athletic trainers interested in undertaking the process of research and publication. The text can be used to introduce undergraduate students to the importance and process of conducting athletic training research. This addresses the National Athletic Trainers' Association Education Council's Health Care Administration teaching objective: "the student will demonstrate the ability to prepare and interpret sample design for scientific research" (Athletic Training Educational Competencies, 3rd Edition, 1999, page 78).

The text can also be used to guide graduate students through the process of conducting a thesis or dissertation. Our philosophical approach is to have students write the first three chapters (i.e., introduction, literature review, and methods) of a traditional thesis. These chapters are then transformed into the introduction and methods of a journal format manuscript. The final product is a manuscript divided into the sections required by most scientific journals – the introduction, methods, results, and discussion. The goal is to present the research at a scientific forum and to submit a manuscript for publication in a refereed journal.

Practicing certified athletic trainers could also use the text as a guide for conducting research in the clinic or laboratory settings. The guidelines for choosing a topic, applying the appropriate research design and statistical procedures, and preparing and submitting a manuscript for publication are the same for students and practicing certified athletic trainers.

The text is divided into six sections. Part I provides an introduction to athletic training research, the types of research commonly undertaken by athletic training scholars, and the keys to choosing a research topic. Part II discusses how to conduct and write a review of the literature. Part III addresses the research process, beginning with guidelines for how to write the introduction. Next, research design issues, the concepts of internal and external validity of these designs, and the importance of reliable and valid measurement in athletic training research are covered. Alternative measures and the important role of survey research in athletic training are addressed. Part III concludes with guidelines for how to write the methods.

Part IV introduces the process of statistical decision-making, and discusses the more commonly applied techniques in athletic training research - analysis of variance, repeated measures analysis of variance, and correlational analysis. We have emphasized the logic behind the use of statistics, rather than the mathematics or formulae addressed in statistics textbooks.

Part V provides guidelines for writing the results and discussion in both thesis chapter and manuscript formats. The process of disseminating the findings of a research project through presentations and a published manuscript is also addressed in Part V.

Part VI addresses important additional issues. Our colleague, Sandra Shultz, PhD, ATC has a special talent for the art of grant writing, and she has addressed the process of identifying and obtaining sources of internal and external funding. Finally, the concept of scientific misconduct and keys to ethical research are discussed.

We have applied several important pedagogical strategies throughout the text. You will find objectives and questions at the beginning of each chapter. We have used actual SPSS printouts to illustrate how to interpret and understand the various statistical techniques. Learning activities that can be undertaken individually or as class projects are presented at the end of each chapter. We have also included student fictional boxes that present many of the problems and solutions our students have experienced during the process of conducting athletic training research.

The research process can appear daunting and overwhelming. Our hope is that this text will help alleviate your apprehensions by providing a step-by-step approach to conducting research. Good luck as you embark on the process of conducting research in athletic training.

Brent L. Arnold
Bruce M. Gansneder
David H. Perrin

Foreword

by Chad Starkey

For many students, thinking about taking a research course is like Dorothy, the Tin Man, the Scarecrow, and the Cowardly Lion anxiety about meeting the Wizard of Oz... a larger-than-life, omnipotent, intimidating, and unforgiving entity. The anxiety of actually meeting the Wizard is worse than actually doing it. Once the Wizard is exposed, he is an approachable – and even likeable – sort. In their text *Research Methods in Athletic Training,* Drs. Arnold, Gansneder, and Perrin pull back the curtain to expose the research process for what it is: predictable, flexible, and masterable.

The quality and quantity of research produced is a benchmark by which professions are judged. Not only does research establish professional identity by adding to our professional knowledge base, it also assists in clinical decision-making, clinical practice, and being well-informed consumers. This text has been structured so it is useful to both producers of research and consumers of research.

The authors have created a precise roadmap for conducting research, from conceptualizing the research topic to submitting the final paper for publication. Although not everyone will see their research project to completion or submit a paper for publication, an understanding of this process lends individual credibility to consumers of research. With the recent emphasis on evidence-based practice, an understanding of the scope and limitations of research will help practitioners make informed decisions.

Part I addresses a question commonly posed to instructors, "What should I do my research on?" The authors help the reader develop a research topic based on personal interests, rather than being "suggested" one by the instructor.

Part II illustrates the process of conducting a literature review and provides practical tips for using common computer-based literature searches. They are then guided through the process of organizing and interpreting these findings and how to incorporate the results into their research project.

Designing the research project and writing the introductory sections of a paper for publication are the focus of Section III. The authors not only describe the mechanics of designing the research project, they also describe the seemingly esoteric language of research and statistics using everyday examples.

The most intimidating material – Statistical Measurement – is discussed in Section IV. At first glance, the output produced by most computer statistical software packages can make the da Vinci

Code seem like the Cat in the Hat. One of the primary features of this text is the inclusion of annotated SPSS-PC printouts that decode the statistical jargon and decipher the statistics produced. The authors identify the key points of the printout and provide an understandable explanation of each.

The authors detail how to write the results and discussion in Section V and provide an overview of the steps required to see the manuscript through the publication process. For those individuals, such as graduate students, who will attempt to attract funding for their research, Section VI discusses methods to obtain funding and ethical considerations in the research process.

This text should be a "must" for all who are enrolled in a research course, are instructing the course, or are conducting research. Although this text is written for the athletic training market, its content and examples are relevant to all professions that have an orthopedic patient base. Although research is complex, it can be mastered and these research Wizards lead us down the right road.

Contents

Preface
Foreword by Chad Starkey

5 Writing the Literature Review 57

Part III

The Research Process 67

6 Writing the Introduction 69

7 Research Design 77

8 Common Measures in Athletic Training. 101

Part VI

20 Ethical Considerations in the Research Process. . . . 351

Index. 391

Part 1
Introduction

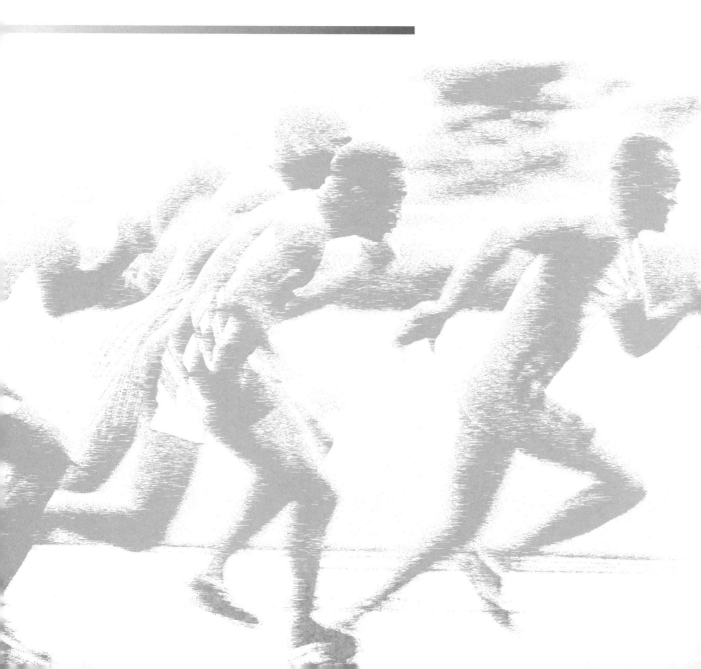

Chapter 1

Introduction to Research in Athletic Training

Objectives

After reading this chapter, you will:

- Understand the role of research in establishment of a profession.
- Understand the importance of a scientific body of knowledge to athletic training clinical practice.
- Become aware of the progress made by the National Athletic Trainers' Association in the areas of research and scholarship.
- Become aware of the overall research process.
- Become aware of the fundamental components of a profession.

Questions

While reading this chapter, think about answers to the following questions:

1. Why should I be involved in research?
2. Where can I learn more about athletic training research and research funding?
3. What is a profession, and how does research contribute to the evolution of a profession?
4. What is my professional organization doing to promote research?
5. What does the process of conducting research entail?
6. How does research in athletic training benefit clinical practice?

What Is a Profession?

Three components are fundamental to the establishment of an allied health profession such as athletic training: practice, education, and research (Display 1–1) (Osternig, 1988). Athletic training has made tremendous strides to become a true profession since the founding of the National

Display 1-1

Three Components Fundamental to All Allied Health Professions

- **Practice:** The application of a particular skill
- **Education:** The formulation and transmission of a particular body of knowledge
- **Research:** The systematic examination and testing of a particular discipline's methods and principles

Source: Osternig, L.R.(1988). Research in athletic training: The missing ingredient. Athletic Training, 23, 223–225.

Athletic Trainers' Association (NATA) in 1950. We have seen especially significant improvements in the areas of clinical practice and education, and more recently we have made remarkable progress in the areas of research and scholarship.

Clinical Practice

You probably chose to study athletic training because you enjoy clinical practice—the opportunity to apply the art and science of an allied health field to physically active people. Clinical practice in athletic training involves the hands-on application of prevention, recognition and evaluation, immediate care, and treatment and rehabilitation of injuries to people who are physically active. The NATA Board of Certification has a validated examination to ensure a minimal level of competence for the entry-level clinical practitioner. This examination is based on a periodically updated athletic training role delineation study, from which the written, practical, and written simulation portions of the examination are administered.

In a 50th-anniversary article in the *Journal of Athletic Training*, Grace (1999) identified the milestones in athletic trainer certification (Display 1–2). Grace explained that the most significant public pronouncement a profession can bestow on an individual is certification. (This should not be confused with states' obligations to certify or license professionals for the purpose of public safety.) This process has undoubtedly enhanced the public's impression of athletic training as a profession.

Display 1-2

Milestones in Athletic Trainer Certification

1969	The decision to begin certifying athletic trainers
1982	External recognition of the Board of Certification
1989	The incorporation of the NATA Board of Certification

Source: Grace, P. (1999). Milestones in athletic trainer certification. Journal of Athletic Training, 34, 285–291.

Display 1-3	**Major Events in the Evolution of Athletic Training Education**

1959	First athletic training curriculum model approved by the NATA
1969	First undergraduate athletic training curriculum approved by the NATA
1972	First graduate athletic training curriculum approved by the NATA
1980	NATA resolution requiring athletic training curriculum major, or equivalent, approved by the NATA
1990	Athletic training recognized as an allied health profession by the American Medical Association (AMA)
1994	First entry-level athletic training educational programs accredited by AMA Committee on Allied Health Education and Accreditation

Source: Delforge, G.D., & Behnke, R.S. (1999). The history and evolution of athletic training education in the United States. Journal of Athletic Training, 34, 53–61.

As in many medical and allied health professions, some of what we do in clinical practice is based on research, yet many of the techniques we apply have little scientific basis. Research will enable us to expand the body of knowledge in our field, which in turn will not only improve clinical practice but also enhance our standing among the other medical and allied health professions.

Education

The evolution of athletic training education has resulted in a well-structured accreditation process for athletic training education programs at the entry and postcertification levels. Presently there are over 400 accredited entry-level athletic training programs throughout the country, and the NATA accredits 13 advanced postcertification programs. In another 50th-anniversary article in the *Journal of Athletic Training*, Delforge and Behnke (1999) outlined and discussed the evolution of athletic training education in the United States (Display 1–3). In this paper, the authors explained that the development of athletic training education programs has contributed significantly to the professionalization of athletic training. Research to validate the techniques we teach—and the instructional technology we use to teach them—will serve to further enhance our standing as a profession.

Research

Research is the process by which we expand the body of knowledge that serves as the basis for athletic training clinical practice. The notion of scholarship is inextricably connected to research and the expansion of our body of knowledge. Knight and Ingersoll (1998) contend that scholarship is what delineates a profession from a trade. Display 1–4 summarizes the reasons

Display 1-4   **Why Scholarship Is Important to Athletic Training**

- Our standing as professionals will be enhanced.
- The standard of care we can provide to physically active people will improve.
- Our reputation, which is determined by what others see (or fail to see) in writing, will be enhanced.
- Change and progress will come because we focus on our problems rather than waiting for others to give us answers.
- We will gain prestige as others look to us for knowledge.
- Our claim as authorities on health care for the physically active will be enhanced.

Source: Knight, K.L., & Ingersoll, C.D. (1998). Developing scholarship in athletic training. Journal of Athletic Training, 33, 271–274.

why scholarship is important to our profession. Learning about the process of research will help you develop your skills in scholarship. You may not build your career around the process of research, but we hope you will develop an appreciation for the role scholarship plays in advancing our profession. We also believe that you will be a more informed consumer of the research articles you read in athletic training and sports medicine journals. Scholarship and research will improve the techniques available to athletic training clinicians.

We also believe that your critical thinking skills as a clinician will be enhanced by learning about the research process. You will be more inclined to scrutinize the techniques you apply in clinical practice for their scientific validity. As you read articles in journals, you will learn to watch for flaws in design and overgeneralizations related to clinical application. You will begin to appreciate the necessity of establishing efficacy of treatment through quality outcomes research. In sum, we hope you will appreciate the value of research to educators, scholars, and clinicians in the athletic training profession.

Throughout the book we feature a series of boxes titled "In the Field" that describes fictional students involved in conducting research projects. These boxes are intended to give you practical examples of the ways in which people employ research in athletic training. We hope that you will benefit from their thought processes, successes, and mistakes. Our first example is Aidan.

Evolution of Research in Athletic Training

Since its establishment in 1950, the NATA has taken several steps to promote research in athletic training. Some of its more noteworthy initiatives include the *Journal of Athletic Training*, the Research and Education Foundation, and the Free Communications session at the Annual Meeting and Clinical Symposia. Developments in graduate-level education have also

In the Field

Aidan is an undergraduate student who is studying to become an athletic trainer. As a former football player, he hopes to become a certified athletic trainer for a college or professional team. He really enjoys his clinical practice classes and does not want to take a research class, believing that it will have no bearing on his future work. What Aidan does not understand is how the process will actually help make him a better clinician. Good clinical practice requires critical thinking. Similarly, the research process demands critical thinking, organization, and structure. Even if Aidan never does research again, the research class will help him learn to synthesize and organize information for his clinical practice. As Aidan begins to further develop his clinical practice, he will be inundated with new techniques and practices. Not all of the techniques will be scientifically sound. By engaging in the research process, he will gain an insider's perspective on what is and is not good research. This will help him sort through the clinical literature and assess the value of new clinical techniques more critically. Like most young professionals, Aidan wants to be part of a dynamic profession that is accepted by all the health professions. Aidan will learn that the distinction between a trade and a profession is the development of its body of knowledge and that research is a necessary activity of a true profession.

advanced research in athletic training. Some of these include the requirement to conduct research as part of many graduate programs in athletic training and the development of doctoral programs designed for certified athletic trainers.

The Journal of Athletic Training

The *Journal of Athletic Training* is the scholarly, peer-reviewed journal of the NATA, and its development has mirrored the growth of athletic training as a profession. Since its inception in 1956, the journal has undergone many changes, including changes in mission, organization, structure, name, and content. In another 50th-anniversary article for the *Journal of Athletic Training*, Knight and Thompson (1999) reviewed the 44-year history of the journal. The present mission of this journal is to enhance communication among professionals interested in the quality of health care for physically active people through education and research in prevention, evaluation, management, and rehabilitation of injuries. The *Journal of Athletic Training* serves as an outlet for the research conducted by many certified athletic trainers, and its quality has improved as the quality of scholarship in our profession has improved. It is now available at PubMed Central (the United States National Library of Medicine's digital archive of life sciences journal literature), which has exposed the *Journal* to other allied health professionals and to the international sports medicine community. A quality peer-reviewed scholarly journal is yet another hallmark of a true medical or allied health profession.

National Athletic Trainers' Association Research and Education Foundation

The Research and Education Foundation of the NATA was founded in 1991 and is a nonprofit body that provides financial support for research in athletic training. The Foundation includes an education committee, a scholarship committee, and a research committee. The education committee conducts the Athletic Training Educators' Conference on a biannual basis. The scholarship committee oversees the process of nominating and distributing undergraduate and graduate scholarships for student members of the NATA. The research committee oversees the review of grant proposals and conducts the Free Communications session at NATA's annual meeting and clinical symposia. These three committees operate under the auspices of the Foundation's board of directors.

The Foundation provides funding under the category of General Grants and also issues Requests for Proposals (RFPs) for research in areas of special interest, such as pediatric sports health care. The Foundation also awards grants for certified members of the NATA who are enrolled as doctoral students. Finally, the Foundation provides education research and program grants to support studies related to clinical instruction and learning styles, educational research, and educational projects and programs.

Several other opportunities exist for athletic trainers to pursue funding to support their research. Some of the state organizations and several of the NATA's districts provide grants to support athletic training research. A whole host of private foundations and federal agencies also provides money to support research in the medical and allied health-care professions. These foundations and agencies will be discussed in further detail in Chapter 19.

Free Communications Session

The Free Communications session of NATA's Annual Meeting and Clinical Symposia is a forum for presentation of original research in athletic training. Authors in Free Communications sessions are required to categorize their abstracts in one of five areas of research funding by the Research and Education Foundation: basic science, clinical studies, educational research, sports injury epidemiology, and observation/informational studies. The opportunity also exists for presentation of clinical case reports, which involves presentation of unique individual athletic injury cases. Each year the Research and Education Foundation issues a call for abstracts. Specific guidelines for preparation and submission of abstracts are provided, and each abstract is carefully reviewed by a committee of experts to determine suitability for presentation at the annual meeting. The abstracts that are accepted for presentation at the Free Communications session are published in the spring supplement of the *Journal of Athletic Training*. The process of preparing and presenting an abstract for the Free Communications session is described in Chapter 18.

Athletic trainers can present their research at other forums. Many athletic training researchers are members of the American College of Sports Medicine who attend and present research at that organization's annual meeting. Some athletic trainers are also credentialed physical therapists or strength and conditioning specialists who present their research at the annual meetings of the American Physical Therapy Association and the National Strength and Conditioning Association.

Development of Doctoral Programs in Athletic Training

One of the more recent and exciting developments in athletic training education has been doctoral programs specially designed for certified athletic trainers. For many years, certified athletic trainers who were interested in careers as curriculum directors and scholars in higher education had to pursue doctoral education in disciplines related to athletic training. Examples of such disciplines included exercise physiology, biomechanics, motor learning, and curriculum and instruction, among others. The advent of doctoral programs in athletic training permits the development of research skills directly related to our discipline. Several universities have developed or are in the process of developing doctoral programs in athletic training, and some are listed in Display 1–5.

Display 1-5

Examples of Universities Offering Doctoral Level Programs in Athletic Training

Indiana State University. Retrieved 3/25/04: *http://www.indstate.edu/athtrn/*
Oregon State University. Retrieved 3/25/04:
   http://www.hhs.oregonstate.edu/exss/graduate/sports-medicine/
Temple University. Retrieved 3/25/04:
   http://www.temple.edu/education/kinesiology/
University of Florida. Retrieved 3/25/04:
   http://www.hhp.ufl.edu/ess/pages/grad_program/grad_index.html
University of Kentucky. Retrieved 3/25/04:
   http://www.mc.uky.edu/rehabsciences/about/about.htm
University of North Carolina at Chapel Hill. Retrieved 3/25/04:
   http://www.unc.edu/depts/exercise/phd_study1.htm
University of North Carolina at Greensboro. Retrieved 3/25/04:
   http://www.uncg.edu/ess/anrl/
University of Oregon. Retrieved 3/25/04: *http://www.uoregon.edu/~ems/ems2.htm*
University of Pittsburgh. Retrieved 3/25/04:
   http://www.shrs.pitt.edu/cdn/degrees/phdsm.htm
University of Toledo. Retrieved 3/25/04:
   http://www.hhs.utoledo.edu/kinesiology/phd_bio.html
University of Virginia. Retrieved 3/25/04:
   http://curry.edschool.virginia.edu/sportsmed/
Virginia Commonwealth University. Retrieved 4/20/04:
   http://www.soe.vcu.edu/depts/exSci/PHD_RehMovSc.htm

The Research Process

The process of conducting research is a complex and lengthy one that requires several steps and usually involves many people. These steps, and the chapters in which they are discussed, are:

- Choosing a topic (Chapters 2 and 3)
- Establishing the research team (Chapter 3)
- Reviewing the literature and writing the literature review (Chapters 4 and 5)
- Designing the study (Chapters 7 through 15)
- Obtaining human investigation committee approval (Chapter 20)
- Collecting pilot data (Chapter 16)
- Collecting actual data (Chapter 16)
- Analyzing and interpreting data (Chapters 12 through 16)
- Writing, presenting, and publishing the study's findings (Chapters 16 through 18)

This book will lead you sequentially through this process. Good luck as you embark on your journey of conducting research in athletic training.

Summary

A profession can be envisioned as a three-legged stool with clinical practice, education, and research as the legs. As a student, you have experienced the first two of these first hand, but you may have not had the opportunity to experience the third. This text is focused on research in athletic training because research is essential to the profession's continued development. Within the past decade, there has been tremendous growth in athletic training research. This is manifested by the evolution of the *Journal of Athletic Training* and the establishment of the NATA Research and Education Foundation and its associated Free Communications session at NATA's Annual Meeting and Clinical Symposium. For students who are interested in research, ample opportunities exist through master's and doctoral programs around the country.

Activities

1. Visit the PubMed website and find the *Journal of Athletic Training* and other journals related to the field of sports medicine.
2. List the reasons why research is important to a profession.

References

Delforge, G., & Behnke, R.S. (1999). The history and evolution of athletic training in the United States. *Journal of Athletic Training, 34,* 53–61.

Grace, P. (1999). Milestones in athletic trainer certification. *Journal of Athletic Training, 34,* 285–291.

Knight, K.L., & Ingersoll, C.D. (1998). Developing scholarship in athletic training. *Journal of Athletic Training, 33,* 271–274.

Knight, K.L., & Thompson, C. (1999). 44 years of "The journal." *Journal of Athletic Training, 34,* 397–406.

Osternig, L.R. (1988). Research in athletic training: The missing ingredient. *Athletic Training, 23,* 223–225.

Bibliography

National Athletic Trainers' Association Research and Education Foundation. Retrieved 3/25/04: *http://www.natafoundation.org*

Journal of Athletic Training, National Athletic Trainers' Association scholarly, peer reviewed journal. Retrieved 3/25/04: *http://www.journalofathletictraining.org*

PubMed Central. Retrieved 3/25/04: *http://www.pubmedcentral.org*

Chapter 2

Areas and Types of Research

Objectives

After reading this chapter, you will:

- Differentiate between basic and clinical research.
- Describe different types of clinical research.
- Describe different types of educational research.
- Describe different methods of qualitative research.
- Describe the strengths and weaknesses of multicenter studies.

Questions

While reading this chapter, think about answers to the following questions:

1. What is the difference between a prospective study and a retrospective study?
2. How does a cross-sectional study differ from a cohort study?
3. When should I think about running a multicenter study?
4. What is the difference among basic, applied, clinical, and educational research?
5. What is meant by qualitative research?

This chapter describes the various types of research conducted or used by athletic trainers, including basic, applied and clinical, multicenter, injury surveillance, meta-analytical, educational, and qualitative. Because of our background and experience, we will focus primarily on applied research, but this does not mean we believe that applied research is more important than the other types. We made a research choice based on our expertise and interests, and as a potential researcher, you will be faced with a similar choice. We encourage you to make your choice, just as we did, based on your personal interests. However, with choices come consequences. In an era with funding to state institutions decreasing, there is increased pressure on researchers to find external grant support that can be used to support university activities—that is, make up for lost state support. Some areas of research are more conducive to procuring large external grants than others (e.g., biomedical versus educational). Therefore, your selection of an area of research may coincidentally affect your ability to secure grant funds and to be successful at larger research institutions.

Although this text will focus predominantly on applied or clinical research, it should be emphasized that this is largely an issue of presentation, not content. The issues of research discussed in this text apply to all forms of research. They are not unique to applied research. For example, the issue of instrument reliability (Chapter 9) is just as applicable to a classroom pencil-and-paper test as it is to a test used to assess a person's balance. Therefore, although we hope that the examples used in this text will address your interests, we encourage you to focus on the issues presented. They remain the same regardless of the type of research. Display 2–1 outlines the types of research.

Display 2–1 | **Types of Athletic Training Research**

Basic Science

Applied and Clinical Studies

- Prospective cohort study
- Retrospective cohort study
- Cross-sectional study
- Case-control study
- Randomized control trial
- Crossover trial
- Case study
- Case series

Multicenter Studies

Injury Surveillance

Meta-Analytical

Educational Research

- Learning styles
- Instructional methods
- Clinical instruction
- Program administration

Qualitative

- Ethnography
- Phenomenology
- Grounded theory

Basic Science Research

Basic science research typically focuses on anatomical or physiological questions that may eventually lead to applied or clinical research. The purpose of basic science research is to establish fundamental mechanisms associated with the biology of the organism. In athletic training, this may mean establishing the function of a ligament to basic joint mechanics. Alternatively, you might be interested in how ultrasound moves medications across the skin into inflamed tissues (i.e., phonophoresis). This is not the same as asking, "Does phonophoresis decrease inflammation?" The latter would be the clinical or applied question associated with the basic research question. Put another way, basic science research is interested in establishing biological plausibility. If your theory is that phonophoresis is effective in treating inflammation because it can move anti-inflammatory medications across the skin into inflamed tissues, there must be basic evidence indicating that this is possible. If it is not possible, you should look for another mechanism to explain the potential effectiveness of phonophoresis. Basic science research is often conducted without specific interest in clinical applicability. Rather, it is used to identify underlying explanations that may lead to clinically applicable research.

Applied and Clinical Studies

Applied and clinical studies are very similar in format, and the overall discussion applies to both. The key difference between the two is the population being studied and the treatment (if applicable) used. Clinical studies examine populations with disorders or the treatments intended for use in these populations. Applied studies fit somewhere between basic and clinical studies. They typically study uninjured populations with the goal of identifying normal values or establishing normal patterns of function. For example, it might be of interest to determine whether men and women have different muscle activation patterns at the hip and knee. Because the subjects are uninjured and the intent is to establish normal patterns of muscle activation, this would be considered an applied study. However, if the subjects were women and men with injured anterior cruciate ligaments (ACLs), the study would be considered a clinical study.

Within the context of clinical studies, several subcategories exist. The remainder of this section will focus on the different types of clinical studies: cohort (both prospective and retrospective), cross-sectional, case-control, randomized control trials, crossover trials, case studies, and case series.

Cohort Studies

The term cohort study refers to studying a preselected group of subjects across time. The fundamental feature of this cohort is that it is representative of the population you intend to study. The purpose of the cohort is to determine whether some factor is more prevalent in individuals with a disorder than in those without it. For example, you may be interested in studying ACL injuries in basketball players. More specifically, you may be interested in determining whether an individual's gender is related to ACL injury. Therefore, the disorder is ACL injuries and the factor of interest is gender. Other questions you might consider when defining your population are:

1. Should I include a variety of ages (e.g., middle school versus high school versus collegiate)?
2. Should I include recreational athletes (e.g., noncompetitive versus competitive)?
3. Should I include contact or noncontact injuries, or both?

Once you determine the population, disorder, and factor(s) of interest, you need to determine whether the study should be conducted prospectively or retrospectively.

Prospective Studies

As the name suggests, prospective studies run forward in time (Figure 2–1). In the ACL study discussed in the previous section, you would identify a group of subjects that fits your population (e.g., men and women who play basketball). Obviously, you immediately know their gender, but let us also

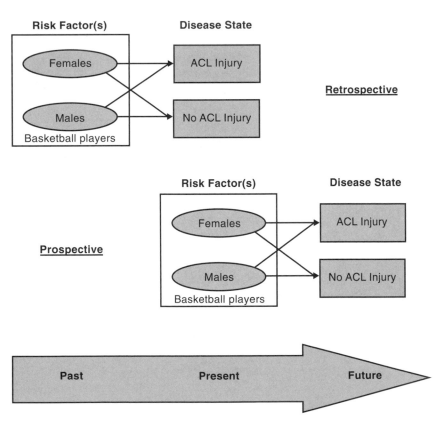

Figure 2–1 Retrospective and prospective designs.

assume that you are interested in knee strength (e.g., hamstring strength measured isokinetically). In the prospective study, you would measure strength before the subjects were injured and then follow them across time. Your expectations might be that women are more susceptible to injury and that women with weak hamstrings are the most susceptible. Assuming that your expectations are proven true, because you measured gender and strength before the study, your hypothesis that weakness and gender are causes of injury is strengthened.

The primary weaknesses of prospective studies are time, effort, and frequency of injury. These studies take a great deal of organization and planning. Similarly, to do one well may take several years. Even if the time interval is rather long, there is always the chance that there would not be enough injuries from which to draw accurate conclusions.

Retrospective Studies

An alternative to the prospective study is the retrospective study (see Figure 2–1). In this case, you would identify an existing group of individuals (e.g., basketball players) and examine previously measured factors (e.g., gender and strength) that may be related to the presence or absence of injury. For example, a group of basketball players would be identified, and their gender, knee strength (before injury), and ACL injury status would be determined. The expectation would be that a greater proportion of ACL-injured players would be women who have weak knees.

Obviously, the advantage of this design is that most of the data have been previously collected. Therefore, the time interval of the study can be dramatically shorter than the time in a prospective study. However, you are also relying on data collected by others. Because of this, you have no control over the quality of that previous data. If, in this case, the knee strength data were not collected correctly (e.g., knee strength was measured at different isokinetic velocities for different individuals), the data would not be useful. It is also possible that data on strength may be missing in some individuals and that other important factors (e.g., balance) were not measured.

Cross-Sectional Studies

Cohort studies follow a group across time; cross-sectional studies examine a group at the same point in time. For example, you might identify a group of basketball players at the end of their season, measure their knee strength, and determine their injury status. The advantage of cross-sectional studies is that they are relatively fast. The disadvantage is that they cannot determine cause and effect. For example, if you found that knee weakness was present in individuals with ACL tears, you would not know whether it existed before or after the injury. For a factor to be a cause of injury, it must always come before the injury, and you must be able to demonstrate that it occurred before the injury.

Case-Control Studies

Case-control studies are probably the most frequently used type of athletic training research study. Instead of identifying factors and then relating them to disorders, as in the cohort study, in this study the disorder is identified first. Once a group of individuals with the disorder is identified, a second group is identified to serve as controls. (The use of the term "control group" is common in medical literature. However, as we point out in Chapter 7, this type of group is better described as a comparison group. A true control group exists only in experimental research, where random assignment is used.) For example, you would select athletes with ankle injuries and a second uninjured group (Figure 2–2). You would then look backward in time at factors that may be associated with ankle instability (e.g., evertor weakness) and examine how the groups differ.

The main weakness of these studies is in selecting the control group. Generally, this is done by trying to match subjects according to common variables such as age, height, and weight. A full description of matching and its pros and cons is addressed in Chapter 7.

Randomized Control Trials

As discussed in more detail in Chapter 7, the studies described in the previous sections can be categorized as nonexperimental clinical studies. The randomized control trial is the experimental design applied to clinical research. In recent years, this has become the workhorse of medical clinical trials research. In general, this design is considered the gold standard

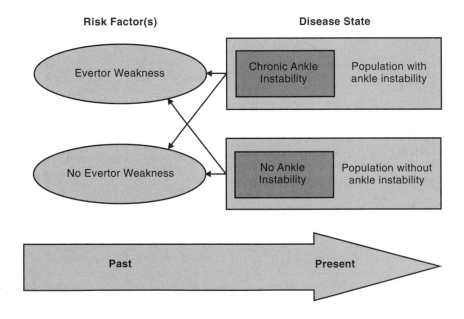

Figure 2–2 Case-control design.

for identifying causal relationships. Chapter 7 provides a more detailed description of the experimental design, its advantages and disadvantages, and its variations.

Crossover Trials

Crossover trials are in some cases identical to the pretest-posttest design, discussed in Chapter 7. In crossover trials, at least two groups each receive all of the treatments included in the study. The advantage is that a smaller number of subjects is required, but carryover effects from one treatment to another are possible.

Case Study and Case Series

The case study, an in-depth study of a single case or subject, is another useful method in clinical research. The goal of the case study is to describe a unique case for the clinical literature. In athletic training you may encounter a rare or atypical injury that is not described in the literature. The injury may be unusual in some feature such as its pathology, mechanism of injury, or response to treatment. Regardless, your emphasis in writing a case study should be on the uniqueness. It should be emphasized that this is not a technique that should be used on common injuries that can be studied as a group. You should reserve case studies for the exception rather than the rule.

An extension of the case study is the case series. You can think of the case series as being multiple case studies (e.g., multiple cases of non-contact ACL injuries). These studies are useful in describing the characteristics of a rare and often new injury. They are also useful in providing a quick description of new injuries or conditions and may anecdotally identify possible risk factors. You should view these studies as useful starting points, not end points for your research.

Multicenter Studies

Multicenter studies probably represent the future of athletic training research. As the name suggests, these are single, large research studies executed at multiple sites. including multiple universities, medical centers, or physician clinics. In all the centers, the same protocols are used to ensure that the same data are collected, the same treatments are implemented, and so on. The advantage of multicenter studies is number of subjects. Often injuries occur in relatively low numbers at a single site. However, if several sites are partnered together, the number of injury occurrences available for study may increase dramatically.

The disadvantage of multicenter studies is the complexity of coordination. Personnel across multiple sites must be trained to ensure that procedures at all sites are followed correctly. Reliability testing (see Chapter 9)

In the Field

> *Terry is interested in studying the effects of post-acute ACL tears on ankle joint proprioception. In checking with her athletic training room, she discovers that only one to five ACL tears occur per year. She would not be able collect enough data to analyze in a single year. To solve this problem, she begins to make contact with other schools. In doing so, she has to make several decisions. Will she collect data at each site or have the athletes come to her athletic training room? If she collects data at other sites, will she travel to do the testing or train others to test for her? Will other athletic trainers and clinicians at the other sites be considered authors? Terry quickly realizes that a great amount of coordination will be required to complete this study.*

should be conducted within and among the sites to ensure that collection procedures are consistent. One site should serve as the central location for the analysis and interpretation of data. With multiple investigators, the criteria for authorship can be complex and should be discussed before the study begins (see Chapter 18). Therefore, although the dividend of conducting a multicenter study is high, it comes with a great deal of effort.

Injury Surveillance

Injury surveillance has been the foundation of much of the research in athletic training. It helps us define the clinical problems we face, for example, whether women suffer more ACL injuries than men. The focus of this type of research is observational in nature. The goal is to establish the occurrence of injury or injuries in a population. These studies take the form of either a cohort or a cross-sectional study. In the cohort design, in which subjects are followed across time, the interest is in determining the incidence of injury. Incidence is calculated as:

$$\text{Incidence} = \frac{\text{Number of new injuries across time}}{\text{Number of people at risk during the same time}} \qquad (2\text{--}1)$$

By using this statistic, you can determine the overall incidence of an injury to a population or you can subdivide the population (e.g., men versus women, or pes planus versus neutral versus pes cavus feet) and calculate the relative incidence for each group. For example, you could calculate the incidence of ACL injuries in men versus women. Dividing the women's incidence by the men's incidence can determine the relative risk of injury for women.

Alternatively, injury surveillance research can be conducted using a cross-sectional study. Because, in this case, subjects are not observed across time but are instead observed at the same point in time, prevalence, not incidence, is studied. Prevalence is calculated as:

$$\text{Prevalence} = \frac{\text{Number of injured people at one point in time}}{\text{Number of people at risk same point in time}} \qquad (2\text{--}2)$$

You will note that this Formula is very similar to Formula 2–1. In fact, the difference is primarily one of logic, not form—that is, measures are taken across time rather than at one point in time. Just as relative risk can be calculated from incidence, relative prevalence can be calculated from prevalence. Therefore, if you studied ACL injuries in men and women at the end of the basketball season rather than across the season, prevalence and relative prevalence would be calculated rather than incidence and relative risk.

Meta-Analysis

Although meta-analysis has been available as an analytical technique for some time, it has only recently been applied to athletic training research (Cordova, Ingersoll, & LeBlanc, 2000). This technique analyzes existing studies rather than creating new data and can be used to assess the clinical efficacy of a treatment (Richy, Bruyère, Ethgen, Cucherat, Henrotin, & Reginster, 2003). It takes the form of both a critical literature review and a statistical analysis. A full description of the technique is beyond the scope of this text. However, the basic premise of meta-analysis is that results from different studies can be transformed into a common metric. For each study, you calculate one or more effect sizes of the variables of interest and then compare the results of the different studies. This method requires many studies (the more the better) of a single topic. Therefore, it cannot be applied to new areas of research. Its strength is that you can numerically synthesize the results of many studies in a very efficient format and make broader interpretations across multiple studies. Meta-analytic results can provide the foundation for evidence-based practice.

Educational Research

Educational research has gained increased popularity recently in the profession of athletic training, probably because of recent reforms in athletic training education as well as a greater number of scholars pursuing this type of research. Although educational research (e.g., examining the best way to evaluate student clinical proficiencies) is not the primary focus of this text, we acknowledge its importance and recognize that many interesting and important questions remain to be answered in this area. Because educational research tends to look very different from clinical and experimental research, it may be perceived as requiring a different set of rules. In our view, this is not the case. Research is a generic form of problem solving and exploration. The same issues exist regardless of whether the research is clinical or educational. For example, regardless of the type of research, your measures and methods should be both reliable and valid (see Chapter 9). Similarly, the research design in most cases should match the designs outlined in Chapter 7 to produce internally and externally valid results. Finally, unless you are performing select types of qualitative research, the statistical analyses outlined in Chapters 12 to 15 should be completed.

Educational research can be divided into several sub-areas. Brief descriptions of common areas are presented in the following paragraphs. However, it should be emphasized that each of these areas may actually be combined with others to address multiple facets of education delivery.

Learning and Learning Styles

Students generally exhibit different learning styles (e.g., visual, auditory, kinesthetic, individual, and group). The purpose of this research is to identify differences in student learning styles and to study and compare techniques that take advantage of those styles.

Instructional Methods

Instructional methods research is a broad area that generally refers to methods used in the classroom to deliver information. The goal is to identify the methods (e.g., the Socratic method versus lecture or problem-based learning versus content-based learning) that are most effective for athletic training instruction.

Clinical Instruction

Clinical instruction research is likely to grow rapidly in the next several years. With the adoption of the Approved Clinical Instructor (ACI) model by athletic training education programs, studies of what characteristics make an ACI effective, what techniques should be used by the ACI to be effective, what general formats of clinical education are most effective, and so on, are surely needed.

Program Administration

Any entry-level education program director will tell you that a great deal of time goes into the daily operation of the athletic training education program. This ranges from clinical assignments, student admissions, student evaluation, instructor evaluation, and program evaluation. How to conduct these activities efficiently and with validity is an area that needs further research.

 # Qualitative Research

Although qualitative research is more a method of research than a type of research, we believe that some discussion of qualitative research is necessary. Hopefully, this discussion will help you contrast the role of qualitative research with that of quantitative research (the primary focus of this text)

and appreciate how the two might be used to complement each other. Qualitative research frequently uses interview and observational techniques to describe an environment, experience, or process from the subjects' perspectives. Within qualitative research, three primary approaches are typically used to answer different questions. They are ethnography, phenomenology, and grounded theory.

Ethnography

Ethnography focuses on describing the cultural environment of the subjects. In education this might be a description of the athletic training room environment and how it, as a cultural setting, affects student learning. From a clinical perspective, the athletic training room culture might be studied for its effect on the patient's recovery.

Phenomenology

Phenomenology is the study of experiences. It seeks to describe how an individual experiences an environment or situation. In the educational environment, this might be how the student experiences teaching of clinical proficiencies. From a clinical research perspective, you might seek to understand how the patient experiences his or her care or how the clinician experiences return-to-play decisions.

Grounded Theory

Whereas ethnography studies culture and phenomenology studies experiences, grounded theory studies process and interactions. For example, you might seek to describe how an athletic trainer's interaction with a coach or administrator affects return-to-play decisions. Another example might be how a student's interaction with a clinical instructor affects skill development.

In the Field

Gene is curious about how return-to-play decisions are made. He realizes that, although the results of functional tests can be quantitative, how the data are used by the clinician is the result of a qualitative process. As a result, Gene decides that in order to study return-to-play decision-making, a qualitative research process would be most appropriate. As a result, he elects to interview 4 certified athletic trainers who each have 10 or more years of experience. In the interview, Gene asks about how the clinicians use clinical data, knowledge about the athlete and coaches, and competition issues (e.g., critical games) in return-to-play decisions. After the interviews, Gene looks for common themes used by the clinicians in describing their decision-making.

Summary

Athletic training research has evolved into multiple forms. Basic research focuses on the biological (anatomical or physiological) mechanisms of injury, pathology, and treatment. Applied and clinical research focuses on factors associated with normal and abnormal function and how those factors might be treated or changed. In contrast, educational research examines the educational process and the most effective means of educational delivery and learning. Finally, although the focus of this text is on the quantitative type of research, certain questions in athletic training research may be more appropriately addressed through qualitative inquiry.

Activities

1. Find a basic and clinical research study related to your research topic.
2. Find a qualitative study in the field of athletic training.
3. Find an example of a case-control study. Redesign the study into a retrospective study.
4. Find an example of a retrospective study. Redesign the study into a case-control study.

References

Cordova, M.L., Ingersoll, C.D., & LeBlanc, M.J. (2000). Influence of ankle support on joint range of motion before and after exercise: A meta-analysis. *Journal of Orthopaedic and Sports Physical Therapy, 30*, 170–182.

Richy, F., Bruyère, O., Ethgen, O., Cucherat, M., Henrotin, Y., & Reginster, J.-Y. (2003). Structural and symptomatic efficacy of glucosamine and chondroitin in knee osteoarthritis. *Archives of Internal Medicine, 163*, 1514–1522.

Bibliography

Hulley, S.B., & Cummings, S.R. (1998). *Designing clinical research*. Baltimore: Williams & Wilkins.

Pitney, W. A., & Parker, J. (2002). Qualitative research applications in athletic training. *Journal of Athletic Training, 37*, S168–S173.

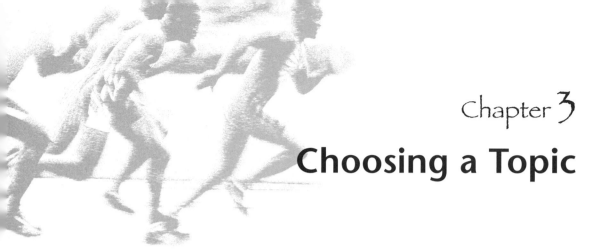

Chapter 3

Choosing a Topic

Objectives

After reading this chapter, you will:

- Understand the importance of creating a personal line of research.
- Learn the factors essential to considering the feasibility of a research topic.
- Appreciate the importance (and limitations) of conducting a thorough review of the literature before embarking on a research project.
- Understand how to draw from the clinical environment in the selection of a research topic.
- Appreciate the role of choosing a research topic and making a contribution to the athletic training body of knowledge.
- Appreciate the value of contributing to an institution or laboratory research agenda.

Questions

While reading this chapter, think about answers to the following questions:

1. How do I match my research interests with the right mentor, program, or institution?
2. Does the research agenda of the faculty or laboratory match my interests?
3. What are the factors important to consider in determining the feasibility of a research topic?
4. How do I determine if the topic is too big or not big enough?
5. How does my athletic training clinical practice relate to the selection of a research topic?
6. How can I make an important contribution to my profession's body of knowledge?

Overview of Selecting a Research Topic

Perhaps the most important phase of the research process is the selection of a topic for research that can be successfully undertaken and completed within the time frame available to you. It is quite common for students to struggle with the selection of a topic, sometimes for weeks on end. You may consider and explore several topics before you and your research mentor agree on a final topic. In this chapter we will provide several guidelines that will help you select a research topic that is of interest, can be completed in a reasonable amount of time, and has the potential to make a contribution to the athletic training body of knowledge.

Factors to Consider in Selecting a Topic

Many factors should be considered in selecting a research topic for your thesis or dissertation. In all probability, your topic will not fit perfectly with every factor described in this section. However, these factors are offered to assist you with selection of a topic that provides the highest probability of your successfully completing the project in a timely manner. For example, clinical trials involving injured populations tend to be far more time intensive and may be more appropriate once you have obtained a faculty position. Display 3–1 provides a checklist of factors to consider in selecting a research topic.

What Is Your Level of Interest in the Topic?

Your topic might fit every other criterion addressed in this chapter, but if you do not have a high level of interest in the topic, the probability of successfully completing the project is diminished. The process of conducting a research project is a lengthy one that will take many months to complete.

Display 3-1

Checklist of Factors to Consider in Selection of a Research Topic

- Is the topic of great interest to you?
- Does the faculty member with whom you will work have expertise in the topic?
- Is the laboratory instrumentation you will need readily available now and under your control?
- Are the subjects you anticipate studying accessible and sufficient in number?
- Is the scope of the project consistent with the time and resources available to you?
- Is the study original?
- Does the study intentionally replicate a previously published study?
- Does the topic have application to athletic training clinical practice?

In the Field

> One of the most important decisions of any young scholar's career is the selection of a dissertation topic. Kevin was trying to select a research question for his dissertation that would be both clinically applicable and timely. He had been studying postural stability for 2 years, and because proprioception was receiving a lot of attention at the time, balance and postural stability after joint injury seemed like a natural direction for him to go. However, Kevin also had an interest in mild head injury, which intensified after his advisor returned from NATA's Mild Brain Injury Summit and shared some of the suggestions the group had identified as needing more attention from the research community. The summary statement following the summit called for more valid ways to objectively measure readiness to return to participation after sports-related concussion. After reading several articles and meeting with faculty members with an interest and expertise in this area, Kevin formed a dissertation committee. He had identified a unique approach to combining his interests in both postural stability and mild head injury in studying "the effect of mild head injury on postural stability."
>
> In going through this process, which took several months, Kevin identified a researchable question for which he had a lot of passion and that was of great interest to the sports medicine community. Because he had chosen a timely topic, it was also a priority for funding agencies. Kevin and his advisor applied for and received a research grant, which allowed their research team to expand the dissertation work into a larger project. Eventually their work was published and has contributed to the changing approach to the management of sports-related concussion.

You will inevitably begin to feel "married" to the project at some point, and therefore a high level of interest at the beginning is essential.

Is the Topic Feasible?

You might have a great research idea, but you need to consider its feasibility in terms of the resources available at your institution. Some of the issues you need to consider include the expertise of your faculty mentor, the availability of laboratory equipment, the accessibility of subjects, and the risk-benefit ratio established by the institution's review board for the protection of human subjects.

Ideally, you have landed at an institution and are working with a research mentor in whose research agenda you have an interest. If your mentor has expertise in the topic you are undertaking, he or she will be better suited to provide timely and appropriate feedback. Your mentor will also be very familiar with the published literature related to the topic and can thus point you in the right direction as your methods evolve. It is very tedious for a faculty member to advise a student about a research project in which the mentor has little expertise or interest. The reality of this fact from the student perspective is that, consciously or unconsciously, you might not receive optimal feedback as you progress through the research project.

It is also essential that the laboratory equipment you need to undertake the project be readily available and accessible. You should consider the degree to which it is being used during the period of time you anticipate collecting data. It is risky to undertake a research project when the equipment you need is expected to be purchased or loaned but is not yet physically present. It is also risky to plan to use the equipment in a facility or laboratory over which you and your mentor have no control. The use of loaned or donated equipment carries many complexities (e.g., potential conflicts of interest, ownership of data, etc.), some of which are discussed in Chapter 20.

You should also carefully assess the accessibility of the subjects you anticipate studying. For example, you might have an interest in studying some aspect of neuromuscular performance in the throwing shoulder of intercollegiate pitchers. However, if the coach of the baseball or softball team has no intention of making his or her athletes available for purposes of data collection, your efforts are likely to be fruitless. Many research paradigms in athletic training study subjects with pathology related to the research question. This, however, carries all sorts of risks for the student interested in completing a research project within a limited period of time. For example, you might be interested in studying the effects of some form of cryotherapy on swelling in subjects with acute ankle sprain. However, you have no control over the number of subjects who might fit your inclusion criteria and who might be available during the period when you expect to collect data.

Is the Scope of the Topic Appropriate?

Everyone who undertakes a research project wants his or her study to make an impact. The risk of this approach is creating a research project that is too excessive in its scope. This carries a high probability of the study never being completed. In reality, very few single research projects make a major impact. Rather, it is the accumulation of several studies around a theme that begins to make a substantial contribution to our understanding of a topic. Similarly, it is often more productive to select a piece of an existing research problem than to invent a new research problem. Expanding into new areas often leads to efforts that are too broad. Our best recommendation in this chapter is to focus, refocus, and focus yet again on exactly what it is you want to study. It is easy to broaden the scope of your study unintentionally as you conduct your literature review and begin to formulate your methods. Even a focused topic naturally becomes bigger than it initially appears, and you do not need to add to this expansion.

It is important that you consider the period of time you have in which to complete your research project. If you are undertaking a master's degree thesis, you probably want to devote no more than 6 months to 1 year to your research project. If you are a doctoral student, you might have 1 to 2 years to devote to your dissertation. The magnitude of the study should match the amount of time you have to devote to the project. An experienced research mentor is invaluable in helping you assess these factors.

Is the Topic Original, or Is It an Intentional Replication?

Some people think that every research project must be completely original. In all probability, your project will be similar to others in some respects. It is essential that you review the literature thoroughly so that you know what has already been studied in relation to your evolving topic. The strategies you learn in Chapter 4 will be invaluable in conducting a thorough literature review.

From the literature review, you will determine what has been studied, what is known, and what is not known about your topic. This information will enable you to develop a topic that does not unintentionally replicate a study that has already been completed. You will also learn a great deal about the methods of other studies, and this information will enable you to capitalize on the strengths of these studies while avoiding the pitfalls that others have experienced.

In some cases, the replication of a published study is very appropriate. This approach might apply when a study's findings are extraordinary and have not been independently corroborated by other researchers. For example, one study might report that a preventive strength and conditioning program significantly reduces the incidence of injury to the anterior cruciate ligament (ACL) in female athletes. This finding would potentially have great clinical application to the athletic training profession. However, before the preventive program is widely adopted by athletic training clinicians, it would be useful to know if independent researchers arrive at the same conclusion.

Even when conducting a thorough review of the literature, the possibility still exists that you will be unaware of a recent study as you formulate your topic. Very recently published papers, or those accepted for publication by a journal but not yet published, will not appear in the electronic databases you will use for your literature search. For this reason, it is a good idea to search the literature repeatedly as you conduct your research project and to review conference presentations, proceedings, and published abstracts for recent research. This is also the reason why it is inappropriate to state in the introduction or discussion sections of your paper that "this is the first study to examine this topic."

Does the Topic Have Good Clinical Application?

One of the distinguishing features of athletic training research is the potential to conduct a study that has immediate clinical application. Indeed, an excellent way to formulate a research topic is to draw from your clinical experience. As you prepare your team for practice, think about what is known and what is not known about the preventive interventions you employ. Does the tape you apply to the ankle sufficiently restrict excessive inversion motion? Will it facilitate proprioceptive feedback so as to prevent inversion ankle sprain? Does the stretching program you prescribe effectively increase and retain muscle flexibility? As you rehabilitate a patient, what is known about the therapeutic modalities you use and the therapeutic exercise interventions you apply? Does the ultrasound you apply sufficiently increase tissue temperature and blood flow? Is it effective in returning the patient to preinjury levels of function faster? Is the functional progression you use to return the athlete to competition an adequate predictor of ability to perform in the given sport?

A similar process can be used to conduct educational research. If you are teaching a laboratory class in athletic training, are the instructional strategies you use known to facilitate effective learning of the psychomotor skills you wish to convey? Are the clinical competencies you teach based on clinical research that has established the efficacy of treatment? These are just a few examples of how you can draw from your athletic training experiences to formulate a research topic.

Does the Research Topic or Theme Have Potential for External Funding?

In Chapter 19, you will learn the importance of finding sources of external funding to support a research program. The ideal research topic is one that is timely and thus has some potential for external funding. One way to assess timeliness is to compare your interest with the interests of funding agencies. If you are a master's degree student, you may need only a small amount of money to support your research project. If your topic is important to the field, you might be eligible for a small grant from a source such as your National Athletic Trainers' Association (NATA) district. The NATA's Research and Education Foundation provides small grants to support doctoral dissertation research. If you are a doctoral student, a timely and important topic could lead to funding from this source. Most funding agencies periodically release requests for proposals (RFPs), or calls for research funding proposals. RFPs are calls for proposals around a central theme or research question. Regardless of which avenue you select for funding, if you need funding, you should begin the process early. The funding process can take time, and therefore planning ahead is essential for success.

The potential for external funding should not be the sole or necessarily the primary criterion in selection of a topic. However, it is one consideration, and it would be helpful to you to review the funding sources available to athletic trainers as your research topic evolves.

The Importance of Building a Research Theme

If you are an undergraduate student, it is unlikely that your first research experience will set the agenda for your career. However, it might help you identify a graduate degree program that you will attend later in your career.

If you are a master's degree student, this project may be the only exposure to the research process you have in your entire career. On the other hand, you may be so fascinated by the experience that it will serve as only the beginning of a career in athletic training education and research. Perhaps you are a doctoral student who is already planning to pursue a career as an athletic training scholar in higher education. In any event, one of the distinguishing characteristics of the best athletic training researchers is the ability to focus one's research around a central theme or agenda. The following paragraphs will address several important factors in building a research theme.

Selecting the Right Institution and Mentor

The process of selecting an institution to pursue your master's or doctoral studies should ideally include a careful investigation of the research for which the school and its faculty are known. To accomplish this task, you can use the Internet, the literature and author search techniques explained in Chapter 4, and a personal visit and interview with the institutions in which you have an interest.

Most athletic training academic programs are thoroughly described in college and university Websites. A careful review of an institution's Website is an excellent way to investigate the institution's research agenda and the topics and themes for which the faculty members are known.

Another effective means of exploring the research for which the faculty are known is to apply the electronic database literature search techniques you will learn in Chapter 4. Using this technology, you can perform an author search on the name of the faculty member or members at the institution you are considering. The list of publications credited to the faculty members will appear, and you can review these books and articles to determine if the topics are consistent with the research you would like to undertake. Another option is to conduct the search using key words associated with your research interests and then review the resulting list of publications and their authors for a good match with your interests. Regardless of how you explore the research interests of the faculty at the institutions you are considering, you will make the best possible impression during an interview if you become very familiar with the research conducted by the faculty with whom you will be interviewing.

A personal visit to the institution to which you are applying for admission is a critical component of the selection process. This is your opportunity to talk with the faculty member who would serve as your research mentor and with the students currently enrolled in the program who will be your colleagues for at least part of your graduate studies. At this time, you can also visit the research facilities to determine if the instrumentation is adequate and an appropriate match for your research interests. Another effective means of exploring the potential of the institution as a good match for you is to obtain a listing of the alumni who have completed their grad-

In the Field

Sandy had been a certified athletic trainer for 13 years, most recently as the associate head athletic trainer at a major Division I university, working with women's basketball. She loved her job, but for some time had been contemplating going back to school to get her doctorate degree. She now thought that this might be a good time in her career to take the plunge. She sought out the advice of a friend who was also on the faculty at the university. "Any advice, George?" she asked. He replied, "Sandy, pursuing a doctorate is a significant commitment. My best advice is to think about the area of research that you are most interested in, then find a program in which at least one of the fac-ulty shares that interest. Matching your interests to that of the faculty does two things: (1) you can be assured that the faculty has the knowledge and expertise in the research designs and methods that you will be using and will be better able to advise and mentor you in the research process, and (2) because they are interested in the same area of research, the opportunities for collaboration will be greater, and you can bet they will be more engaged and enthusiastic about your work." Sandy carefully considered George's advice, and it made a lot of sense to her. She knew that this would be a big commitment and that research would be a large part of her doctoral studies. Because she hadn't done a thesis with her master's degree, she knew she needed a good research mentor.

Sandy already knew what she wanted to study; she just didn't know where. Clinically, she had worked with a number of female athletes over the past few years who had injured their ACLs, and she really wanted to understand why women were more prone to this type of injury. After researching the various institutions that offered doctoral degrees in sports medicine, she did a literature search on the faculty at each institution to learn more about the type of research they were doing. She found two programs that appeared to have a strong research agenda related to neuromuscular risk factors in ACL injury. Ultimately, she applied and interviewed with both programs, and both granted her admission. It was tough to choose between the two because both programs had excellent facilities and faculty, but she ultimately decided on the one that felt like the best fit for her both personally and professionally. Although it took her considerable time and effort to investigate potential doctoral programs, her "initial research project" paid off, and she never once regretted her decision.

uate studies at the college or university. You can then contact them to ask them about their level of satisfaction with the program and of the quality of the research mentoring they received and if they were able to complete their research and program of study in a timely manner. Additional considerations for selecting an institution might include location, cost, curriculum, funding opportunities, and the option of clinical opportunities.

Selecting Your Personal Research Theme

If you are interested in exploring a career as an athletic training scholar in higher education, you will ultimately learn a great deal about the process of promotion and tenure. Normally, the criteria for promotion and tenure include sufficient productivity and competence in teaching, research, and service. The degree to which productivity in these three areas is valued in the review process varies according to the level of an institution's research rating. For example, institutions rated by the Carnegie Classification of Institutions of Higher Education as Doctoral Research Extensive or Intensive place a great deal of emphasis on research (Display 3–2). Institutions rated lower in the research classification in all probability place greater emphasis on classroom teaching and individual student advising. One of the key elements of assessing a faculty member's productivity in research is the degree to which he or she has established a credible and recognized research agenda.

Display 3-2

Carnegie Classification of Research Institution

The 2000 Carnegie Classification includes all colleges and universities in the United States that grant degrees and are accredited by an agency recognized by the United States secretary of education. The 2000 edition classifies institutions based on their degree-granting activities from 1995–1996 through 1997–1998. For definitions and detailed information on classification procedures, refer to the Technical Notes. In addition, important limitations are documented in The 2000 Carnegie Classification: Background and Description.

Doctorate-Granting Institutions

Doctoral/Research Universities—Extensive

These institutions typically offer a wide range of baccalaureate programs, and they are committed to graduate education through the doctorate. During the period studied, they awarded 50 or more doctoral degrees per year across at least 15 disciplines.

Doctoral/Research Universities—Intensive

These institutions typically offer a wide range of baccalaureate programs, and they are committed to graduate education through the doctorate. During the period studied, they awarded at least 10 doctoral degrees per year across 3 or more disciplines, or at least 20 doctoral degrees per year overall.

Master's Colleges and Universities

Master's Colleges and Universities I

These institutions typically offer a wide range of baccalaureate programs, and they are committed to graduate education through the master's degree. During the period studied, they awarded 40 or more master's degrees per year across three or more disciplines.

Master's Colleges and Universities II

These institutions typically offer a wide range of baccalaureate programs, and they are committed to graduate education through the master's degree. During the period studied, they awarded 20 or more master's degrees per year.

Continued

Display 3-2	**Carnegie Classification of Research Institution** *(Contd.)*

Baccalaureate Colleges

Baccalaureate Colleges—Liberal Arts

These institutions are primarily undergraduate colleges with a major emphasis on baccalaureate programs. During the period studied, they awarded at least half of their baccalaureate degrees in liberal arts fields.

Baccalaureate Colleges—General

These institutions are primarily undergraduate colleges with a major emphasis on baccalaureate programs. During the period studied, they awarded less than half of their baccalaureate degrees in liberal arts fields.

Baccalaureate/Associate's Colleges

These institutions are undergraduate colleges where the majority of conferrals are below the baccalaureate level (associate's degrees and certificates). During the period studied, bachelor's degrees accounted for at least 10 percent of undergraduate awards.

Associate's Colleges

These institutions offer associate's degree and certificate programs but, with few exceptions, award no baccalaureate degrees. This group includes institutions where, during the period studied, bachelor's degrees represented less than 10 percent of all undergraduate awards.

Specialized Institutions

These institutions offer degrees ranging from the bachelor's to the doctorate and typically award a majority of degrees in a single field. The list includes only institutions that are listed as separate campuses in the 2000 Higher Education Directory. Specialized institutions include:

- *Theological seminaries and other specialized faith-related institutions*: These institutions primarily offer religious instruction or train members of the clergy.
- *Medical schools and medical centers*: These institutions award most of their professional degrees in medicine. In some instances, they include other health professions programs, such as dentistry, pharmacy, or nursing.
- *Other separate health profession schools*: These institutions award most of their degrees in such fields as chiropractic, nursing, pharmacy, or podiatry.
- *Schools of engineering and technology*: These institutions award most of their bachelor's or graduate degrees in technical fields of study.
- *Schools of business and management*: These institutions award most of their bachelor's or graduate degrees in business or business-related programs.
- *Schools of art, music, and design*: These institutions award most of their bachelor's or graduate degrees in art, music, design, architecture, or some combination of such fields.
- *Schools of law*: These institutions award most of their degrees in law.
- *Teachers' colleges*: These institutions award most of their bachelor's or graduate degrees in education or education-related fields.
- *Other specialized institutions*: Institutions in this category include graduate centers, maritime academies, military institutes, and institutions that do not fit any other classification category.

Carnegie Classification of Research Institution *(Contd.)*

These colleges are, with few exceptions, tribally controlled and located on reservations. They are all members of the American Indian Higher Education Consortium.

©2004, The Carnegie Foundation for the Advancement of Teaching. Reprinted with permission. Retrieved 8/9/04 from The Carnegie Classification of Institutions of Higher Education website: http://www.carnegiefoundation.org/Classification/CIHE2000/defNotes/Definitions.htm/

Most institutions become known for the line of research conducted by its faculty. The information illustrated in Figure 3–1 is an example of one institution's research agenda. This kind of presentation of a research agenda

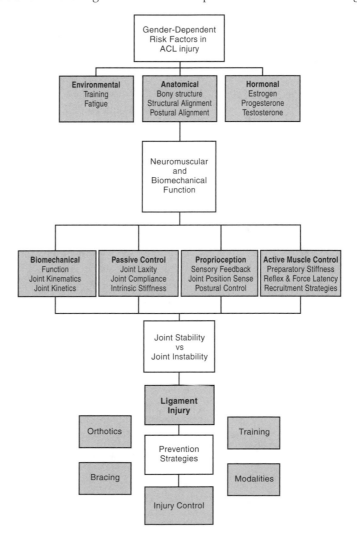

Figure 3–1 One institution's laboratory musculoskeletal research agenda. This agenda could be used as a guide to select a topic that helps to advance the lab's research program, falls under the expertise of the research mentor, and uses instrumentation readily available for the student's research project.

could be used to assist with selection of an institution at which to pursue your graduate studies. It could also be used to help with selection of a topic that would help to advance the institution's research agenda and one that presumably falls within the field of expertise of the mentor with whom you will study. As suggested in the previous section, matching your interests with those of your potential mentor and the agenda of the research laboratory are essential for a rewarding and productive graduate experience.

Summary

The formulation of a viable research topic is the first step in undertaking a successful research project. It is a phase of the study that should not be taken lightly because embarking on a project that does not meet the criteria discussed in this chapter carries a higher probability of failure. The checklist in Display 3–1 will help you formulate a topic that is feasible in terms of the time and resources available to you.

Activities

1. Using your clinical experience as a foundation, identify a treatment protocol or rehabilitation technique that is commonly used but has not been validated through the research process.
2. Choose a research topic and explore the literature for researchers and institutions performing research in that area.
3. Review requests for proposals (RFPs) from granting agencies to identify potentially fundable topics in which you may have an interest.

Bibliography

Applied Neuromechanics Research Laboratory Website at the University of North Carolina— Greensboro. Retrieved 3/25/04: *http:www.uncg.edu/ess/anrl*

Grants.gov home page. Retrieved 3/25/04: *http:www.grants.gov*

National Athletic Trainers' Association Research and Education Foundation. Retrieved 3/25/04: *http://www.natafoundation.org*

Part 2
The Literature

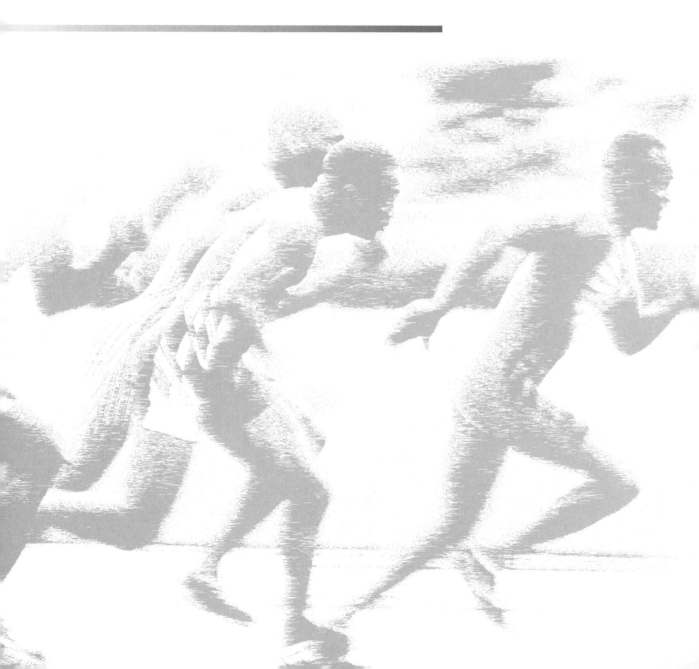

Chapter 4

Reviewing the Literature

Objectives

After reading this chapter, you will:
- Appreciate the importance of a literature review.
- Demonstrate how to complete an electronic database search.
- Be able to perform nonelectronic database searches.
- Demonstrate how to organize a comprehensive literature review.
- Demonstrate how to identify and collect articles for your literature review.

Questions

While reading this chapter, think about answers to the following questions:
1. Why do I need to perform a literature review?
2. How do I find the articles that I need?
3. What is the difference between a primary and secondary source?
4. Can I use secondary sources?
5. How should I organize my material?
6. When I read an article, what am I looking for?
7. How many sources do I need?
8. How do I know I have everything?

Importance of the Literature Review

The primary purpose of your literature review is to build the foundation for the proposed research. Essential elements of the literature review are establishing the need and the theoretical model for the research. For example, if the purpose of the research is to study a specific injury's mechanism, pattern, or treatment, you can best accomplish this by including epidemiological evidence. Epidemiological studies provide the most efficient way of establishing the need for your research by identifying the incidence of and potential causes of injury.

Your literature review should also establish the theoretical model of your research. This includes reviewing the biomechanical, physiological, and/or psychological factors associated with the research problem. The theoretical model will have a greater emphasis if the research focus is not directly related to an injury. For example, studies examining the effectiveness of ultrasound will be more dependent on the theoretical model than on epidemiological evidence. Regardless of the topic or purpose, your theoretical model should establish the biologic plausibility of your study.

The literature review should also help you identify deficiencies or gaps in the literature. Often these deficiencies (or unresolved issues) assist in directing you to logical starting points. Your goal should be to identify important issues that have not been studied. Conversely, you can avoid unintended duplication by identifying issues that have already been studied. Exact replication of an existing study is typically not the best use of a researcher's time. If two studies have identical methods and results, the second study may be considered unimportant by the scientific community. Consequently, journal editors may choose not to publish the study because it does not make a significant contribution to the literature. Intentional replication, on the other hand, can play an important role in the scientific process. If existing studies are contradictory or equivocal, replication is sometimes necessary to establish a specific finding. Intentional replication is most efficiently accomplished as part of studies examining new issues. This allows you to confirm or refute existing studies as well as make a new contribution to the literature.

The literature review can also assist you in developing appropriate research methods and establishing the reliability and validity of the dependent measures. Put another way, you do not need to reinvent the methods. It is very appropriate to use the methods of other researchers. In fact, this can be a strength because it makes your study directly comparable to other studies. Additionally, using other researchers' methods can save considerable time by avoiding having to develop new methods and subsequently establishing the reliability and validity of the dependent measures.

Electronic Databases

The first step in developing the literature review is identifying the literature needed for the review. Fortunately, this has been made easier with the advent of electronic databases. These databases are typically available at university and college libraries or through the Internet. With practice, these databases provide you with a fast and efficient mechanism for identifying important journal articles, theses or dissertations, and in some cases books.

Medline, PubMed Central, and PubMed

Medline (National Library of Medicine, Bethesda, Maryland) is an electronic database operated by the National Library of Medicine (NLM). This database is the electronic version of Index Medicus and contains basic, applied, and clinical science journals related to health science. You will find this database very useful for basic science research and medical research outside the area of athletic training. However, several athletic training and exercise science journals (e.g., *Journal of Athletic Training* and *Journal of Sport Rehabilitation*) are not included in Medline, and therefore you should not consider Medline searches comprehensive.

PubMed Central is the digital archive of the NLM. For a journal to be included, it must have at least three editors or editorial board members who are principal investigators of national (e.g., the National Institutes of Health) or international research grants, and it must be willing to provide an online version of the journal to the NLM. Medline journals are included (provided that they are in an online format) as well as journals currently not indexed on Medline (e.g., the *Journal of Athletic Training*). Finally, PubMed is the online retrieval system for biomedical journals operated by the NLM. Medline and PubMed Central journals are included as well as citations that precede a journal's selection for Medline.

Sport Discus

Sport Discus (SilverPlatter Information Inc., Norwood, MA) is an electronic database containing journal articles specifically related to exercise science and athletic training (Display 4–1). It is a useful first source for athletic training research and contains most of the exercise science and sports medicine journals found in Medline (e.g., the *American Journal of Sports Medicine* and the *Journal of Orthopedic and Sports Physical Therapy*), plus many that are not (e.g., the *Journal of Athletic Training* and the *Journal of Sport Rehabilitation*). One drawback to using Sport Discus is that it contains mostly applied research. Therefore, if you need basic science research for your literature review (e.g., joint proprioceptor physiology), Medline should also be used.

Other Databases

Several other databases may also be useful. The Cumulative Index to Nursing and Allied Health (CINAHL) of CINAHL Information Systems, Glendale, California, has many of the same references as Medline but is more focused on allied health. The Educational Resource Information Center (ERIC) of the United States Department of Education, Office of Educational Research and Improvement, Washington, DC, is the world's

Display 4-1 | **Partial Output from a Sport Discus Search for Ankle Sprains**

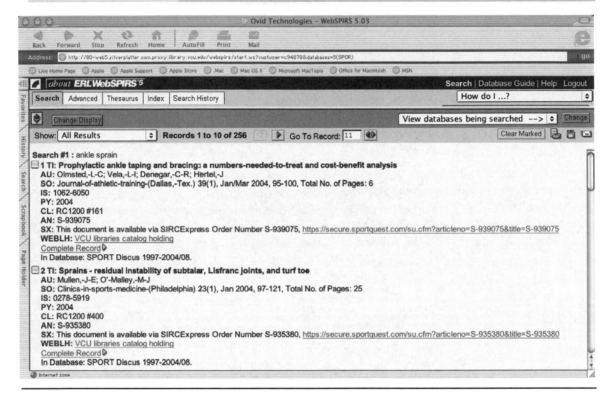

largest education database and is useful for education rather than health science research. Finally, Dissertation Abstracts of ProQuest Information and Learning, Ann Arbor, Michigan, is an indexing source for doctoral dissertations and master's theses. This database includes American and European dissertations and theses on all topics.

Database Fields

Although each electronic database contains different information, the basic structure of all databases is similar. For example, each entry in the database (i.e., each journal article or book listed in the database) contains at least five fields. These are title, author, key words, journal, and year of publication. In addition to the five primary fields, some databases include an abstract field containing the abstract printed with the article, a language field indicating the language of the publication, and a level field indicating the difficulty level of the article (with "basic" indicating a lay publication and "advanced" indicating a research publication).

Search Strategies for Electronic Databases

Because the databases are structured into fields, they can be searched by those fields, making database searches very versatile. Examples of the various types of searches according to field are given in the following paragraphs.

Keyword Searches

Keyword searches are the most generic searches. The keyword can be a single word (e.g., ankle) or a string of two or more words (e.g., ankle injuries). When using a keyword search, the database will look for the selected terms in all the fields of the database. Therefore, this type of search is likely to produce the greatest number of potential references, but it is also most likely to produce irrelevant information, especially if the search term is too broad. For example, if you keyword search for "cruciate," topics such as "anterior cruciate" and "posterior cruciate" will result. If you are interested only in anterior cruciate studies, this search will give you too many references. One solution to this is to use word strings such as "anterior cruciate" to narrow the search. This appears to be a very useful way to limit a search and, in fact, will produce articles containing the word string "anterior cruciate." However, because the database searches for that exact combination of words, word combinations such as "cruciate injuries" will not be found, and information will be missed. This can be avoided by conducting searches in stages and then combining searches (see Boolean Searches further on in this section).

Subject Searches

Subject searches are searches of specific topics established by the database. These subjects are established differently for each database. For example, Medline uses Medical Subject Headings (MeSH), established by the National Library of Medicine (Display 4–2). Similarly, Sport Discus uses subject headings specifically established for sport sciences. Most databases contain a thesaurus or listing of subjects that will help you identify topics that may be used in a search. Subject searches are most useful for well-established topics such as "strength" or "proprioception," in which you expect large amounts of information. If you are unfamiliar with a topic, browsing the thesaurus can give you a helpful perspective on the scope of your topic. The shortcoming of subject searches is that if the topic of interest is not in the subject field, the search will yield no results.

Display 4-2 | **Medline Subject Categories Resulting from a Subject Search for Ankle Sprains**

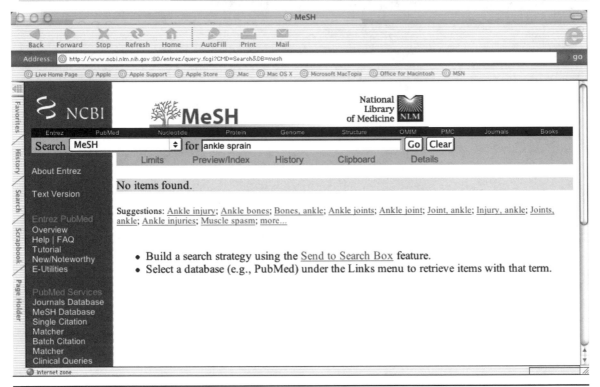

Author Searches

Author searches are also possible with electronic databases. These can be very useful if you are looking for an article written by a specific person. Searching for the author will produce all of the author's publications, allowing you to select the needed references. Obviously, this also makes it possible to collect sets of publications by authors, including those that are listed after the first author. Finally, because an author search produces all publications by authors of the same name, knowing the initials of the author is useful in narrowing your search.

Title Searches

Title searches are another option and are limited to the title only. This type of search is useful when you know the exact title. However, it produces limited results as a general search because titles may not represent the full content or important concepts of an article.

Journal Searches

Searching for a specific journal is also made possible by searching the journal field. By itself, this is not particularly useful because it will locate all issues of the journal. However, you will find it useful for narrowing a search when you know the journal in which the article was published or use it in combination with other searches.

Boolean Searches

Boolean searches are a useful way of building complex searches. There are several ways in which you can build these searches, but they all use the same three logical operators: AND, OR, and NOT. The strength of these operators is that you can use them to search for word combinations in any field or to combine searches of different types, for example, an author search with a journal search.

The OR Operator

You can use OR to limit a search to either of two words but not necessarily both words. For example, a title search for "peak OR torque" will produce "Quadriceps peak torque production," "Torque produced during cycling," and "Peak EMG activity during walking" (Figure 4–1).

The AND Operator

The most common way of building searches is to combine searches with AND. When you use AND, you limit the search to publications that contain both words but not necessarily both words adjacent to each other. For example, a title search combining "peak AND torque" will produce titles

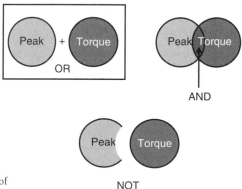

Figure 4–1 Visual representation of Boolean searches.

such as "Peak power as a function of muscle torque" and "Quadriceps peak torque production." To avoid getting the first example, more complex combinations including the command OR can be created. See Figure 4–1 for a visual representation of an AND search.

The NOT Operator

One possible way to narrow the search further is to use the NOT operator. For example, the search "cruciate" would produce articles for both the anterior and posterior cruciate ligaments. By contrast, the search "cruciate NOT posterior" would eliminate all references to the posterior cruciate. However, it would also eliminate all references that contain the word posterior, including appropriate references such as "Anterior and posterior knee motion following ACL injury." This search could be better refined as follows: "cruciate NOT posterior cruciate." In this case, only references containing "posterior cruciate" would be eliminated (see Fig. 4–1).

Combining Searches with Parentheses

You can also create combinations using parentheses, with items in the parentheses taking precedence over the other items. The combination "(peak OR average) AND torque" will produce peak torque, average torque, and "Peak EMG as a function of muscle torque." An alternative combination could be "(anterior AND cruciate) OR ACL" which would produce anterior cruciate, ACL, and "Anterior and posterior drawer test results associated with posterior cruciate injuries." Another advantage of combining search terms is that it enables you to identify the most relevant references. For example, if you are interested in ACL injury prevention, searching for ACL would produce thousands of citations, mostly related to ACL reconstruction. However, combining ACL and prevention might generate fewer than 100 references, but these would be more relevant to your topic.

Search Problems

As you can see, combining searches often produces undesired results. Unfortunately, narrowing a search to exactly your interests is never possible. Therefore, your goal should be to narrow the search electronically as much as possible and select references from the remaining items. Other typical problems include using the wrong keywords. It often takes several failed attempts to find the words needed to produce desirable results.

If you are new to database searches, you will probably make the common mistake of searching for concepts rather than words. For example, "injury" might be mistakenly used to find publications describing injury mechanics. Although the search may do exactly that, it will also find any occurrence of the word "injury" and produce many undesirable items (often hundreds to thousands). An efficient researcher thinks in terms of how concepts might be described with words and searches for those words, not the concepts.

Finally, two other problems with electronic databases are unlisted journals (as with Medline) and update frequency. Databases are typically updated only every 3 to 6 months. Unfortunately, the only way to counter these problems is to know the limitations of the database with which you are working and to visit the current periodicals section of the library.

Nonelectronic Sources

It is tempting to use only electronic databases in performing a literature search or to believe that electronic searches are the only way of conducting a literature search. However, if electronic databases are not available, you can conduct effective searches with nonelectronic sources. In fact, several very good nonelectronic sources should be used. The obvious limitation of nonelectronic databases is that they require manual retrieval of information, which creates the potential for mistakes.

Review Articles

Probably the best nonelectronic resource is the review article. Review articles are typically written by experts and summarize a large volume of research in a specific area. They will provide you with both information and references. For an investigator starting in a new area, review articles can provide excellent direction. They frequently outline and elaborate on important issues related to the selected topic.

Although they are excellent resources, review articles are secondary sources (meaning they are dependent on other publications) and therefore have several disadvantages. For example, the authors may have misinterpreted the research included in the article. Therefore, the information may be inaccurate. This is probably rare, but it can happen. Similarly, you may find inaccurate source citations, which can frustrate your efforts to locate important material. Finally, the review may be incomplete. This is likely if the article is several years old and new research has been published subsequently. You can avoid these problems by retrieving the original (i.e., primary) sources and supplementing the review article with a complete up-to-date literature search.

Journal Article References

You can also obtain references from journal articles. These references often have significant impact on a literature search. For example, say that you conduct an electronic database search for "os trigonum fractures" and find three related articles. This is insufficient for a literature review. However, if each of these articles has three additional, different articles, you now have 12 articles related to os trigonum fractures. In other words, one article often leads to several others, producing a domino effect. This is a normal process and is fundamental to a thorough literature review.

Dissertations and Theses

Dissertations and theses are also useful but frequently overlooked reference sources. However, you should keep in mind that theses and dissertations have not gone through the scientific review process. This means that you should not give them the same level of importance as journal articles. If the dissertation or thesis is several years old, it is likely that the author has since published portions of the work in a scientifically reviewed journal. If parts of the dissertation have been published, you can conduct an author search on an electronic database to locate the article(s). Keep in mind that dissertations are never published in their entirety, are often published as several different articles, and are rarely published with the same title. Therefore, some effort may be needed to match the correct article(s) to the dissertation.

Nonscientifically Reviewed Publications

You should generally avoid sources that have not undergone the rigor of the scientific review process required for a manuscript to be published in a refereed journal. These sources include abstracts, newspaper articles, lay publications, Websites, and professional publications that do not use the scientific review process. These publications are not considered valid research by the scientific community. Many scientific journals now have Websites and have placed their journals online. These are valid sources. In some cases, these sources may provide references to scientifically reviewed

In the Field

John has had difficulty conducting a successful search for his research topic. However, he has been able to find one article related to his topic in an issue of the Journal of Athletic Training. Using the references from that article, he was able to find four other articles related to the topic. From this small set of articles, John did three things. First, he continued using the references of each article to build his reference list. Second, using the authors' names, he conducted an author search. From this search he was able to find several related articles published by most of the authors. Third, at the end of each article's abstract, he noted the keywords listed. Using these, he performed a keyword and subject search of the electronic databases. When he completed these steps, the number of articles for his review greatly expanded.

sources, which can then be used. The citation of abstracts should be avoided unless the information presented is very recent and there are no published manuscripts on the topic.

Critical Review of the Literature

Once you have collected the literature, your next step is to conduct a critical review of it. Implicit in this review is your obligation to collect the original articles (i.e., primary sources) and read each of them. You may be tempted to rely on the comments and interpretations from other journal articles (i.e., secondary sources) that used the primary source. This is an unacceptable shortcut because an author may misinterpret the findings of other studies. Therefore, if you rely on another author's erroneous interpretation, you may reproduce previous errors.

Trying to organize a literature review can seem overwhelming. However, you will find the task more manageable if it is divided into a gross examination and an in-depth examination of the literature.

Gross Examination

The primary purpose of the gross examination is identifying important issues and sorting the literature into categories. You should examine each article for important features without scrutinizing the details too closely. We suggest that you write the key issues on the face page of each article to permit quick identification and easy sorting of the articles. When you identify important issues, at least three broad categories should be developed. The first consists of issues related to the research problem. As you develop this category, subcategories will evolve and/or should be created. The second category is research methods. For example, in the area of proprioception/kinesthesia, researchers often measure the ability to reposition a joint to a specified angle either actively or passively. This may be important when you develop your methods. The final category is the reliability and validity of measures (see Chapter 9). It is important for you to have measures that are reliable and valid as part of the research. Therefore, studies that have demonstrated the reliability and validity of your measures (or similar measures) should be identified. Finally, you should recognize that some studies might belong to multiple categories. A study of balance may have also measured strength. In this situation, the article should be listed in both categories.

Once you have identified the important issues, you should begin to identify common themes. This may be done around common research issues, research methods, and so on. As you identify themes, you will find it useful to structure these themes into subcategories and begin developing a topical outline (Display 4–3). Doing this early will help you organize the information, keep you focused on the topics, and simplify your writing later.

Display 4-3 | **Example of a Topical Outline for Ankle Instability**

I. Ankle/Foot Kinesthesia

A. **Kinesthesia during Traumatic Inversion**
Bahr 94
Robbins 97

B. **Cutaneous Input**
Magnusson 90
Robbins 88 (jte), 88 (msse)

C. **Muscle Receptors**
Gregory 88

D. **Following Exercise**
Robbins 95

E. **With Tape/Support**
Feuerbach 93
Firer 90
Robbins 95

II. Neurologic Injury

Freeman 65
Garn 88
Kleinrensink 94
Levine 85

Nitz 85
O'Connor 85
Simoneau 96
Van den Bosch 95

III. Function Instability

A. **Definition**
Freeman 65

B. **Mechanical Instability**
1. General
Bernier 97
Black 77
Bosien 55
Brand 77
Clayton 68
Conlin 89
Freeman 65 (etiology, instability)
Kristiansen 82
Tropp 85
Freeman 65 (etiology)
Nitz 85
Nitz 87
Vaes 98

2. Surgical Repair
Black 77
Brostrom 66
Conlin 89
Evans 84
Freeman 65 (treatment)
Prins 78
Staples 72,75

C. **Muscular Weakness**
Bernier 97
Bosien 55
Lentell 90,95

Tropp 86
Wilkerson 97

D. **Neuromuscular Response**
Beckman 95
Ebig 97
Grillner 72
Isakov 86
Karlsson 92
Konradsen 90,91,97
Lofvenberg 95 (prolonged)
Louwerens 95
Nawoczenski 85

E. **Kinesthesia/Proprioception**
Appleburg 79
Freeman 67
Garn 88
Glencross 81
Gross 87
Kennedy 82
Lentell 95
Lundberg 78

F. **Balance**
Bernier 97
Cornwall 91
DeCarlo 86
Forkin 96
Freeman 65 (etiology)
Friden 89
Fuerbach 93
Garn 88
Gauffin 88
(Continued on following page)

Guskiewicz 96
Konradsen 91
Leanderson 96
Lentell 90
Magnusson 90
Tropp 84 (factors)
Tropp 84
  (stabilometry)
Tropp 85
Tropp 86
	Tropp 88
	
	G. Stiffness
	Grillner 72
	Louwerens 95
	
	H. Synovial Hypertrophy/
	   Capsular Lesion
	deAndrade
	Ferkel 91
	Freeman 65 (instability)

IV. Training/ **Treatment**	
Bosien 55 Freeman 65 (etiology) Gauffin 88 Hoffman 95 Mattacola 97	Johnson 93 Milch 86 Nashner 76 Prins 78 Sheth 97

In-Depth Examination

Once the gross examination is completed, each article must be read in complete detail. Under no circumstances should the review of the literature be conducted and written after reviewing only the abstracts of published articles. This process appears daunting, but it can be simplified if a specific routine is followed. That routine should include identifying the purpose, the independent and dependent variables, the participant characteristics, the research methods, the experimental design and statistical methods, the results and conclusions, and recommendations for future research (Fig. 4–2). We recommend this order of procedure because it is typically the most efficient. However, you should select an order that matches your goals.

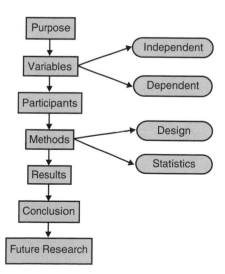

Figure 4–2 Flow chart of an in-depth examination of the literature.

Purpose

Identifying the purpose will help you put the study in the appropriate context. It should help you determine whether the study is related to your research topic. In addition, it should suggest what the hypothesis is and may indicate the type of methods that were used. However, stated purposes do not always match the actual purpose. Therefore, you will need to be cautious about using the purpose to determine an article's appropriateness.

Independent and Dependent Variables

Independent variables are variables manipulated by the researcher (e.g., ice versus no ice). Dependent variables are the variables that are measured by the researcher (e.g., pain) and are modulated by the independent variables. In other words, the independent variable is the input, and the dependent variable is the output

Identifying the independent and dependent variables is important. You may discover that they are not consistent with your interests or goals. For example, if you were interested in the effects of ankle rehabilitation on ankle strength, a study that measures only kinesthesia would not be appropriate. Similarly, if your independent variable of interest was strength training, studies using balance training would not be appropriate. However, eliminating articles from your literature search because the variables do not match yours should be done cautiously. Sometimes, variables (e.g., center of pressure and center of balance [Grabiner, Lundin, & Feuerbach, 1993]) are similar enough that, although they are not identical, they measure the same or highly related variables. Finally, when identifying variables, remember that more than one independent or dependent variable may have been studied.

Participant Characteristics

Participant characteristics include height, weight, age, gender, injury status, percent body fat, and so on. The first four of these should be reported with every study, and other characteristics should be reported when relevant. You should use participant characteristics to determine the appropriateness of the participants for the study. For example, if researchers had been interested in balance deficits in individuals with acute ankle sprains, including individuals with 3-week-old sprains would not have been appropriate. You should also consider whether the participant sample would generalize to the appropriate target population. It is important that the participant pool match the goals of the study. If applying the results to a broad population was the goal, researchers should have included a broad sample of individuals (e.g., men/women, young/old) in their study. However, if only young, healthy men were used in the study, the results would not apply to an older or female population. In this case, it would not be possible to generalize from the participant sample to the larger population.

Methods, Experimental Design, and Statistics

As with participant characteristics, you should determine whether the methods, experimental design, and statistics match the goals of the study. Instruments, treatment and measurement protocols, and statistical methods should be identified. Differences among study results may occur because of different methods used. Identifying these differences may be important in explaining differences among studies. Furthermore, if statistical analyses were performed incorrectly, the reported results may not be valid.

Results/Conclusions

In examining the results of the study, you will want to note the magnitude of the measures. This will give you a sense of what your results should be. You should also compare the magnitude of the measures with other studies. Large inconsistencies in magnitude may suggest that the measures are unreliable or that individual studies are not valid. You should also closely compare the results with the conclusions of the study. The results should support the conclusions. If they do not, the conclusions are not valid. Novice investigators often make the mistake of relying on the reported conclusions rather than critically reviewing the results. This should be avoided because investigators occasionally misinterpret or overinterpret results. It is also possible that the conclusions are invalid because statistical analyses have been applied incorrectly. Another mistake that is occasionally made is drawing conclusions from descriptive data that are not statistically supported. If you find a researcher has drawn conclusions without statistical support, these conclusions should be disregarded. Finally, as you read the conclusions from a set of articles, you should begin to determine how the articles are related to each other and identify important issues discussed in the articles. This will help you to organize and develop your own discussion.

Future Research

Finally, you should examine each article for suggestions for future research. This is often helpful in providing direction for your research, or it may direct you away from unproductive lines of research. However, suggestions for future research should not be considered comprehensive, and you should use your own judgment based on what you have learned from your literature search.

Organization

Once you have collected and read each article, the next step is to organize the articles. This is best done by establishing how the articles are related to each other. They may be related by methods, subjects, pathology, and so on. Depending on the purpose, it may be appropriate to organize your articles

In the Field

> Tom has managed to collect more than 50 articles for his literature review on ankle strength after an ankle sprain. He now faces what seems to be a daunting task: organizing the articles. As he reviews the literature, he notices two common themes. The first is postacute versus chronic sprains. In other words, some articles studied strength loss after an acute sprain, and others studied strength in individuals with chronic sprains. The second theme is the method of strength testing. Some studies used manual muscle testing, whereas others used isokinetic testing. Tom notes both of these themes on the front page of each article. He now sorts the articles into two piles, acute and chronic, and begins his detailed review. As he reads the articles, he realizes that he is really interested in chronic ankle injuries and fine-tunes his review by setting aside the postacute injury articles. As he studies the articles further, he notes that they can be further subdivided. Isokinetic strength testing can be done in multiple directions and speeds, and chronic ankle sprains can be sorted into the broad categories of giving way and other chronic symptoms. Based on this, he adds additional labels to his articles and begins building an outline similar to that in Display 4–3.

based on any of these characteristics. However, usually it is best and most efficient to organize articles based on their results. There is no single rule for organizing the articles in your literature review, but by using the results, you will build stronger connections among similar studies and clearer distinctions among differing studies. Initially, you should identify studies whose results are similar and support each other, but you will also want to identify discrepant studies. Discrepancies among studies may represent exceptions to the general consensus. If this is the case, you should try to identify the reasons for the differences. These differences often represent important departures in methods, subjects, or other characteristics that you will want to consider as you develop your own research project. Explanations for differences among studies are often the most important feature of your literature review.

Solutions to Common Problems

Organization of Material

The most common problem faced early in the literature review process is organization. The best way to solve this problem is to build your topical outline with abundant subheadings. Under each of these subheadings, you should place the author names and year of publication of the relevant article(s). One strategy in building the outline is to use a published literature review as a guide. However, you should be cautious not to plagiarize the review. Use it only to develop the topics (adding and deleting subheadings as needed) and identify articles that belong under each subheading. To avoid plagiarizing the review, be sure to read each article and take your own notes.

Material Collection

As you begin collecting articles, you will find that keeping track of the articles that you have and the articles that you need is tedious and frustrating. To avoid this, you should keep a running list of the articles for quick reference. Because you will rarely find two or more articles with the same first author and year, the easiest way to do this is to list only the first author and year of each article. However, if two articles do have the same first author and year, include the second author or the first two to three words of the title to distinguish between the articles.

We highly recommend photocopying articles for later reference. To prevent frustration, be sure to take the following steps. First, always check the front page of the article for all of the reference information (i.e., journal title, volume number, pages, and year). This information is often found at the top or bottom of the page or under the abstract. If you cannot find this information, copy the title page or cover of the journal to have a record of this information. Second, be sure to copy all the reference pages. To save time and money, you will be tempted not to copy these pages. However, inevitably the missing page or pages will contain a reference that you want. Finally, double-check for all of the pages. It is very easy to miss a page while photocopying. Accurate and complete photocopying can save you from return trips to the library.

Source Selection

While searching for articles, ask yourself at least three questions: How do I select the articles? How many articles do I need? and How old is too old? When you are selecting articles, it is best to make your decision from reading the abstract or full paper. Titles can be misleading or incomplete and therefore are not very useful in making the final decision. There is no clear answer to the number of articles you will need. However, a good indicator that you have reached the end of the search process is redundancy. In other words, when the reference lists of articles begin to refer to articles you already have, you are probably done. Finally, deciding if an article is too old can be difficult. If relevant references are older than 10 years, we recommend obtaining only the foundational articles regardless of how old they are. Typically, a few foundational articles will establish the knowledge base of a topic, and other articles will confirm and support the results. Therefore, obtain these older articles, but maintain your focus on more recent references.

Failure to Obtain an Original Article

Failure to obtain original articles is a common mistake made by novice researchers. If an article you are reading refers to the results of another article that is of interest, you should obtain the original and not rely on information provided in the referring article. By obtaining the original, you can avoid misinterpretations by others and erroneous references. If you do not obtain the original, you may perpetuate such errors as well. A citation error repeated across several different articles is a good indicator that the researchers have taken shortcuts.

Summary

Collecting your literature can be a daunting task. It includes not only finding the literature you need but also reading and organizing your materials. Fortunately, using a combination of electronic and print sources will make your search easier. Once you have obtained your materials, examining them in a systematic way and organizing them in a meaningful way are essential to your success. The most effective way of organizing your literature review is to create a detailed outline.

Activities

1. Using your own research topic, conduct an electronic literature search.
   • Perform both a keyword and a subject search.
   • Perform an author search using an author from the keyword or subject search.
2. As part of the electronic search, conduct a Boolean search to refine your search.
   • Use AND to combine two keywords.

Reference

Grabiner, M.D., Lundin, T.M., & Feuerbach, J.W. (1993). Converting Chattecx Balance System vertical reaction force measurements to center of pressure excursion measurements. *Physical Therapy, 73*, 316–319.

Bibliography

Day, R. (1995). *Scientific English: A guide for scientists and other professionals* (2nd ed.). Phoenix, AZ: Oryx Press.
Day, R. (1988). *How to write and publish a scientific paper* (3rd ed.). Phoenix, AZ: Oryx Press.
Iverson, C., Flanagin, A., Fontanarosa, P.B., et al. (1998). *American Medical Association manual of style* (9th ed.). Baltimore: Williams & Wilkins.

Chapter 5

Writing the Literature Review

Major Components of the Literature Review

After collecting your literature, organizing it, and writing your topical outline, the next step is to write the literature review. In a thesis or dissertation, the literature review is formally known as Chapter 2. Because the literature review is fundamental to the remainder of the research process, we recommend writing it before other parts of the thesis. There are four main components in a literature review:

1. The introduction
2. The body
3. The summary
4. The references/citations

Each component has a different structure and/or purpose that should be followed to make the literature review effective. The components are described in the following sections.

Introduction

The introduction to the literature review should be one paragraph in length. It outlines the general purpose of the review as well as the content and order of the body. In other words, it provides your reader with a guide to what follows. An example of an introduction is shown in Display 5–1.

Body

The body is the major portion of the literature review. It is the foundation for your study, and in it you should discuss all the fundament topics related to your research. To accomplish this, use your topical outline to establish a logical progression for the review. When you construct the body, we recommend beginning with epidemiological studies when they are available. They are the best way of establishing the need for your research. Next, discuss the etiological and/or pathological information related to your study. These factors will help you identify the factors that should be the focus of your research. Finally, biomechanical or physiological rationales should be discussed. We believe that research without biomechanical or physiological rationales (i.e., biological plausibility) is the equivalent of guessing. Our experience has shown that researchers who fail to develop these rationales often propose inappropriate hypotheses and are subsequently frustrated when the results contradict their expectations. For example, a researcher might hypothesize that hamstring stretching will decrease postural sway. In fact, just the opposite is more likely because stretching would increase the length of the muscle spindle (making it more difficult for the muscle to sense changes in length). Had the researcher spent more time establishing the biologic plausibility of the study, a different hypothesis might have been proposed.

Display 5-1	**Example of an Introduction**
Introduction	Ankle injuries are frequent in athletics. Common outcomes of ankle sprains are chronic and functional ankle instability. The reasons for these conditions are unclear, but several factors, including strength, mechanical instability, and neuromuscular response, have been suggested. Therefore, the purpose of this review is to distinguish between chronic and functional ankle instabilities and discuss the roles of strength, mechanical instability, and neuromuscular response in producing these conditions.

One goal of the literature review should be to establish the scientific consensus. Your examination of the literature should reveal a general agreement among studies. For example, if you were interested in anterior cruciate ligament injuries in women, you would want to use the literature to establish the primary cause. Previous researchers should have established a consensus for a single cause, but unfortunately, this is not always the case. When there is no consensus, examine the literature for a set of causes that have been suggested.

In your literature review, you should also compare and contrast studies. Often a lack of consensus about a topic is the result of methodological differences among studies. Emphasizing points of agreement and disagreement can reveal why no consensus exists or why studies disagree with the consensus. You will seldom find total agreement on a topic. However, it is important that you present and understand research that agrees and disagrees with the consensus. It is also important that you present and discuss research that disagrees with your theoretical model. You should not focus only on research that supports your theory and hypotheses. If you do, you may overlook important research or not be prepared for rebuttals and criticisms.

Finally, you should address relevant design issues (e.g., reliability and validity of measures) and identify limitations in existing literature. By doing this, you can avoid mistakes made by others and improve your research design. Better research is almost always built by studying the strengths and weaknesses of previous research. It is important to identify these when you are critiquing an article.

In the Field

Carl is interested in strength and ankle instability. In reviewing the literature, he discovered that the studies conflicted. Some studies showed strength deficits and others did not. In consulting with his advisor, he was told to focus on the methods used in each study because different methods can have differing results. Carl discovered that the chief difference between studies was that some used repeated episodes of instability as an inclusion criterion, whereas the others used chronic symptoms, including pain and swelling. He then grouped studies into those that limited inclusion to subjects with chronic instability and those that also included pain and swelling. On re-examination, the consensus was that evertor strength deficits between chronically unstable and stable ankles were apparent when inclusion criteria were limited to multiple sprains and/or complaints of giving way. However, these deficits were absent when broader inclusion criteria such as chronic pain or swelling were added. Based on this, he concluded that it would be important for him to use a stricter set of exclusion criteria and exclude individuals with chronic pain or swelling.

Summary

Your final section of the literature review should be a one- to two-paragraph summary. A summary is necessary because the body of your literature review has covered a great deal of information on a variety of issues. At this point, the reader may have lost the main point of your review. Therefore, the summary is your opportunity to create a coherent synthesis of the most important elements of your literature review. Even if your readers read only the summary, they should have a clear sense of the important issues of your research and how these issues are interrelated.

References/Citations

The reference section has the most specified format of all the sections. In constructing you reference list, two factors must be kept in mind. The format of the references will be specified by the journal in which you intend to publish. This means that you have limited creative input. So, before you begin, check the journals' authors' guide to get the correct format. Otherwise, you'll waste a lot of time reformatting the references. Second, your reference list should contain only materials cited in the text. Other "supplemental" references should not be included.

Writing the Literature Review

Formatting

Format refers to the physical structure of the literature review and includes margin setting, type spacing, type justification, type size, citation/reference format, and so on. Acceptable formats vary greatly. However, you should select one format to use throughout the literature review (as well as the other sections of your document). The American Medical Association's (AMA) (Iverson et al., 1998) and the American Psychological Association's (APA) (1994) formats are the most frequently used in athletic training research. Which you select is mostly a matter of choice, but most journals

In the Field

Denise is preparing her manuscript for submission to the Journal of Athletic Training. As part of this process, she begins searching for the authors' guide for the journal. To do this, Denise's first step was to go to the National Athletic Trainers'Association Website, http://www.journalofathletictraining.org/. At the bottom of the page, she found the section "Other Useful Information related to JAT." Under this section, the link "Authors' Guide" took her to the guide, which she was able to read and print for her records.

and publishers specify which format they accept. Therefore, it is useful to identify your target journal/publisher early and follow the prescribed format. This information is available in the authors' guide of the journal/publisher.

Preparing to Write

As you prepare to write, you will find it useful to convert your topical outline to a sentence outline (Display 5–2). The sentence outline is a more detailed version of the topical outline. In a sentence outline, your major

Display 5-2 **A Sentence Outline and the Resulting Paragraphs**

Sentence Outline

I. 85% of ankle injuries occur to lateral ligaments
  A. Degree of severity varies
  B. Produce high incidence of chronic instability
    1. Affects length of rehabilitation
    2. Affects level of participation
    3. Attributed to joint laxity, muscle weakness, and proprioception deficits
II. Sprains produce trauma to ligaments, musculature, and sensory nerve endings.
  A. Sensory fibers damaged by joint capsule disruption
    1. Feedback from joint mechanoreceptors assist joint stabilization during locomotion
    2. Individuals may compensate for ligamentous loss with cues from:
      a) Spindle
      b) Cutaneous
      c) Vestibular
      d) Visual
  B. Muscle spindle is stimulated by vibration producing a sensation of movement
    1. Sense of movement occurs in the direction of vibrating muscle.
    2. Corresponds to the direction of muscle stretch.
    3. Therefore, muscle mechanoreceptors may aid in controlling joint motion.
    4. Rehabilitation may improve sensitivity

Resulting Paragraph*

"Inversion ankle sprains are the most common ankle injury with over 85% of all ankle sprains occurring to the lateral ligaments (Diamond, 1989). These injuries vary in their degree of severity and have been reported to produce a high incidence of chronic ankle instability that can affect both length of rehabilitation and level of participation in sports-related activities (Bosien, Staples, & Russel, 1955; Freeman, 1965). Ankle instability has been attributed most frequently to joint laxity, muscle weakness, and proprioception deficits (Lentell, Katzman, & Walters, 1990)."

"It has been suggested that ankle sprains not only produce trauma to joint ligaments and supporting musculature, but also to sensory nerve fibers within the joint capsule (Freeman, Dean, & Hanham, 1965). These nerve fibers provide feedback from the joint mechanoreceptors to assist stabilization of the ankle during locomotion. Individuals with ankle sprains that result in ligamentous laxity may compensate by relying on muscle spindle, cutaneous, vestibular, or visual cues. One possible mechanism of compensation is provided by the muscle mechanoreceptors. It has been shown that muscle and tendon vibration produce a sensation of joint movement (Goodwin, McCloskey, & Matthews, 1972). Specifically, movement is sensed in the direction that a vibrating muscle would have been stretched. This indicates that muscle mechanoreceptors may aid in controlling joint motion, and suggests that ankle rehabilitation might alter the sensitivity of these receptors."

*Quoted from Docherty, C. L., Moore, J. H., & Arnold, B. L. (1998). Effects of strength training on strength development and joint position sense in functionally unstable ankles. *Journal of Athletic Training, 33*, 310–314.

headings represent the topic sentence of a paragraph, with sentences or brief statements from which to construct sentences included below it. As with the topical outline, we recommend using many subheadings and being very detailed. Detailed sentence outlines are useful in avoiding awkward transitions.

Writing Style

Writing style refers to the way in which the text is written. As with the format, style varies by journal/publisher, and you will want to consult the author's guide. However, most publishers prefer use of the active voice. In the active voice, the subject acts. For example, "Participants performed a maximum quadriceps muscle contraction" is an example of active voice. Conversely, "A maximum quadriceps contraction was performed by the participants" is an example of passive voice. In the passive voice, the subject is acted upon. You can recognize the passive voice because the verb phrase includes a form of "to be," such as am, is, was, were, are, or been.

It is also preferable to use first person rather than third person. For example, "I/we instructed participants to..." is preferred to "The researcher(s) instructed participants to...." Other considerations are to write simply, to include one idea per paragraph, and to avoid direct quotes. If you use direct quotes, you must include the quote exactly as it occurred in the original source. Therefore, direct quotes require greater precision than does paraphrasing. Regardless of whether you are using direct quotes, paraphrasing, or summarizing others' work, it is essential to carefully reference your source to avoid plagiarism, a serious example of scientific misconduct (see Chapter 20).

Keys to Good Writing

In our experience, writing is a very individual experience, and there is no one way to accomplish the task. However, we have found at least three ways to make the process easier:

1. First, outline in detail. Detailed topical and sentence outlines can make the actual writing process more mechanical. If you have constructed your outlines well, the creative and intellectual processes are mostly completed, and all you have left to do is connect the ideas.
2. Second, work on one section at a time. This will help you maintain your focus and avoid being distracted with side issues.
3. Finally, we suggest that you "talk it out." Verbalizing material as if you were trying to explain it to a friend often helps clarify your writing. This is especially true with sections that you are finding difficult to write. If you can explain it, you can write it.

Referencing

Text Referencing

Ultimately, text referencing (i.e., citation) formats are determined by a journal/publisher's authors' guide. For example, if you use AMA style, citations are numbered in order of occurrence in the manuscript. In contrast, APA style uses the authors' names and publication year in place of numbering. See Display 5–3 for examples of AMA and APA styles. You should consult the appropriate style manual for specific guidelines.

Despite these differences, some general conventions exist. Specifically, citation placement in the text is uniform across styles. You should place citations either with the authors' names or at the end of the sentence. For example, either of the following would be acceptable: "Arnold, Gansneder, and Perrin (1) reported that inversion is the most common form of ankle sprain" or "Inversion has been reported as the most common form of ankle sprain. (1)" Following this convention puts your citations as close as possible to the referenced information.

If you are using a format that requires citations to be numbered, you will find it frustrating to maintain the numbering while you write. Typically, as you rewrite and edit, you will add, delete, and move references, thus changing their numbers. To avoid this dilemma, we recommend using a modified APA style while writing. Specifically, insert the first author's name and the date of the reference in parentheses. After you have completed writing, replace the name and date with the appropriate reference number and construct your reference list. (This can be easily done with a word-processing application's find-and-replace feature.)

Display 5-3 | **Comparison of AMA and APA Text Reference Styles**

AMA Method	APA Method
In the body of the text:	
Inversion ankle sprains are the most common ankle injury. (1–3) These injuries vary in their degree of severity. (4)	Inversion ankle sprains are the most common ankle injury (Jackson, 1995; Monk, 2002; Rowe, 1998). These injuries vary in their degree of severity (Arnold, 2001).
In the reference section:	
1. Jackson …	Arnold …
2. Monk …	Jackson …
3. Rowe …	Monk …
4. Arnold …	Rowe …

Display 5-4 | **Comparison of AMA and APA Reference List Style**

	AMA Style	APA Style
Journal Article	Docherty CL, Moore JH, Arnold BL. Effects of strength training on strength development and joint position sense in functionally unstable ankles. J Athl Train. 1998;33:310–314.	Docherty, C. L., Moore, J. H., & Arnold, B. L. (1998). Effects of strength training on strength development and joint position sense in functionally unstable ankles. *Journal of Athletic Training, 33,* 310–314.
Book	Arnold BL, Gansneder BM, Perrin DH. Research methods in athletic training. Philadelphia, FA Davis, 2005.	Arnold, B. L., Gansneder, B. M., & Perrin, D. H. (2005). *Research methods in athletic training.* Philadelphia: F. A. Davis.
Book Chapter	Jones LA. The senses of effort and force during fatiguing contractions. In: Gandevia SC, Enoka RM, McComas AJ, eds. Fatigue: Neural and muscular mechanisms. New York: Plenum Press; 1995:305–313.	Jones, L. A. (1995). The senses of effort and force during fatiguing contractions. In S. C. Gandevia, R. M. Enoka, & A. J. McComas (Eds.), *Fatigue: Neural and muscular mechanisms* (pp. 305–313). New York: Plenum Press.

Reference Lists

As with citations, reference list styles are also determined by the journal/publisher. Therefore, you should consult the authors' guide or style manual for the correct format. Display 5–4 shows examples of the AMA and APA reference list styles. The references in this book are in APA style, which is the style preferred by our publisher.

Reference Management

Managing your citations and reference list can be tedious. Therefore, we believe that reference management programs such as Endnote (Niles Software, Inc., Berkeley, California) and Reference Manager (Research Information Systems, Inc., Carlsbad, California) are worth the investment. These programs are database programs specifically designed for referencing. They also have several automated features. For example, they automatically insert citations into your document, and once the citations are in the document, they automatically format the citations and reference list to any journal style (e.g., AMA or APA) you select. (Most journal formats are preloaded into the programs, and others can be created.) Our favorite feature is the ability to reformat the citations and reference list. This can be done after inserting new references to produce an updated reference list or after changing styles (e.g., AMA to APA) to produce citations and references based on the new style. Our experience indicates that these programs can save you significant time and frustration with the citation process.

Solutions to Common Problems

Abstracting

One of the most common problems we see with novice writing is the abstracting of articles. Abstracting involves writing a brief summary of each article and then sequencing these abstracts one after another. This can have the effect of producing incoherent and tedious paragraphs in literature reviews. Instead of abstracting, your goal should be to summarize the results of related studies and synthesize a consensus from these studies. Your end product should be a review of articles that have been combined on the basis of common themes.

Author/Date Focus

A second problem that you should avoid is organizing articles by the authors or publication dates. Again, this typically occurs when you fail to organize your information along topics and/or do not use a topical outline. As with abstracting, writing this way is either incoherent or tedious to read.

Summary

The key to writing an effective literature review is topical organization. Organizing and writing with a sentence outline structured around appropriate topics will make your writing easier. When writing, be careful to adequately and correctly reference materials to ensure accuracy and avoid plagiarism. You should also plan ahead and determine what format/style is required by the journal to which you intend to submit your research. Finally, keep in mind that the literature review is the foundation of all subsequent work. The better it is written, the easier your work will be later.

Activities

1. To obtain feedback on your writing style, write a two-page literature review containing three to five articles. Make sure to organize the review topically.
2. To establish the organization and completeness of your literature review, submit a topical outline of your literature review.
3. Submit a first draft of your literature review.

References

American Psychological Association. (1994). *Publication manual of the American Psychological Association* (4th ed.). Washington, DC: American Psychological Association.

Bosien, W. R., Staples, O. S., & Russel, S. W. (1955). Residual disability following acute ankle sprains. *Journal of Bone and Joint Surgery, 37A,* 1237–1243.

Diamond, J. (1989). Rehabilitation of ankle sprains. *Clinics in Sports Medicine, 8,* 877–889.

Docherty, C. L., Moore, J. H., & Arnold, B. L. (1998). Effects of strength training on strength development and joint position sense in functionally unstable ankles. *Journal of Athletic Training, 33,* 310–314.

Freeman, M. R. (1965). Treatment of ruptures of the lateral ligament of the ankle. *Journal of Bone and Joint Surgery, 47B,* 661–668.

Freeman, M. R., Dean, M. E., & Hanham, I. F. (1965). The etiology and prevention of functional instability of the foot. *Journal of Bone and Joint Surgery, 47B,* 678–685.

Goodwin, G.M., McCloskey, D. I., & Matthews, P. B. C. (1972). The contribution of muscle afferents to kinaesthesia shown by vibration induced illusions of movement and by the effects of paralysing joint afferents. *Brain, 95,* 705–748.

Iverson, C., Flanagin, A., Fontanarosa, P. B., Glass, R. M., Glitman, P., Lantz, J. C., et al. (1998). *American Medical Association manual of style* (9th ed.). Baltimore: Williams & Wilkins.

Lentell, G. L., Katzman, L. L., & Walters, M. R. (1990). The relationship between muscle function and ankle stability. *Journal of Orthopaedic and Sports Physical Therapy, 11,* 605–611.

Bibliography

Day, R.A. (1998). *How to write and publish a scientific aper.* Phoenix: Oryx Press.

Day, R.A. (1992). *Scientific English: A guide for scientists and other professionals.* Phoenix: Oryx Press.

Huth, E.J. (1990). *How to write and publish papers in the medical sciences.* Baltimore: Williams & Wilkins.

Knight, K.L., & Ingersoll, C.D. (1996). Structure of a scholarly manuscript: 66 tips for what goes where. *Journal of Athletic Training, 31,* 201–206.

Knight, K.L., & Ingersoll, C.D. (1996). Optimizing scholarly communication: 30 tips for writing clearly. *Journal of Athletic Training, 31,* 209–213.

Strunk, W., & White, E.B. (2000). *The elements of style.* Needham Heights, MA: Allyn & Bacon.

Part 3
The Research Process

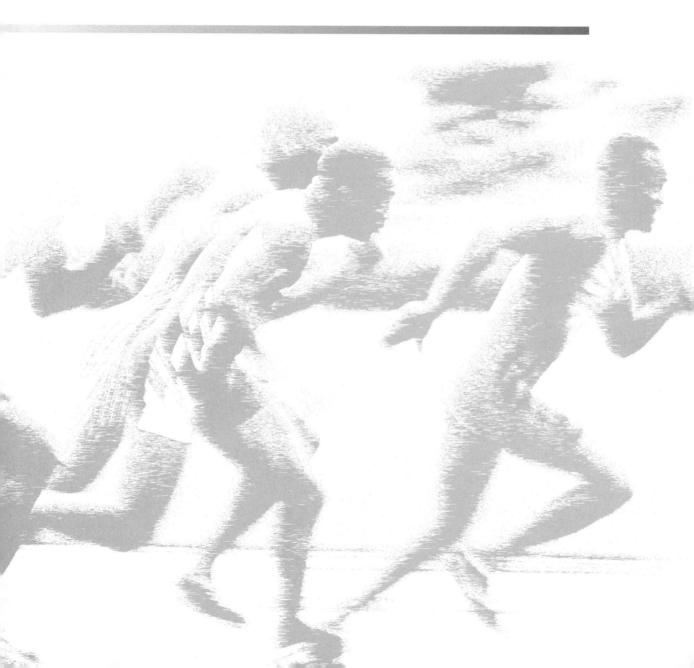

Chapter 6

Writing the Introduction

Objectives	*After reading this chapter, you will:*

Objectives

After reading this chapter, you will:

- Write Chapter 1 of your thesis.
- Write operational definitions.
- Identify appropriate assumptions, limitations, and delimitations for your research.
- Distinguish between limitations and delimitations.
- Write a research problem statement.
- Select and write appropriate research and statistical hypotheses.
- Distinguish among and select appropriate independent, dependent, and control variables.

Questions

While reading this chapter, think about answers to the following questions:

1. How do I distinguish between an operational definition and a standard definition?
2. What is the purpose of an operational definition?
3. How do I establish the delimitations for my study?
4. What is an assumption?
5. When should I use assumptions?
6. On what should I base the assumption?
7. Do limitations lead to assumptions?
8. What is the difference between a purpose statement and a problem statement?
9. What is the difference between a research hypothesis and a statistical hypothesis?
10. What is the difference between an independent variable and a dependent variable?
11. What is a control variable?

The Purpose of Chapter 1 (Your Introduction)

The purpose of Chapter 1, or the Introduction, of a thesis/dissertation is to outline the total research project. As part of this chapter, you should develop important technical components and definitions for the research. Additionally, your Introduction will establish the scope of your research and identify your hypotheses. Your first chapter should include several different sections and should be based on your literature review, which should be mostly complete before starting. Chapter 2 of the thesis will contain this review.

Introductory Paragraphs

The first section of Chapter 1 is three to five paragraphs that highlight important previous research. Unlike your literature review, they do not have to be comprehensive. Rather, these paragraphs should address the specific studies that establish the merits of your research. These studies should identify important factors related to the research. There is no limit on the number of studies to be included, but we recommend 8 to 12 studies. If you need more, you probably have not focused on the problem sufficiently, and if you have fewer studies, your review probably will not be adequate. The introductory paragraphs for Chapter 1, along with your problem statement, should be ultimately appropriate to use for the introduction of your journal format manuscript (see Chapter 16, Organizing and Writing the Results).

Operational Definitions

Operational definitions constitute the second part of your Introduction and are fundamental to your research methods. Operational definitions are not theoretical definitions, but rather definitions that precisely describe concepts or measures. Your operational definitions may not be identical to those used by other researchers. Instead, they may be modifications of previous researchers' definitions that are more specific to your purpose or instrumentation. Examples of standard and operational definitions are given in Display 6–1.

Delimitations

Delimitations are limits chosen by yourself to set the boundaries for your study. Common delimitations include participant age, gender, and injury status. Other examples include treatment and testing parameters such as ultrasound application time and wattage or isometric versus isokinetic strength testing. How you delimit your study will depend on your goals. However, in choosing your delimitations, you should base them on the

Display 6-1	**Comparisons between Standard and Operational Definitions**	
	Standard Definition	**Operational Definition**
	Joint reposition sense: A measure of proprioception	*Joint reposition sense:* The ability to actively reproduce 30° of ankle inversion after having the ankle passively placed at 30° for 15 seconds and returned to neutral
	Strength: A measure of muscle force production	*Strength:* The highest peak torque of 3 trials performed isokinetically at 60° per second

results or methods of previous studies or on clinical or theoretical considerations. If you establish your delimitations arbitrarily, you may exclude important factors. It is seldom possible to include all the relevant factors in a single study, but you should be prepared to justify the factors you have included and those you have excluded.

Limitations

In contrast to delimitations, which are under your control, you will identify other factors that are not under your control (e.g., uniform application of athletic tape). This lack of control may or may not represent a significant flaw in your study. If there is previous evidence suggesting that a factor does not need to be controlled, the lack of control can be justified with an assumption (as defined in the next section). If no justification is available, the lack of control becomes a limitation. In other words, limitations result from factors that should be controlled but are beyond your control. Common reasons for limitations include lack of necessary instrumentation, lack of appropriate participants, and physiological parameters that are very difficult to measure.

Assumptions

With almost every research project, researchers make assumptions regarding particular aspects of the study. Assumptions are aspects of the study that researchers cannot or choose not to control but believe to be true. When you make assumptions, you should base them on accepted theory and/or the results of previous research. More specifically, these theories or results should suggest that there is little or no need to control a particular aspect of a study. For example, underwater weighing is the ideal method for determining percent body fat, but research supports a strong relationship between skinfold measures and percent body fat. Therefore, you might make the assumption that skinfold measures adequately represent percent body fat and choose to not use underwater weighing techniques.

Display 6-2	**Examples of Theory- and Research-Based Assumptions**	
	Issue	Assumption
Theory Based	Neuromuscular system protection may be a subconscious process. Joint reposition sense, as a measure of neuromuscular control, is a conscious measure.	The researcher assumes that conscious processes are an accurate estimate of unconscious processes.
Research Based	Quadriceps femoris has been shown to activate as a single unit.	Rectus femoris EMG is representative of the quadriceps femoris.

Because assumptions are foundational, invalid assumptions will lead to invalid results. Therefore, you should use assumptions only when procedures are unavailable or impossible and alternate procedures are equally good. You may also need to make assumptions when procedures are too invasive to be feasible or needed instrumentation is unavailable. Examples of research- and theory-based assumptions are shown in Display 6–2, and a delimitation/limitation/assumption decision tree or flowchart is in Figure 6–1.

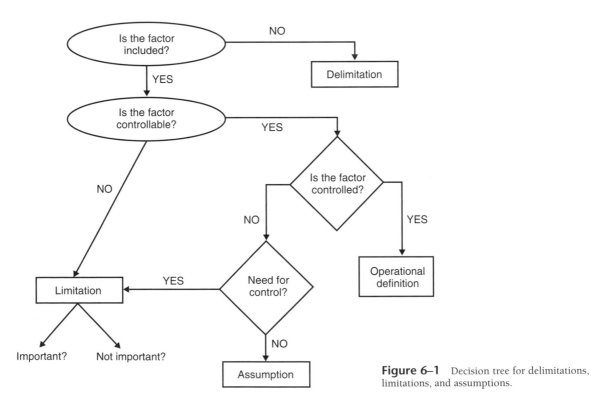

Figure 6–1 Decision tree for delimitations, limitations, and assumptions.

Statement of the Problem

The problem statement states the purpose of your study. It should begin, "The purpose of this study is…." In some cases, you may have subproblems that may be described within the context of the main purpose or discussed separately from the main purpose.

Hypotheses

Your hypotheses should be next. Hypotheses are statements of your expected results. There are two general types of hypotheses: research and statistical. Each has particular features that are important to the research process.

Research Hypotheses

Your research hypotheses should state very specifically what you are expecting, planning, or attempting to find. It is important that research hypotheses be stated directionally. From your review of the literature, you should be able to state that you expect to see a change, for example, "Ice applications will decrease the volume of ankle swelling" or "Hot packs applied to the hamstring will increase hamstring length." In developing your hypotheses, you should base them on theory or previous findings in the literature. Otherwise, your hypotheses are just guesses. Depending on the complexity of your research, you may have several hypotheses. However, you may find that trying to test one hypothesis interferes with testing another. This may be because treatments interfere with one another, participant learning effects develop as part of the measurement procedures, or other reasons. Because of this, you should judiciously select the hypotheses you choose to test.

Statistical Hypotheses

All researchers start with research hypotheses. However, research hypotheses are never directly statistically tested. Rather, it is the statistical hypotheses, corollaries to the research hypotheses, that are tested. Statistical hypotheses are mathematical in form and can be stated verbally or represented with mathematical symbols. For example, assume that you have conducted an experiment with three groups: a control group (C), a strength training group (S), and a balance training group (B). Also assume that balance is what you are trying to change. Your possible research and statistical hypotheses based on this experiment are shown in Display 6–3. You will note that there are a null and an alternate statistical hypothesis. Each statistical hypothesis begins with H_n, with the n representing the number of

Display 6-3

Comparison of Research and Statistical Hypotheses

Research	Null	Alternate
The balance group's (B) mean balance will be better than the control (C) group's mean balance.	$H_0: \mu_C = \mu_B$	$H_1: \mu_C \neq \mu_B$ $H_2: \mu_C \neq \mu_S$ $H_3: \mu_B \neq \mu_S$

*H_n: is the hypothesis number and μ is the population mean from which each group is drawn.

the statistical hypothesis. Also, μ is used to represent the population mean from which each group is drawn. This indicates that the real purpose of statistical testing is to determine differences among population means, not group means. This will be explained in more detail in Chapter 12. For this simple experiment, there are three hypotheses, one for each pair of means (or comparison).

Observe that the research hypothesis is directional, whereas the statistical hypothesis is not. We could also test a directional hypothesis ($_C <_B$). If you state the hypothesis in this form, you are stating that you expect the changes to occur in the specified direction and that you are testing for differences in only that direction. Your use of directional or nondirectional hypotheses depends on your goals. However, directional hypotheses have more statistical power than nondirectional hypotheses and for that reason may be preferred (see Chapter 12).

Dependent Variables

The next section of Chapter 1 should be a listing of your dependent variables. Dependent variables are measured variables such as swelling, strength, and balance. They are the variables that you expect to change as the result of the experimental treatments. In other words, they represent your experimental outcome.

In the Field

Darin is interested in the increased incidence of ACL injuries in women. He suspects that women have more knee injuries because, as they become fatigued, they are unable to maintain enough joint stiffness to stabilize the joint. Therefore, he writes the following hypothesis: "Knee stiffness in women will be less than that of men following a repetitive squatting exercise." His statistical hypothesis would read $H_1: \mu_{female} < \mu_{male}$. Conversely, his null hypothesis would read $H_0: \mu_{female} = \mu_{males}$. In stating his hypothesis in this manner, he has specified a direction for the hypothesis.

Independent Variables

In contrast to the dependent variables, independent variables are the variables you manipulate (e.g., frequency of stretching) or use to represent different groups (e.g., gender). In some cases, the independent variable may represent a clinical treatment. In athletic training research, independent variables might be the length of ice application, ultrasound wattage, therapeutic exercise programs, or the clinical condition.

Control Variables

Some experiments will also have control variables. The purpose of a control variable is to account for extraneous factors. For example, if you believe that men and women may respond differently to an exercise program, you may want to control this effect. You could control the gender effect by including only one gender in the experiment or by including gender as a control variable. If you are interested in differences between men and women, gender would be an independent variable. If you are not interested in gender differences, gender is a control variable.

Solutions to Common Problems

Most researchers have two problems when writing the Introduction. First, they confuse the delimitations, limitations, and assumptions. The best way

In the Field

Melanie is interested in how balance is affected by differences in proprioception. However, she also realizes that balance is affected by age. In other words, as people get older, their balance generally declines. She is now faced with the dilemma of how to address this. Using the Figure 6–1 , she realizes that she could eliminate age as a factor (by using a small age range for her subjects) and list age as one of the study's delimitations. However, she believes that age may be an important factor. So she decides to include it. Again using the decision tree, she realizes that age is a controllable factor and that she needs to control it. Because of this, she must now develop an operational definition for age. Consulting with her advisor and re-examining the literature, she decides to define age as chronological years grouped into 10-year blocks. Therefore, her operational definition might read, "Age is defined as chronological years grouped as 18 to 27, 28 to 37, 38 to 47, 48 to 57, and 58 to 67 years." In most cases, information from other studies will suggest where the breaks should occur. The literature might also suggest that the range of ages included in each group should be smaller or larger. Finally, blocking the ages in this fashion suggests that each group will have the same number of subjects. Therefore, the more groupings used, the greater number of subjects needed. (See Chapter 7, "Nonequivalent control group," and Chapter 12.)

to avoid this is to follow the flowchart in Figure 6–1. The second common mistake is to be too general in your operational definitions. To avoid this problem, you need to think in terms of tasks, not theory. If it is a treatment, how are you going to apply the treatment? If it is a measure, how will you perform the measure? If you write from this frame of reference, your operational definitions will have the correct amount of detail.

Summary

The purpose of the Introduction is to begin laying out the more technical details of your study. Although published research papers do not include all of the information in Chapter 1 of the thesis, writing the Introduction will help you sharpen your focus and translate abstract ideas into definable ideas that can be subsequently measured. In the process of creating your Introduction, you will often find gaps in your thinking that would otherwise lead to fatal flaws for your study. Detecting the flaws early can lead you back to the literature to solve any problems you have. Finally, because Chapter 1 should be based on your knowledge of the literature, it should be completed after Chapter 2 despite the numbering of the chapters.

Activities

1. Identify and be prepared to discuss your independent and dependent variables.
2. Identify and be prepared to discuss your research hypotheses.
3. Submit a first draft of your Introduction.

Bibliography

Day, R. (1995). *Scientific English: A guide for scientists and other professionals* (2nd ed.). Phoenix, AZ: Oryx Press.

Day, R. (1998). *How to write and publish a scientific paper* (3rd ed.). Phoenix, AZ: Oryx Press.

Iverson, C., Flanagin, A., & Fontanarosa, P.B. (1998). *American Medical Association manual of style* (9th ed.). Baltimore: Williams & Wilkins.

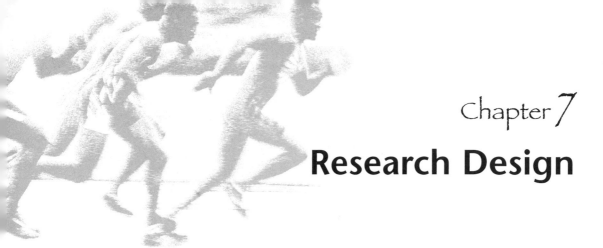

Chapter 7

Research Design

Objectives

After reading this chapter, you will:

- Understand experimental internal and external validity.
- Understand the threats to internal and external validity.
- Apply controls for internal validity.
- Distinguish between experimental and nonexperimental research designs.
- Understand the appropriate usage of alternative research designs.
- Understand the advantages and disadvantages of experimental and alternative research designs.

Questions

While reading this chapter, think about answers to the following questions:

1. What is an experiment?
2. How do I establish cause and effect?
3. Why do I need a control group?
4. Can I randomly assign injured and uninjured subjects in an experiment?
5. Are there designs I can use if I only have a small group of subjects?
6. How do I control for fatigue and practice effects?

Internal Validity

The fundamental purpose of conducting experiments is to determine if a treatment actually produces a change. To use a simple example, assume that you are interested in knowing whether hamstring stretches increase knee range of motion (ROM). Let us also assume that this ROM has increased.

The question that can now be asked is "Was the increase in ROM a result of the stretching?" If all other causes for the change can be ruled out and stretching remains the only explanation, your experiment is considered internally valid. To say that an experiment has internal validity is to say, in this case, that the treatment (stretching) caused an effect (increased knee ROM) to the exclusion of all other plausible explanations.

Threats to Internal Validity

There are several threats to internal validity (Campbell & Stanley, 1963; Cook & Campbell, 1979). In this section, we will describe and give examples of these threats. As you will see in the subsequent section, careful planning of your research design can control threats to internal validity.

History

History refers to the intervention of unexpected events during the course of the experiment. In the case of the stretching experiment, assume that the stretching treatment is conducted over an extended period of time, such as several weeks. Also, assume that your experiment participants are part of an athletic team, and the coach includes stretching as part of his or her warm-up program. Was the change that you found a result of the stretches you had the athletes do, the ones that the coach had them do, or a combination of the two? Obviously, it is impossible to know.

Maturation

Maturation refers to natural changes that occur to participants over time. As the name suggests, the obvious example is maturation with aging. In athletic training, however, it might also include skill performance decrements caused by fatigue or the natural healing process that occurs after an ankle sprain. In your stretching experiment, maturation might be expressed as changed fitness levels across the sport season. The difference between history and maturation is that history refers to a specific event or events, whereas maturation refers to a change within the individuals being studied. Natural changes can occur more rapidly in adolescents. For example, in a study on childhood obesity, changes in body composition that are believed to be a result of fitness training could simply be a result of the adolescent's maturation.

Testing

Testing, or the actual measuring process, can also interfere with your results. This applies when testing is done before the treatment. In athletic training, testing effects are commonly the result of learing or practice.

Memory is a factor when knowledge gained from the pretest either influences the treatment or is carried over to a posttest. Similarly, the pretest is a form of practice. Thus, pretesting skills that improve with practice can be affected by the pretest.

Selection Bias

If you form groups by some method other than random assignment, you run the risk of producing a selection bias. When this occurs, it is possible to have differences between groups that result not from the treatments but from the selection. For example, assigning men and women to separate groups will produce strength differences between the groups that has nothing to do with any treatment. In other words, the strength difference that you find may be the result of differences in muscle size associated with gender. Another example common in athletic training research is assigning individuals to groups based on injury (e.g., individuals with ankle sprains versus uninjured individuals). Another hazard frequently found in our research is the use of volunteers. Under society's current ethical framework, all research participants must be volunteers. This is certainly appropriate. However, people who volunteer may not be the same as those who do not volunteer in their motivations, interest levels, perceived gains, and so forth. Therefore, with research using volunteers, some caution must be exercised in applying the results to individuals who refuse to volunteer.

It should be emphasized that establishing groups based on criteria having a special relevance to the research question (e.g., individuals with ankle sprains) may be important. However, you must consider the fact that these groups may be different in other important ways. Individuals with ankle sprains may have poor balance. For example, in a study on ankle sprains, a researcher finds that individuals with ankle sprains have poorer balance than those without ankle sprains. The researcher concludes that an ankle sprain is a result of poor balance. However, the fact may be that an ankle sprain is a result of a deficit in joint reposition sense, not balance.

Statistical Regression

Statistical regression (i.e., shifting of data toward the mean) is a result of two things: extreme group scores and the reliability or unreliability of measures. When a group scores very high, a ceiling effect is created. On the second measurement, scores are likely to remain the same or go down (i.e., be closer to the mean). When a group scores very low, a floor effect is created. On the second measurement, scores are likely to remain the same or go up (i.e., be closer to the mean). Less reliable measures result in more error and therefore will increase regression to the mean. This is an added reason why reliability of measures is so important. A perfectly reliable measure would not change at all (when there is no treatment) and therefore there would be

In the Field

Shelby has decided to study the effect of ACL surgery on single leg balance. To do this she must recruit injured participants as well as uninjured individuals. She has partnered with an orthopedist and has put up fliers at the university's fitness center. However, she learned that in order to put up the fliers she first had get the flier approved by her university's human investigation committee and then had to get permission to post the fliers from the fitness center manager. Shortly after posting the fliers, several people began to call to volunteer for the study. She scheduled the first few people to visit the lab for testing, but once they arrived, she realized that several did not meet the qualifications of the study. This was a waste of both their time and her time. Following this, she began asking more detailed questions on the phone to make sure that the individuals qualified for the study. After identifying several patients who did qualify for the study, she began scheduling them to visit the lab. However, approximately a third of these individuals didn't show up at the lab. Now, 4 weeks into the scheduled data collection period, she has collected data on only 6 of her 40 injured subjects. In frustration she contacts her advisor to ask what to do. Her advisor suggests that on the day before testing she call the subjects to remind them of their appointment in the lab. The advisor also suggests that subjects who missed their first appointment after being reminded the day before should be rescheduled, and these individuals should be reminded the morning of their second appointment. Shelby implemented these techniques and found that approximately 90 percent of the individuals showed up for their first appointment. While this was a much better rate, Shelby was still frustrated with the subjects who didn't make their appointment. Her advisor pointed out that this type of attrition is normal for the research process and that it is almost always the case that more subjects will be recruited than are actually used.

no statistical regression regardless of group characteristics. In athletic training research, statistical regression potentially results when groups are selected or created based on some measured characteristic. For example, you are interested in whether pes planus feet are related to tibial stress fractures. One way to measure pes planus feet is with navicular drop during standing. This is done by placing the foot in subtalar neutral, measuring the height of the navicular tubercle from the floor, asking the person to relax the foot, and remeasuring the distance between the floor and the navicular tubercle. The difference between the neutral and relaxed measures is the "navicular drop." Based on this measure, you could then categorize people as having flat feet (large navicular drop scores) or high arches (small navicular drop scores) and would eliminate people with average or intermediate navicular drops. The result is two extreme groups. The problem of statistical regression becomes obvious if you measure navicular drop on a second occasion (Fig. 7–1). On the second day, the navicular drops of both groups have moved closer (i.e., regressed) toward the average of both groups. Why did this happen? The complexity of measuring navicular drop has the potential

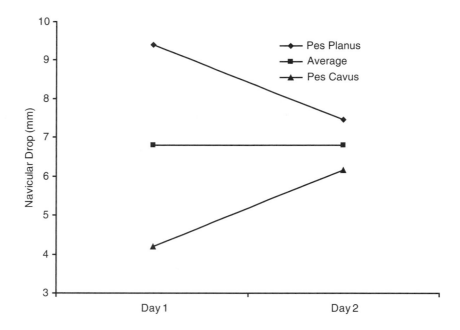

Figure 7–1 An example of navicular drop scores regressing toward the mean.

of measurement error. Consequently, measurement of subjects with extremes of pes planus or pes cavus has the potential of exhibiting regression toward the mean on subsequent measurements.

Remember that statistical regression can occur with any measure used to create extreme group scores. Any extreme score is likely to be caused by extraneous factors, and whenever that measure is repeated, the odds are in favor of the second score being closer to the average.

Experimental Mortality

Experimental mortality refers to the loss of subjects during the course of the experiment. Mortality can occur for a variety of reasons. Sometimes participants get bored, dislike a treatment, favor a treatment, and so forth. Any experiment is likely to have some mortality. When it occurs, you should analyze only the data for subjects who have completed the experiment.

Instrumentation

In athletic training, research instrumentation error typically refers to the calibration of instruments (e.g., an isokinetic dynamometer). However, instrument error can also occur in standardized tests, clinical observations, analysis of physical movement, and interviews about educational or clinical practices. This is called observer (or interviewer) drift. Obviously, if your instrument does not measure the same on two different days, this can have negative effects on your data. If this change is systematic (e.g., all measures are increased on the second measure), this could create the misinterpretation that there was a change from one time to the next. The best way to control this is to know your instrument well and calibrate it as often as is necessary. Similarly, observations and interviews should be monitored periodically.

You should also be aware that instrumentation errors can occur because the person giving the test gets better or worse over time. For example, if you are measuring knee ROM on many people and are not well practiced with the goniometer, it is likely that during the experiment you will get better at using the goniometer. Therefore, you will be better at measuring the people you measured last. This probably means that you are more accurate later in the experiment. This too can adversely affect your data.

Selection Interactions

Selection interactions can compound the effects of history, maturation, mortality, and instrumentation. An example of a selection-history interaction might be sorting men and women into separate groups. If you make measurements over the course of a month or longer, female hormonal fluctuations as a result of the menstrual cycle may create data fluctuations that do not exist in men. This may create differences between the groups that are incorrectly attributed to differences in experimental treatments. Therefore, you can see that some thought must be given to the special characteristics of selected groups and how the groups might change across time. An example of a selection-mortality interaction might be more participants dropping out of one group than another. For example, assume that you conducted an experiment in which you had the experimental and control groups perform eccentric muscle contractions to produce delayed-onset muscle soreness. Also assume that one group received a compression wrap after exercise with the goal of determining whether the wrap helped reduce soreness. What if the wrap actually increased the soreness of people who were the most sore, and what if these people decided to drop out of the study because they didn't want to wear the wrap? In this case, by the end of the experiment, only the less sore people would remain in the wrap group. This would mean that the wrap group had decreased soreness, not because the wrap worked but because the individuals with the most soreness had dropped out. This would make it appear that wearing the wrap worked, when the result was actually caused by mortality.

Strategies to Counteract Threats to Internal Validity

A variety of strategies can be used to counteract threats to internal validity. The first fundamental strategy for experimental designs is random assignment to control and treatment groups.

Random Assignment

A control group provides a baseline by which you can compare all other groups. For example, in a stretching experiment, you might have 3 groups: a control group receiving no treatment, a 30-second stretch group, and a 45-second stretch group. In this case, your control group serves as the baseline with which to test whether stretching was better than nothing.

Control groups are created by random assignment. By randomly assigning participants to control and treatment groups, you create a theoretical equality between or among the groups. When this equality is established, the threats to internal validity have an equal chance of occurring in all groups.

Occasionally it is not possible to assign individuals randomly to groups. An example would be comparing a group of individuals with ankle sprains to an uninjured group. In this case, the uninjured group would serve as a comparison group, not a control group.

Statistical Controls

Another option is statistical control. Special statistical procedures can be used to equalize groups on some characteristic such as strength. For example, we typically normalize strength by dividing strength by body weight to account for differences in body size. Alternatively, analysis of covariance can be used to statistically remove the effect of body weight on strength. These types of procedures are less desirable than random assignment because statistical controls can unintentionally eliminate other important factors. For example, age is related to strength. Therefore, statistically equalizing groups for strength may also eliminate important effects resulting from age.

Matched Pairs

Another way to equalize groups is the use of matched pairs. With matched pairs, individuals are assigned to each other based on some characteristic (e.g., isokinetic quadriceps strength). The individuals of the strongest pair are randomly assigned to the control and experimental groups. Then individuals of the next strongest pair are assigned to the experimental and control group, and so on, down to the weakest pair. In the end, each group would, on average, have the same strength. This procedure has the same weakness as a statistical control. It potentially controls factors other than strength. Strength is related to body size (more specifically, muscle mass) and age. By controlling for strength, you are also controlling for body size and age, which may or may not be desirable. The point is that when you control one factor, you often control others, which may not be desirable, and even worse, you may control unknown factors that bias your results.

Placebos

Another important control is the use of a placebo. A placebo is any intentionally ineffective intervention that is used in place of a treatment that is believed to be effective. As we all know, people can believe that they get better when they receive a placebo. Therefore, you may find it important to test the psychological effects of receiving a placebo against the effects of actually receiving a treatment. However, keep in mind that a placebo is not the same as a control. The placebo is a treatment by itself. This means that your experiment will still require a control group. You might find that there is no difference between the group receiving a placebo and the control group, meaning that there is no psychological effect, but you cannot assume that the two are equivalent.

Blinding

Finally, blinding is another control. Blinding comes in two forms: single blind and double blind. In a single-blind study, the participants are unaware of which of the groups they have been assigned to, but the researcher is aware of the assignment. This prevents the participants from becoming

In the Field

Ted is studying the effects of two different hamstring stretching techniques (assisted-stretch with a clinician stretching the subject and self-stretch with the subject doing their own stretching) on knee extension. To do this he has established three groups: two stretch groups and a control group. However, the two treatment groups are not told about how the other group is stretching nor told which treatment is suspected of being better. Ted has hypothesized that assisted stretch will be more effective than self-stretch and believes that self-stretch will be the same as the control. For economy, Ted has decided to be the clinician who does the stretching as well as be the individual who measures hamstring flexibility. Thus, Ted has created a single-blind study. Without realizing it, Ted has potentially biased his study because he knows who is in which treatment group. Thus, there are at least two ways he can influence the study as the researcher. First, he may apply more rigorous stretch than another clinician who is unaware of treatment expectations. Thus, the assisted-stretch may be more potent than self-stretching because the researcher is making the treatment more potent. Second, even if the treatments were equal, since Ted knows who is in each group, he may inadvertently bias the measurement process. For example, he may more strongly encourage subjects in the assisted-stretch group to extend their knee as far as possible. This would have the potential effect of producing range of motion that is greater than that actually produced by the treatment. Thus, the assisted-stretch group's range of motion would be greater even though the self-stretch group's treatment was equivalent.

overeager to participate in a specific treatment group or frustrated by not receiving the treatment. In the former situation, participants may work harder and increase the treatment's effect (e.g., strength training). In the latter situation, discouraged participants may drop out, thus increasing the experimental mortality rate.

In double-blind studies, both the participant and the researcher are blind to which group is getting the real treatment. This procedure has the same effect as that of the single-blind study, with the added effect of preventing the researcher from contaminating the experimental data or treatment. Although researchers do not intentionally contaminate the data or treatment, if they know who is getting the treatment, they may give those individuals more encouragement, expect them to work harder, and so on. These unintended manipulations are often very subtle and are done without the researchers' recognition. Without double blinding, it is also possible that the researcher might "tip off" participants to their group assignment and unintentionally contaminate a single-blind study.

Subject Characteristics

A final form of control frequently used in athletic training is restrictions on subject characteristics. For example, you may find it desirable to restrict subjects to those having no injuries in the past 3 months. Obviously, the intent is to prevent unwanted factors, such as injury, from inappropriately influencing your results.

Summary of Strategies to Increase Internal Validity

As you can see, there are several threats to the validity of your results and several strategies to combat those threats. Which one you use depends on the specific circumstances of your study. However, the most powerful strategy is random assignment. This strategy controls for most of the internal validity threats. The following section describes several basic research designs that either use or do not use these controls. Each of the descriptions that follow will discuss the strengths and weaknesses of the design in relation to its statistical control or lack of control.

Basic Research Designs

There are several different types of research designs you can use in athletic training research. Research designs differ in four major ways: (1) how many groups (e.g., one or more than one) are studied; (2) how subjects are assigned to groups (i.e., randomly or not); (3) when the measures are taken (e.g., after the treatment or before and after the treatment); and (4) how many measures are taken (e.g., a single measure or a number of measures across time). Choices regarding these features allow you to make comparisons that are appropriate for answering your research questions. If you understand these four features, you can correctly choose an appropriate design from common designs. You can also vary these features to create entirely new designs.

The most common is the experimental design. An experimental design includes random assignment of subjects (as described previously) and explicit control of the treatment. The researcher exercises control over the treatment in three ways: First, the researcher specifies the exact nature of the treatment and implements the treatment exactly that way. In a strength-training study, the researcher specifies the exact amount of weight, number of sets, and the number of repetitions for subjects. Each subject within the treatment has exactly the same treatment. Second, the researcher controls the exact time at which the treatment is introduced. It does not occur before the researcher wants it to begin or last after the researcher wants it to stop. For example, subjects do not begin weight lifting before they are supposed to, and they are admonished not to do any other weight lifting. Third, the researcher controls the duration of the treatment. It might be for 10 minutes, 2 weeks, or 10 weeks. In any case, it is no longer or shorter than the researcher wants it to be. In an experimental study, strong conclusions can be made about the effect of the treatment. In this example, the researcher can draw conclusions about the effect of this specific weight-training program on strength.

In contrast, in nonexperimental studies, the researcher may have few or none of these controls. For example, weight training might occur as a part of preseason activities. Subjects are not randomly assigned to the training. They may do more or less of the training than they are supposed to. Even if the researcher collects data before and after the time of the training and finds strength changes, only very weak conclusions can be made about the effect of the training.

We will spend most of our time discussing experimental design and its variations. However, other designs, such as pre-experimental, quasi-experimental, and nonexperimental, can be very useful. Table 7–1 recaps the most common research designs. By convention, treatments are usually identified with a T and observations (i.e., the dependent measure) with an O. To be consistent, we use the same convention in Table 7–1. More specifically, in the left column is the name of the basic design. The second column identifies which groups are treatment and control groups, and the third column is a schematic of the design.

Pre-experimental

Designs are considered pre-experimental when participants are not randomly assigned to either a control or an experimental group. As explained in the following discussion, if you fail to assign participants randomly, many confounding factors affect the experiment.

Table 7–1 • **Pre-experimental, experimental, and quasi-experimental designs.**

Name	Group	Design								
Pre-experimental										
One-Shot	Treatment					T*	O†			
One Group Pretest-Posttest	Treatment				O_1	T	O_2			
Static Group	Treatment					T	O_1			
Comparison	Comparison						O_2			
Experimental										
Randomized 2-Group	Treatment			R‡		T	O_1			
	Control			R			O_2			
Randomized 2-Group	Treatment			R	O_1	T	O_2			
Pretest-Posttest	Control			R	O_3		O_4			
Quasi-Experimental										
Nonequivalent Control	Treatment				O_1	T	O_2			
Group	Comparison				O_3		O_4			
Time Series		O1	O2	O3	O4	T	O5	O6	O7	O8
Reversal		O1	O2	T1	O3	O4	T2	O5	O6	

* Treatment
† Observation,
‡ Randomized

One-Shot

The one-shot design includes only one group of individuals that receive a treatment and then are measured. For example, if you were to conduct a one-shot study, you would recruit a group of participants, stretch their hamstring (treatment), and then measure how flexible they are with a goniometer. Now assume that you found a large amount of flexibility. Was this caused by the treatment? The obvious problem is that you really do not know if the treatment worked because you have nothing to which to compare it. Maybe the participants were very flexible before the treatment or maybe not. You have no way of knowing. Thus, in our opinion, the one-shot design should be considered a research mistake, not a research design.

One-Group Pretest-Posttest

The problem with the one-shot design can be partially resolved by the one-group pretest-posttest design. This design consists of the one-shot design with a pretest added. Therefore, in the case of the stretch experiment, you would measure flexibility before and after the treatment. Now you have a basis for comparison. This apparently solves the comparison problem but creates another one. How do you know that something other than the treatment produced the change between the first and the second measures? You don't! In the case of your stretching experiment, there probably is little chance of something interfering between the two flexibility measures (but it could). However, if the treatment was a series of stretches done across days or weeks, it is possible that something else may have caused the change. For example, if the stretching also occurs as part of preseason conditioning, it is impossible to determine whether the changes were a result of the overall conditioning program or the stretching. Therefore, this design falls short of being a good design as well.

Static Group Comparison

The final pre-experiment design is the static group comparison. Again, this is an extension of the one-shot design that includes a comparison group. Typically, the comparison group is formed such that it is intended to represent normal, uninjured, or untrained individuals. For example, you may select a group of individuals for your stretching group and another for your comparison group. Are your two groups equal? Probably not. Maybe the comparison group is less (or more) flexible than the stretch group. If this were the case, any changes between groups pre-existed and were not a result of the stretching. Hopefully, it is clear that this design is inadequate as well.

Experimental

Experimental designs are considered the benchmark for cause-effect relationships. These designs are the only designs that can establish cause and effect between the treatment and the measurement of interest. Essentially, they are extensions of the pre-experimental designs, with two key features. First, there is a control group for comparison, and second, participants are randomly assigned to the treatment and control groups. To use an experimental design, participants must be randomly assigned to the groups. Only when you randomly assign subjects does the term control group apply. If your groups are formed by some other method, (e.g., whether individuals are injured or not), the noninjured group is a comparison group, not a control group. (With a comparison group, the design becomes pre- or quasi-experimental.) As we will see, the use of random assignment and control groups solves many problems that can be associated with experimental research.

How does one randomly assign subjects to groups? The easiest way is to use a random numbers table. Random numbers tables are just that, tables that include a large set of random numbers arranged in columns and rows (Table 7–2). To find a starting place, we usually use a pair of dice to determine at what row and column to enter the table. Once you find your starting place, you proceed along the row and use each number to assign participants to groups. If you're using two groups, odd numbers would

Table 7–2 • **Random Numbers**

18	44	65	21	95	26	41	26	81	87	68	57	21	37	24	21	73	07	71	48
65	56	78	92	83	39	06	47	38	85	94	19	20	15	87	31	10	95	37	95
98	88	07	51	59	28	07	38	18	02	39	64	41	05	65	17	73	02	47	51
61	35	16	31	22	88	84	29	05	82	61	03	45	22	92	87	28	17	68	70
72	17	83	06	94	34	63	87	66	91	98	80	84	20	72	84	49	62	29	70
39	90	51	86	63	38	76	93	11	59	19	85	60	53	58	55	76	96	89	29
49	79	81	37	40	86	86	15	45	71	19	16	50	53	90	33	49	30	36	38
60	63	82	35	87	80	44	43	33	38	30	71	35	26	76	92	84	62	14	54
75	98	70	91	45	15	95	15	25	16	25	56	93	08	91	68	34	04	46	85
45	25	52	82	66	48	56	29	89	12	88	08	98	45	21	20	81	87	25	09
93	38	58	09	47	07	66	89	94	73	03	86	10	59	41	94	70	33	79	04
96	19	61	23	24	16	28	32	29	41	45	43	38	07	59	94	12	22	62	20
87	37	86	68	60	08	63	39	21	29	03	90	00	48	63	68	03	01	06	68
36	84	13	20	80	61	02	59	68	22	13	89	83	81	40	70	98	88	75	43
88	68	18	71	81	98	11	01	15	86	93	22	45	09	76	77	88	16	77	51
44	32	96	01	68	57	38	13	41	87	43	72	24	35	12	08	66	26	53	64
89	75	86	38	79	56	86	97	33	79	40	95	07	83	97	71	85	58	83	52
81	72	22	37	19	46	79	81	59	76	50	71	39	98	52	23	63	60	95	15
57	96	65	96	27	09	21	32	84	95	08	41	05	88	90	45	88	13	08	27
01	61	34	25	37	82	31	40	38	34	43	19	56	71	79	84	82	63	68	22
79	77	31	43	43	15	35	35	21	97	06	19	95	22	70	30	49	90	39	02
81	89	89	43	28	51	25	63	02	78	44	08	03	76	48	40	91	17	60	64
00	66	00	43	56	43	62	72	56	66	61	57	67	75	47	28	51	46	63	95
90	60	23	96	41	29	80	14	78	15	46	73	64	40	93	43	74	15	39	64
64	16	77	58	87	59	91	58	61	63	14	34	87	99	54	30	71	95	94	47
24	54	29	82	76	47	24	97	26	93	20	80	18	15	12	61	10	84	44	27
65	66	56	03	53	84	67	30	19	95	61	65	92	82	31	11	35	07	68	30
62	47	20	26	50	68	02	46	35	30	87	33	79	69	11	24	76	62	66	43
38	16	35	43	50	53	74	31	60	70	44	70	18	96	77	33	65	82	04	96
43	82	50	08	58	86	34	23	83	91	54	93	08	87	47	70	81	20	36	73
87	51	35	18	51	43	88	19	97	50	06	80	07	28	88	94	14	74	35	02
67	99	88	94	91	94	89	03	44	47	34	53	15	41	63	97	54	95	32	80
08	79	90	78	51	67	99	87	60	10	91	40	33	97	25	42	53	78	49	72
97	60	13	14	55	26	31	11	85	92	99	84	31	50	40	23	03	78	70	21
24	44	54	72	43	77	69	89	18	89	57	13	87	32	13	07	83	88	82	38
25	56	66	64	37	54	34	50	47	08	78	36	51	29	74	94	42	32	19	67
87	67	78	42	63	12	41	40	20	91	77	51	30	90	26	66	52	60	11	21
63	80	52	49	32	48	42	81	91	98	47	61	18	49	52	39	46	14	27	80
50	52	59	91	06	92	03	12	56	64	90	87	17	97	02	76	30	19	46	45
25	85	67	87	79	37	94	34	66	25	69	95	57	52	80	56	27	74	73	67
31	11	94	43	10	80	61	96	76	16	10	33	56	13	82	94	32	84	91	65
12	29	69	74	89	31	65	69	28	56	18	59	19	48	68	76	86	69	73	83
79	50	86	43	61	00	89	88	33	49	77	49	61	31	56	89	12	84	37	57
58	58	05	01	65	27	10	00	04	77	33	25	55	35	09	26	27	06	78	87
79	85	21	73	80	48	68	50	17	66	25	30	81	04	55	28	78	18	36	94
27	86	76	41	32	63	13	31	41	26	78	82	55	37	42	15	09	31	08	18
30	09	66	64	91	17	93	33	11	47	93	33	89	42	99	08	42	16	38	41
73	42	63	80	08	71	61	05	42	06	04	03	08	25	22	50	60	60	02	90

Table generated using Micorsoft Excel RAND function.

assign people to one group and even numbers would assign them to the other. If you have three groups, numbers ending in 1 to 3, 4 to 6, and 7 to 9 can be used to assign groups (in this case zeros are skipped). Similar schemes can be developed for any number of groups.

Randomized Group

The most basic design is the randomized group design. This design can be used for any number of groups, but in Table 7–1 we have limited it to two-group designs. You will notice that we have added an R to the table for these groups. This indicates that, because the groups were randomly assigned, the design is an experimental design. The purpose of this design is to test whether the treatments are different from the control group and from each other. Therefore, in the example of the stretch study, the two-group design would be used. You would randomly assign your participants to one group or the other; the experimental group would receive the hamstring stretch; and after the treatment the two groups would be compared on hamstring flexibility. If a difference is found between the two groups, you could conclude that the difference was a result of the treatment. For the results to be interpretable, it is important that the control group not receive any other treatments that might interfere with their hamstring flexibility (e.g., hot packs). Otherwise, the difference between groups might be more attributable to the hot packs than the stretch.

Pretest-Posttest Randomized Groups

You can extend the randomized group design by adding a pretest. As can be seen from Table 7–1, this design looks similar to the previous design, except that a pretest (i.e., a test measuring hamstring flexibility before stretching) has been added. This measure must be the same measure as used in the posttest, and both groups must get the pretest. At a glance, it may seem that pretesting the control group is unnecessary. However, as has been discussed, a pretest can produce a treatment effect by itself. Thus, both groups must get the pretest to keep this effect similar for both groups. The benefit of this design is that you assess your treatment's effect twice: once in the comparison of the stretch and control groups' posttest results, and second by whether the difference between pretest and posttest is greater for the stretch group than the control group. It also gives you the advantage of comparing your groups' pretest scores for equivalence. The disadvantage is that pretests can interfere with the treatment (see Testing), may be more time consuming, and may be too expensive.

Quasi-experimental

Quasi-experimental designs attempt to apply experimental principles to the field setting. Because of the rigorous controls needed for true experimental designs, controlled settings such as the laboratory are needed. However, sometimes the most interesting questions can be answered only in the field. Therefore, Cook and Campbell (1979) have proposed the use of quasi-experimental designs. The hallmarks of these designs are multiple groups and multiple observations after a single treatment.

Nonequivalent Control Group

The nonequivalent control group design is simply the two-group pretest-posttest design, except that assignment to the groups is not randomized. This design is frequently found in athletic training research. For this design to work well, the two groups must be formed so that they are as similar as possible. This can be tested with the pretest, which permits you to determine whether the two groups are the same on your measure of choice (e.g., hamstring flexibility) before any treatment. If they are the same at the pretest and different after the treatment, you have a good justification for concluding that the treatment (i.e., stretching in our example) worked. However, it should be emphasized that being equal on your measure of choice does not mean that they are equal on all things. It is possible that some other confounding factor such as relaxation, stress, or fatigue may be present at pretest and coincidentally increase or decrease during treatment. Therefore, these other factors may explain the result rather than the actual treatment.

This design is common in athletic training because many groups we study are naturally occurring groups. The most obvious example of this is groups by gender, but other examples include injured versus noninjured, age groups, limb dominance, and so on. When these types of factors are studied, the static multigroup pretest-posttest design is your only option. Therefore, this design is acceptable provided that you are aware that other factors can account for any differences you find and that you should identify and control these factors if possible.

Time Series

The time series is another potential design for the field setting. As depicted in Table 7–1, this design consists of a single group measured multiple times before a treatment and multiple times after. The plan of this design is to determine a baseline for the group, implement a treatment, and determine whether the data pattern after the treatment differs from the baseline. Figure 7–2 illustrates a typical data pattern for this design. The arrow marks the implementation of a stretching protocol. As you can see, before the treatment a very steady baseline was established, and after the start of treatment there was a progressive improvement in ROM. The significant question is whether the treatment or something else caused the change. The answer is really unknown. However, the strategy is to have the baseline long enough to be convincing that the ROM was stable before treatment and to

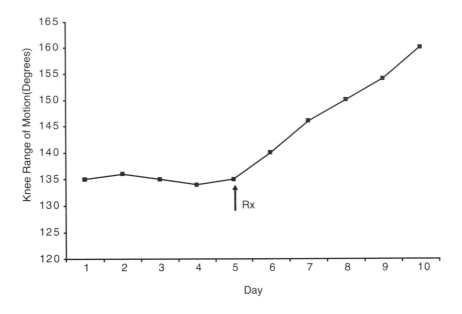

Figure 7–2　Typical data pattern for a time-series design.

have the posttreatment phase long enough to be certain that the observed effect was not a coincidence (i.e., a history effect). The results of this type of design are more convincing if it can be repeated on another group, especially if that group is different than the first (e.g., linemen versus running backs).

Reversal

To counter the history effect of the design, a reversal design can be used (see Table 7–1). Figure 7–3 depicts a reversal design, which is a variation on the time-series design. The main feature of this design is the withdrawal (i.e., reversal) of the treatment (represented by the downward arrow). In this case, the knee ROM begins to decline. Whenever an apparent treatment effect can be reversed by withdrawing the treatment, this strengthens the conclusion that the treatment was effective. The obvious drawback to this design is that it can only be used with treatments that are susceptible to reversal. For example, if this were a strength-training study, you would not expect to see an immediate decline in strength with the completion of training. Similarly, you would not expect a learning effect to reverse. Because of this, the reversal design has limited applications in athletic training research.

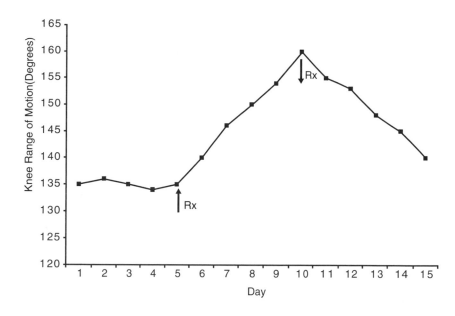

Figure 7-3 Typical data pattern for a reversal design.

Single-Subject Designs

Single-subject designs are another research alternative. Although a full explanation of these designs is beyond the scope of this book, we feel that a brief introduction is warranted. If you have an interest in these designs, we recommend the text by Kazdin (1982). In their most basic form, single-subject designs are identical to the time-series and reversal designs except that individuals rather than groups are studied. However, despite the name, these designs rarely involve one individual. Instead, they generally focus on two to five specific individuals who usually have a clinical condition of interest (e.g., an ankle sprain) (Mattacola & Lloyd, 1997). The premise behind single-subject research is that the clinical condition being studied does not occur in sufficient numbers to be studied through the research designs described previously. Therefore, you may find these designs more useful in the clinical environment. You should be cautioned against thinking these designs are easier because of smaller number of subjects. Our experience is that maintaining experimental control in these designs is more difficult than in group designs. Finally, we should emphasize that these designs are not replacements for group designs. Whenever possible, group designs are preferred, and single-subject designs are good alternatives when a group design is not possible.

Nonexperimental Designs

Nonexperimental designs are also an important form of athletic training research. These designs are centered on establishing the relationship between two variables. This is typically done through various statistical techniques such as correlation and multiple regression (see Chapter 15). Unlike experimental designs, these methods cannot establish a cause-and-effect relationship because they do not use randomization and control groups. However, sometimes cause and effect are not of interest. For example, maybe you are interested in determining whether there is a relationship between age and injury rates. Clearly, it is not logical to believe that age causes injury, but it would be reasonable to think that older people might be injured more often because their bones are weaker or their mobility has decreased. Therefore, nonexperimental research is useful in determining what factors may relate to injury and lead the way to more controlled experimental studies.

External Validity

In contrast to internal validity, external validity refers to whether your results are applicable outside of your study. As indicated previously, internal validity refers to whether your results are from the experimental treatment you have provided. If not, and the results are from other extraneous and/or uncontrolled factors, the experiment is not internally valid. Determining whether your results are applicable beyond the study is equally important. In other words, are your results clinically applicable or do they apply only to the research setting? Similarly, do your results apply to all individuals like the ones you studied or just the ones you studied? For example, if strength training improves strength in young healthy basketball players, you cannot assume that it will work as effectively in older sedentary individuals. The applicability of your results to target population, other people, or other situations is referred to as generalizability.

Threats to External Validity

Campbell and Stanley (1963) have identified four threats to external validity. Each of them has the potential effect of limiting generalizability to other populations or conditions. These threats may change the treatment effect (either increasing or decreasing it). Accordingly, study results may be limited to conditions in which those threats are present.

Multiple Treatment Interference

In studies in which multiple treatments or multiple independent variables are being delivered, the effects of one treatment or independent variable

In the Field

Joe is interested in studying the effects of compression on swelling. To do this he elicits elbow swelling by having subjects perform eccentric biceps curls with a randomly selected elbow. Within 48 hours all subjects have swollen elbows. These subjects are then randomly assigned to receive a compression wrap or to the control group. Joe also places each subject in an arm sling to reduce pain but to also reduce any muscle pump effect. Once a day subjects report to the lab where Joe measures the swelling using a volumetric tank. At the end of the study, Joe determines that the swelling reduced more rapidly in the compression wrap group than in the control group. When Joe submits his study for publication, one of the reviewers commends him on a well-controlled, internally valid study. However, the reviewer expresses concern that eccentrically induced swelling is not the same as joint swelling. In response Joe acknowledges that his results may not generalize to joint swelling (i.e., be externally valid to other types of swelling) and that the study should be extended to other types of swelling in the future.

may change the effect of subsequent ones. This is common in clinics when patients are given multiple treatments. In experimental studies, you might study two or more independent variables. An early variable may alter the effect of a later one. To reduce this effect, researchers either study single treatments or ensure that the ordering of the treatments is not the same for every subject. Even when possible ordering effects are removed, the overall study effects may be dependent on the presence of multiple treatments. For example, when manual muscle testing the quadriceps at multiple points through the knee joint's ROM, you may choose to first assess isometric strength near complete extension, then at 45 degrees of flexion, and finally at 90 degrees of flexion. The patient's familiarization with the manual muscle test near extension could affect the subsequent measurement at 45 degrees of flexion. If you are interested in the effects of exercise on ankle circulation but, as a course of treatment, you also include ice before the exercise, the effects could be caused by the interaction between ice and exercise. Thus, you could not generalize your results to a treatment of only exercise or combined heat and exercise.

How is this different from internal validity? Specifically, there is nothing wrong with the experimental treatment of ice and exercise. In combination, they produce a potent treatment. Therefore, an experiment of this type would be internally valid. However, if your intent was to make a generalization about the effects of exercise on circulation, your results would not support this generalization because they are based on using ice before exercise. Other frequently encountered factors that create treatment interactions include fatigue and learning. For example, balance assessments may require individuals to stand on one leg for an extended period of time. If this is done multiple times, fatigue may become a factor. If you are assessing the effects of orthotics on balance, fatigue and the orthotic may combine to produce an unintended effect. Thus, your results would generalize only to situations in which fatigue existed. Similarly, if you have participants complete multiple balance tests, the multiple tests may produce learning or act as practice trials producing improvement across time. If this were the case, your results would not apply to single trials, in which learning or practice would not have occurred.

Interactive Effects of Testing

A testing-treatment interaction is very similar to the testing effect. It suggests that the treatment effect may not have occurred or not been as strong without the presence of the pretest. Pretesting participants often sensitizes them to the treatment and/or the experiment. Therefore, a participant may react differently to the treatment after the pretest than if there were no pretest. In athletic training research, these effects are most likely to occur if the pretest produces fatigue or permits practice.

Selection-Treatment Interaction

Similar to selection bias, selection-treatment interactions result when the treatment has an effect specific to the group studied. The careful selection of subjects in athletic training research may work to decrease the generalization of results to other populations. If you studied a strength-training program in untrained individuals, you would probably see a very marked improvement in strength, but the same program applied to Olympic weightlifters might have little to no effect. Therefore, the effects seen in the untrained individuals cannot be generalized to Olympic athletes. We should emphasize that studying select groups is not a bad thing. You may want to determine the specific effects of orthopedic bracing on basketball players' ankle sprains (in prevention or treatment). However, you should be cautious in applying those results to other athletes, such as soccer players.

Reactive Effects of Experimental Arrangements

Finally, as suggested previously, many results can be produced only in the laboratory (i.e., the experimental arrangement). Because laboratories are generally "foreign" environments, your participants may be apprehensive in the laboratory, and this may affect the results. Similarly, your participants may perceive the experiment as very important and be more attentive to the activity than otherwise. In general, anything that is inconsistent with the participants' natural expectations and natural environment may alter the treatment effect, producing results that will differ from those obtained in the field environment. Thus, generalizing laboratory findings to field settings can be difficult. Subjects may change their behavior just because they are being studied. They may try harder to produce results. For example, they may stand differently, altering postural measures. The laboratory is an artificial place in which unusual demands (equipment, etc.) are placed on subjects. Laboratory behavior may not generalize to performance in other settings. Although the physiological nature of research variables in athletic training limits this threat, generalizing laboratory findings to field settings can still be difficult. Without the laboratory, some things cannot be studied. The important thing is to understand the limitations and advantages of both the laboratory and field settings.

 ## Solutions to Common Problems

How Do I Control Fatigue and Practice Effects?

Controlling fatigue and practice effects in athletic training research is a common problem. You will often be interested in how something changes across time. For example, assume you are interested in whether postural sway changes with orthotic use. To test this, you might have participants balance on one leg while first wearing no orthotics and immediately after putting orthotics in their shoes. To do this it is common to have participants do multiple balance trials (e.g., 3 no orthotic and 3 orthotic trials). This is done to improve the reliability of the test (see Chapter 9). However, by conducting multiple trials it is also possible to fatigue the muscles at the ankle, knee, or hip, decreasing performance across trials. If the no orthotic condition always comes before the orthotic condition, you may get increased postural sway from fatigue during the orthotic condition. Therefore, you might wrongly conclude that orthotics increase postural sway. To counter the effect of fatigue (i.e., maturation effect), you should make sure that appropriate time intervals occur between trials and between the no orthotic and orthotic conditions to allow recovery from any fatigue that occurs.

In addition to fatigue, multiple trials can result in learning and practice effects. In this case, the no orthotic trials may serve as practice for the subsequent orthotic trials. Thus, you may have improvements from the no orthotic condition to the orthotic condition that are due to practice and not the orthotic itself. One way to counter this is to have training trials before the research begins (e.g., familiarization sessions). This assures that learning the task is complete and people are good at the task before measurements are taken.

As a supplement to providing rest and practice to control fatigue and practice effects, respectively, we recommend counterbalancing. Counterbalancing refers to alternating the order of treatments or measures to insure that they occur equally at all time points. For example, in the orthotic study you would select half the participants to receive the orthotic condition first followed by the no orthotic condition, reversing the order for the second half of the participants. By counterbalancing the conditions, the effects of fatigue and practice are evenly distributed across the experiment. It should be emphasized that with counterbalancing the effects of fatigue or practice are not eliminated. Practice or fatigue may still impact your results; however, that impact should be equal across the entire experiment.

Finally, counterbalancing is not limited to fatigue and practice effects. Counterbalancing is an appropriate control any time you believe that the order of treatments or measures may impact your results. The only exceptions to this would be if studying order effects were the focus of your research or if it were impossible, for other reasons, to apply counterbalancing.

Counterbalancing versus Random Assignment

An alternative to counterbalancing treatments is to randomly assign the order of treatments. Because of the emphasis in experimental research on random assignment, this is often perceived as the research panacea. The assumption is that by randomly assigning treatments, the order will be evenly distributed as with counterbalancing. In fact, this may or may not occur. For example, if you toss a coin, the probability of heads is 50 percent, i.e., 5 out of 10. However, experience will tell you that sometimes you will get heads 7 out of 10 times, and on rare occasions you may even get all heads. This is also true of randomizing treatments. Using the orthotic study, if you randomize the orthotic and no-orthotic conditions, on average, half the time the orthotic condition will be first, and on the other half the no-orthotic condition will be first. However, based on the coin example, you should see that other possibilities exist. In other words, it is possible that random assignments will not produce the same balance of treatments as counterbalancing will. It is because of this that we prefer counterbalancing.

We should also point out that with several treatments (e.g., more than 5) counterbalancing may become cumbersome. For example, to counterbalance 5 treatments, you need at least 5 participants (Table 7–3). Clearly this is too few participants for a good study. To maintain counterbalancing, participants must be added in groups of 5. Thus, the next smallest number of participants is 10, then 15, and so on. You should see that including more than 5 treatments rapidly compounds the number of participants you need. In cases where the number of treatments is large, random assignment of treatments may be necessary. However, if you use random assignment, we suggest that you keep track of the frequency of the order of each treatment, i.e., how many times did the orthotic condition occur first.

Table 7–3 • Minimum Counterbalancing for 5 Treatments

Participant	Time 1	Time 2	Time 3	Time 4	Time 5
P1	T1	T2	T3	T4	T5
P2	T2	T3	T4	T5	T1
P3	T3	T4	T5	T1	T2
P4	T4	T5	T1	T2	T3
P5	T5	T1	T2	T3	T4

Can Randomization Fail?

You may ask whether randomization can fail. The answer to this is no, but random assignment by its nature does not ensure that the groups will be exactly the same. It ensures that any differences that do exist are random. For example, if you were conducting a strength study and you randomly assigned participants, men and women, to control and strength-training groups, it is possible that more men would be assigned to the training group than women. In this case, the training group will start off being stronger than the control group. Thus, at the end of training, the training group might be stronger than the control group simply because they started stronger. From a probability point of view, this type of bias cannot be avoided. However, in some circumstances it can be minimized. For example, in the case of strength training involving both men and women, you should randomly assign men and women separately (called stratified random assignment). This maintains random assignment but ensures equal numbers of men and women in each group.

When Should I Blind a Study?

As previously explained, blinding refers to either participants (single blind) or participants and researchers (double blind) being unaware of who is receiving the experimental treatment. Blinding the participants should occur any time a placebo (or psychological) effect is expected. Similarly, researchers should be blinded if they could have an effect on the treatment or be biased by knowledge of the results. In sports medicine, an example of this might be with studying rehabilitation protocols. If, for example, participants are post-surgical knee patients assigned to a standard rehabilitation (control) or a "progressive" rehabilitation protocol (experimental), which you favor, it might be possible that you would spend more time with or encourage participants in the progressive group more than those in the control group. This does not mean that the additional encouragement was intentional. An example of intentional encouragement would be an additional intervention. Rather, blinding prevents unintentional interventions. Sometimes as a researcher you are more enthusiastic about some treatments than others. This enthusiasm can influence the study in unintended ways. Thus, by being ignorant of who was receiving which treatments (and sometimes what the preliminary results are), you protect the study from unintentional influences.

Summary

As a researcher, your goal is to design studies that are not susceptible to alternative explanations of the results. The first concern is to identify whether the results have internal validity. We have reviewed a number of threats to internal validity that can make us less certain that treatments cause outcomes. We also reviewed research design strategies (especially random assignment and the use of control groups) that can help us be more certain about causes. Finally, we reviewed a number of factors that, if present, can limit the generalizability of our findings and discussed solutions to common problems such as how to control fatigue and practice effects.

Activities

1. Submit a randomized group experimental design.
2. Submit a pretest-posttest randomized control design.
3. Develop a scheme to counterbalance two treatments across 20 subjects.

References

Campbell, D. T., & Stanley, J. C. (1963). *Experimental and quasi-experimental designs for research*. Boston: Houghton Mifflin Company.

Cook, T. D., & Campbell, D. T. (1979). *Quasi-experimentation: Design and analysis issues for field settings*. Boston: Houghton Mifflin Company.

Kazdin, A. E. (1982). *Single-case research designs*. New York: Oxford University Press.

Mattacola, C. G., & Lloyd, J. W. (1997). Effects of a 6-week strength and proprioception training program on measures of dynamic balance: A single-case design. *Journal of Athletic Training, 32*, 127–135.

Bibliography

Bordens, K.S., & Abbot, B.B. (2002). *Research design and methods: A process approach*. Boston: McGraw-Hill.

Iverson, C., Flanagin, A., & Fontanarosa, P.B. (1998). *American Medical Association manual of style*. Baltimore: Williams & Wilkins.

Myers, J.L., & Well, A. D. (2003). *Research design and statistical analysis*. Mahwah, N.J.: L. Erlbaum Associates.

Chapter *8*

Common Measures in Athletic Training

Objectives

After reading this chapter, you will:

- Recognize typical measures of strength.
- Recognize typical measures of proprioception and kinesthesia.
- Recognize typical measures of balance and stabilometry.
- Recognize typical measures of joint range of motion and arthrometry.
- Understand the importance of instrument calibration and standardization of procedures.

Questions

While reading this chapter, think about answers to the following questions:

1. What is a good measure? And how do I select one?
2. How can I measure strength?
3. How can I measure proprioception and kinesthesia?
4. What is the difference between center of pressure and center of balance?
5. What is the difference between a goniometer and an inclinometer?
6. How often should I calibrate my instruments?
7. Why should I standardize my procedures and instructions?

 Common Measures

Because of the variety of measures used in athletic training research, it is not possible to provide a comprehensive list of measures or completely describe each one. As you begin to review literature, you will find that measures are seldom defined one way. Thus, part of your challenge will be to discern the differences among similar measures and determine whether these differences affect the results of your study. The following discussion should alert you to some of the subtle differences that can occur when the researcher tries to measure strength, proprioception and kinesthesia, balance and stabilometry, range of motion, arthrometry, and volumetrics.

Strength

Measures of strength are probably the most commonly used measures in athletic training and seemingly easy to define and measure. Unfortunately, that is not the case. In fact, there are differences among kinesiologists and others as to how to measure strength. At a fundamental level, some kinesiologists prefer to measure strength with only isometric measures (Enoka, 1994). The argument for isometric strength measures is that by preventing joint motion, factors such as the muscle force-velocity, length-tension, and stretch-shorten relationships as well as motor coordination can be eliminated. In contrast, dynamic measures, such as isokinetics, have been suggested as useful, provided the velocity of testing is specified (Knuttgen & Komi, 1992). Which you should use probably depends on your goals. However, one reasonable rule of thumb is to use the same measure as similar studies. By doing so, comparisons among studies are easier.

In the Field

Jay is interested in studying muscle strength at the ankle. However, it occurs to him that there are several ways of measuring strength. He considers manual muscle testing, isometric testing using a hand dynamometer, and isokinetic testing. He is uncertain which measure is best and decides to consult with his advisor. His advisor points out that manual testing is good for the clinical setting, but that the grading system is probably too imprecise for this type of research. Isometric testing might be appropriate if there were evidence in the literature that one point in the range of motion was more important than another. In this case, isometrics could test that specific point. In contrast, if a more general measure of strength is required, isokinetics might be better because it can measure strength throughout the range of motion and there is ample evidence for its reliability. Jay's advisor has one other suggestion. Jay is told he should review the literature for the measure that is commonly used. As part of the research process, it is useful to be able to compare your results with those of others. Thus, selecting measures (provided that previous measures are good measures) that have been used in other studies is often an important consideration.

Sherrie has a similar problem. She is interested in balance after a mild concussion. After reviewing the literature, she identifies several tests such as the stork-stand and wobble board. Again, she wonders which is best. Like Jay, she consults with her advisor. In addition to considering the advice given to Jay, Sherrie also notes that some of her measures distinguish between individuals with and without mild concussion, while others do not. It occurs to her that it would be best to limit her measures to those that have been shown to distinguish between injured and uninjured individuals.

Joint Torque

Joint torque is one of the most common strength measures in athletic training research. It can be measured either isometrically or dynamically, and represents the interaction of muscle force production and the muscle's lever arm. The typical unit for torque is Newton meter (Nm). However, you will occasionally find foot pounds (the English equivalent of Nm) in the older literature. When joint torque is measured dynamically, you should be aware that the torque measured is the net torque of the joint's co-activating muscles, gravity, and inertia. For example, during a dynamic knee extension, the measured extension torque is the net result of the extensors producing extension, the flexors trying to counter the extension, the downward effect of gravity, and the limb's inertial resistance to movement. The effect of muscle co-activation is most pronounced at the joint's end ranges of motion, where antagonists begin deceleration in preparation for the change in direction. The force of gravity is most prominent when the limb is horizontal to the floor, but can be corrected with gravity correction procedures. Inertia is more difficult to account for, but remains constant for a given limb. Thus, dynamic joint torque should not be interpreted as only the torque produced by the agonists. Instead, it is the combined effect of all these factors. If you are only interested in agonist force production, you should use an isometric test rather than a dynamic test.

Isokinetic testing is probably the most common dynamic strength test used in athletic training research. However, you will find that methods of isokinetic testing vary greatly. (For discussions on appropriate isokinetic procedures see Dvir [1995], and Perrin [1993].) The most common isokinetic measure is peak torque (PT). PT is the highest joint torque produced by muscular contraction. There are a variety of methods for calculating PT, and most are reliable (Arnold & Perrin, 1993). Thus, the method you choose may depend on your goals and factors such as limiting fatigue.

In assessing joint torque isometrically, you will need to decide the joint angle at which to measure the torque. Which angle you choose depends on your goals. Depending on your research question, the test angle may represent the normal functional angle of the joint. However, you may also want to establish your angle based on the length-tension relationship (Knapik, Wright, Mawdsley, & Braun, 1983a) and select the angle producing the greatest amount of torque.

One-Repetition Maximum

An alternative to measuring joint torque is to measure the one-repetition maximum (1RM) of a joint. The 1RM is the maximum amount of weight that can be moved by a joint or multiple joint system (e.g., a squat exercise) only one time. To find the 1RM participants must lift a series of increasing weights until the 1RM is reached (Berger, 1963). In a one-joint system, the

1RM is an approximation of joint torque. Because the external load is fixed with the 1RM, the 1RM only represents the maximum load lifted by the weakest point in the range of motion. Thus, the 1RM is never the true maximal joint torque. In a multiple joint system, the 1RM never represents a single joint's torque.

Conclusion

Strength is not easily defined, and there are a variety of techniques and measures available to evaluate it. Which you use should depend on the goals of your research. It is well established that each of these measures will produce different results within the same individual (Knapik, Wright, Mawdsley, & Braun, 1983b). Furthermore, strength changes following strength training are best detected using measurement techniques similar to training techniques (Coyle et al., 1981; Moffroid & Whipple, 1970; Pearson & Costill, 1988). Thus, your selection of a strength measure may affect your results. We recommend selecting a strength measure similar to the strength-training techniques used in your study. If participants in your study are not strength training, select a measure from studies similar to yours to permit direct comparisons among the studies.

Proprioception and Kinesthesia

Our review of the literature has revealed at least four different measures of proprioception and kinesthesia. Some of these measures are different methods of measuring the same perceptual response, whereas others measure different perceptual responses.

Joint Position Sense

Joint position sense (JPS) is defined as the nomination of changes in joint angle (Clark, Burgess, Chapin, & Lipscomb, 1985). Nomination simply means that the subjects name the change from a restricted set of choices. For example, the joint is either passively moved (typically very slowly) from a start position or is maintained at the start position, and subjects must correctly nominate the change in joint angle as flexion, extension, or none. This procedure is followed for several trials (typically 10), and the number of correct responses is used as the dependent measure.

Joint Reposition Sense

Joint reposition sense (JRS) involves the reproduction of target joint angles with either the same joint (Docherty, Moore, & Arnold, 1998) or the contralateral joint (Ferrell, Gandevia, & McCloskey, 1987). The difference (or error) between the target angle and the actual angle is used as the dependent measure. These procedures may be done either actively or passively.

Passive testing limits the influence of motor activity on JRS. However, since joint position is primarily important during locomotion, active tests may be more appropriate.

Joint Movement Sense

Joint movement sense (JMS) has been represented in the literature with three distinct methods. The first is similar to JPS and requires subjects to correctly nominate the sensation of movement (Goodwin, McCloskey, & Matthews, 1972). The second is identical to JPS but includes JPS testing of a single position across a range of velocities with differences among velocities representing JMS (Clark et al., 1985). The third requires subjects to report sensations of movement produced by electrical nerve stimulation (Macefield, Gandevia, & Burke, 1990). Which of these is the preferred method is unclear. It is also unclear whether each of these methods is measuring the same sensory modality and how much JMS overlaps with JPS and JRS.

Threshold to Detection

Threshold to detection is defined as the angle at which slow joint movements are initially detected (Lentell et al., 1995) or the smallest angle detected 70 percent of the time with JPS procedures (Refshauge & Fitzpatrick, 1995). The first of these two procedures has been widely used in recent years by athletic training researchers (Lephart, Kocher, Fu, Borsa, & Harner, 1992; Lephart, Warner, Borsa, & Fu, 1994). Unfortunately, both procedures require specialized equipment to control the velocity of movement, and thus, may make it unrealistic for many researchers to use.

Conclusion

As you can see, perceptual measures require a great deal of instrumentation. Which of these you select should depend on instrumentation availability and your interest in a particular perceptual response. Furthermore, we encourage you to select the perceptual response based on the physiological principles of each response and the impairment expected from the injury or medical condition of interest.

Balance and Stabilometry

Balance and stabilometry refer to measures of sway or stability during stance. These measures are either conducted using both legs (double leg) (Horak, Nashner, & Diener, 1990) or a single leg (Arnold & Schmitz, 1998; Schmitz & Arnold, 1998). Additionally, stabilometry has been performed with a variety of instruments and procedures. These include force plates (Tropp, Ekstrand, & Gillquist, 1984; Tropp, Odenrick, & Gillquist, 1985), clinical instruments (e.g., Chattecx Balance System, Chattecx Corp., Hixson, TN) (Bernier, Perrin, & Rijke, 1997; Guskiewicz & Perrin, 1996a), and balance tests (e.g., Rhomberg test) (Guskiewicz & Perrin, 1996b). Which instrument or procedure you select will depend on your goals and availability.

Center of Pressure

Center of pressure (COP) is arguably the gold standard in stabilometry and is the theoretical basis for many of the current clinical devices. COP is defined as the "point of application of the resultant ground reaction force" (Enoka, 1994) and is typically measured by a force plate. As an individual stands quietly, the human body will naturally sway, producing muscular responses (detected as forces on the force plate) to the sway. These muscular responses as well as the force produced by gravity on the body's center of mass will produce changes in the COP's location on the force plate. Variations in the COP's location can then be used as a measure of postural sway (Friden, Zatterstrom, Linstrand, & Moritz, 1989; Tropp et al., 1984; Tropp & Odenrick, 1988).

Center of Balance and Postural Sway

An alternative to center of pressure is center of balance (COB). COB is measured by the Chattecx Balance System (Chattecx Corp., Hixson, TN) and is a variation of COP. "Normal" center of balance is an idealized position in which a person standing on four load cells, one under each heel and one under the metatarsal heads of each foot, has the weight evenly distributed among the load cells (Chattanooga Group, 1992). The center point among the four load cells is used as the reference. Using the "normal" COB as the reference point, the Chattecx Balance System calculates an individual's true COB as the average X and Y distance away from "normal." Using the true COB, the postural sway index is calculated as the standard deviation of a person's sway from the true COB. The utility of using COB rather than COP is unclear. A high relationship between postural sway and COP excursions has been found (Grabiner, Lundin, & Feuerbach, 1993), suggesting that both methods measure the same postural response. Thus, your selection of one or the other may be based on availability and ease of use.

Wobble Boards and the Biodex Stability System

Alternatives to devices that measure COP and postural sway are wobble or balance boards (DeCarlo & Talbot, 1986; Ryan, 1994). These boards can be used in at least two different ways. First, you can measure the time in balance (TIB). TIB is the length of time an individual can keep the edges of the board from contacting the ground. The TIB can be determined as the time to first touch or the cumulative time over a fixed interval; e.g., 30 s. The former of these two procedures is the simplest, with the latter requiring more complicated instrumentation to be accurate. Second, instead of measuring TIB, the number of touches during a fixed time interval can be counted. This procedure is not recommended because during a 30s test, two touches of 15s each would get the same value as two 1s touches.

The Biodex Stability System (Biodex, Inc., Shirley, NY) is an instrumented wobble board (Arnold & Schmitz, 1998). Simultaneously tilting along axes through the frontal and sagittal planes, the Biodex Stability System (BSS) measures the degrees of tilt from horizontal. From this information, stability indexes are calculated for medial/lateral tilt and anterior/posterior tilt. How the BSS measures are related to other balance measures is unclear. However, similar to COP measures (Tropp et al., 1984; Tropp et al., 1985), the BSS is capable of detecting differences in individuals with ankle injuries (Rozzi, Lephart, Sterner, & Kuligowski, 1999).

Clinical Tests

Finally, clinical balance assessments can be performed by having subjects stand on one leg or perform a version of the Rhomberg test (Forkin, Koczur, Battle, & Newton, 1996; Garn & Newton, 1988; Guskiewicz & Perrin, 1996b; Lentell, Katzman, & Walters, 1990). Typically, these tests are evaluated qualitatively, with time in balance or with touch counts. Since qualitative tests have been shown to detect only 52 to 53 percent of ankle injuries (Garn & Newton, 1988; Lentell et al., 1990), our preference is for one of the latter measurement techniques. However, the same limitations associated with wobble boards apply. Clearly, these tests provide an easy means of assessing balance, but we are unaware of studies examining the relationship between these tests and instrumented tests. Thus, the validity of the tests is uncertain.

Conclusion

To assess balance, you have a wide range of possibilities. However, most of these techniques require complex, expensive instrumentation. Simple clinical tests are available, but their validity and ability to assess functional performance is uncertain.

Range of Motion

If you are interested in assessing therapeutic effectiveness, measuring changes in joint range of motion may be of interest. If so, you have at least two common options available: goniometry and inclinometry.

Goniometry

Goniometry refers to the use of the standard clinical (i.e., universal) goniometer. Proper use of goniometers is well established, although the instrument is not always used correctly (Norkin & White, 2003).

When using these devices, you should follow standard clinical procedures for stabilization and measurement. However, for joints of the lower extremity, especially the knee and hip, we recommend attaching dowels to each goniometer arm to extend the length of the arm. By extending the length of the arms, you will find it easier to align the goniometer with anatomical landmarks.

Inclinometers

Depending on the circumstances, you may find inclinometers a useful alternative to goniometers. Inclinometers are special goniometers that use the force of gravity to establish the baseline of measurement. Essentially, inclinometers act as plumb bobs attached to a protractor. The inclinometer's advantage is that it can be attached directly to the limb, does not require alignment with multiple anatomical landmarks, and can be faster to use. The disadvantage is that to provide a valid measure, limbs must be initially aligned in a meaningful reference to gravity. To accomplish this, goniometers are often required. Thus, your accuracy with the inclinometer measures may depend on your accuracy with the goniometer. Nevertheless, with appropriate standardization of the measurement protocol, we prefer inclinometers to goniometers.

Conclusion

Joint range of motion can be measured with either goniometers or inclinometers. Either should give you accurate results provided that you use them correctly. Which you use will depend on your task. Inclinometers are useful when the measure can be made in reference to gravity and are easier to use. However, when gravity cannot be used as a reference, a goniometer is the appropriate choice.

Arthometry and Volumetrics

In assessing joint injury, you may find it useful to measure injury severity using arthrometry, volumetrics, or both. While very different measures, they each can provide useful information about injury severity.

Joint Arthrometry

Joint arthrometry is another frequently used instrument in athletic training research. Arthrometers such as the Telos (Austin and Associates, Fallston,

MD) and KT-1000 and KT-2000 (MedMetric, San Diego, CA) are typically used to measure displacement normally limited by joint ligaments. The two most commonly tested motions are anterior translation of the knee and talar tilt of the ankle joint. In addition to displacement, load-deformation curves can also be plotted to establish joint compliance and stiffness. The Telos has the capability of testing multiple joints, but requires radiographs or computer interfacing to measure joint displacement. Conversely, the KT-1000 and KT-2000 do not require radiography or a computer interface, but are limited to measuring only anterior and posterior knee displacements.

Volumetrics

The effectiveness of treatments on traumatic injuries or inflammatory conditions may be assessed with volumetrics. Swelling is typically measured using volumetric measures. Specifically, swollen joints or limbs are immersed in water-filled tanks, causing the tanks to overflow. The overflow is collected, and its volume or weight is measured. Increases or decreases in the overflow after treatment indicate increases and decreases in swelling, respectively. When using volumetric tanks, you should carefully standardize your immersion procedures to insure that the depth of immersion remains constant for all trials. Volumetric tanks for the extremities are easily constructed with materials from the local hardware store. However, these tanks can be bulky, and separate-sized tanks for different joints are often necessary.

Conclusion

Arthrometers can provide a direct measure of damage to joint ligaments. Depending on the nature of your research, this may be very helpful. However, ligament damage may be only part of the story. Inflammation following injury may be another useful indicator. Thus, volumetrics may add another dimension to your assessment of injury severity.

 # Calibration

Calibration refers to the process of checking the accuracy of your instruments. For example, an isokinetic dynamometer should accurately measure a torque applied to it. To establish this, you would apply a variety of known torques to the dynamometer and measure the dynamometer output. If the calibration is correct, the measured torque will match the known torque you applied. If not, the dynamometer must be adjusted to measure the correct torque. Each instrument you use will have procedures for calibration. If the device was commercially manufactured, the manufacturer will provide you with calibration procedures. If you have constructed the device, you will need to develop your own procedures.

In the Field

Holly has been collecting isokinetic hamstring strength data for approximately 3 months. As part of this process, she has been extracting strength values as she collected data. She entered the data into her database and completed an initial statistical analysis. She then took her data to her advisor. Upon examining the data, her advisor recognized that the hamstring torque data for some individuals was greater than that previously reported in the literature. Holly and her advisor reviewed her procedures but nothing appeared incorrect. At that point her advisor suggested that the calibration of the isokinetic dynamometer should be checked. Although the dynamometer had been calibrated at the start of the study, recalibration of the system revealed that known weights were producing torque values 20 Nm greater than expected. This was consistent with Holly's data. It was concluded that the dynamometer had lost its calibration at some point in the study. Since Holly couldn't be sure from the data whether this was a sudden or gradual change, she couldn't be certain which data were good and which weren't. As a result Holly had to recollect her strength data for all of her subjects. As a safety precaution, she also recalibrated the dynamometer after every third subject.

Commercial instrument manufacturers will provide guidelines on how often to calibrate the instrument. You should follow these guidelines as a minimum and recalibrate more often if you find large differences between calibrations. If you have constructed the device, calibrations should be done frequently to establish the stability of the calibration. If you find your instrument maintains its calibration every day for a week, then calibrating only once per week may be necessary. Similarly, if the calibration is maintained across several weeks, then monthly calibrations may be adequate. The exact calibration schedule will depend on your or others' experience with the instrument.

Standardizing Instruments and Instructions

In addition to calibrating your instruments, you should standardize how the instrument is used in your experiment as well as any instructions to be used. By standardizing, you can maintain uniformity in your procedures. This reduces mistakes and increases your measures' reliability, validity, and precision. For example, you may want to write out the instructions you give to subjects and then read these instructions. By giving each subject the same instructions, you will reduce the chances that you will give slightly different instructions to different subjects. Similarly, you may want to write out a checklist for the setup for an instrument, such as an isokinetic dynamometer. This will ensure that your setup is exactly the same each time. Once you develop these instructions, you need to pilot test them to be sure that your protocols are correct and your instruments are calibrated.

Solution to a Common Problem

Know Your Measure

It is essential that you understand the correct values for your measures of interest. This will enable you to recognize mistakes in the data. For example, if you use an isokinetic dynamometer to measure strength, you should be familiar with normally expected values. By knowing what to expect, you can immediately detect values that are outside the normal range. When this happens, it is likely that there was an error in procedures. Values outside the normal expected range rarely occur. To avoid this problem, you should use your literature review to establish a normal range for your measures. If you are using a new measure without established normal values, you should use similar measures to establish a general guideline for expected values.

Summary

As you can see, the field of athletic training uses a wide variety of different measures, and those presented do not represent an exhaustive list. Clearly, your research will not use all and probably not most of these measures. Which measures you select will depend on your research needs, the quality of the measure, the availability of instrumentation, and the measure's use in the literature. Regardless of which measure you use, it is important for you to understand the measure. You should at least know its normal values, how reliable it is, and whether the measure is considered valid.

Activities

1. Find several studies using your measure of interest. What is the range of values for each study? What is the range of values across studies?
2. Identify the means for each study. Are they similar? What is the range of means across studies?
3. Identify the standard deviations of the measure in each study. Are they similar? What is their range across studies?
4. Were different measures used across studies? What are the units of each measure? Do they differ across studies?
5. Plot the range of scores across studies.
6. Plot the means across studies.
7. Plot the standard deviations across studies.

References

Arnold, B. L., & Perrin, D. H. (1993). The reliability of four different methods of calculating quadriceps peak torque and angle-specific torques at 30°, 60°, 75°. *Journal of Sport Rehabilitation, 2*, 243–250.

Arnold, B. L., & Schmitz, R. J. (1998). Examination of balance measures produced by the Biodex Stability System. *Journal of Athletic Training, 33*, 323–327.

Berger, R. A. (1963). Comparison between static training and various dynamic training programs. *The Research Quarterly, 34*, 131–135.

Bernier, J. N., Perrin, D. H., & Rijke, A. (1997). Effect of unilateral functional instability of the ankle on postural sway and inversion and eversion strength. *Journal of Athletic Training, 32*, 226–232.

Chattanooga Group. (1992). *The balance system: Clinical desk reference.* Hixson, T.N.: Chattanooga Group.

Clark, F. J., Burgess, R. C., Chapin, J. W., & Lipscomb, W. T. (1985). Role of intramuscular receptors in the awareness of limb position. *Journal of Neurophysiology 54*, 1529–1540.

Coyle, E. F., Feiring, D. C., Rotkis, T. C., Cote, R. W., III, Roby, F. B., Lee, W., et al. (1981). Specificity of power improvements through slow and fast isokinetic training. *Journal of Applied Physiology, 51*, 1437–1442.

DeCarlo, M. S., & Talbot, R. W. (1986). Evaluation of ankle joint proprioception following injection of the anterior talofibular ligament. *Journal of Orthopaedic and Sports Physical Therapy, 8*, 70–76.

Docherty, C. L., Moore, J. H., & Arnold, B. L. (1998). Effects of strength training on strength development and joint position sense in functionally unstable ankles. *Journal of Athletic Training, 33*, 310–314.

Dvir, Z. (2004). *Isokinetics: Muscle testing, interpretation, and clinical applications* (2nd ed.). Edinburgh: Churchill Livingstone.

Enoka, R. M. (1994). *Neuromechanical basis of kinesiology* (2nd ed.). Champaign, IL: Human Kinetics.

Ferrell, W. R., Gandevia, S. C., & McCloskey, D. I. (1987). The role of joint receptors in human kinesthesia when intramuscular receptors cannot contribute. *Journal of Physiology, 386*, 63–71.

Forkin, D. M., Koczur, C., Battle, R., & Newton, R. A. (1996). Evaluation of kinesthetic deficits indicative of balance control in gymnasts with unilateral chronic ankle sprains. *Journal of Orthopaedic and Sports Physical Therapy, 23*, 245–250.

Friden, T., Zatterstrom, R., Linstrand, A., & Moritz, U. (1989). A stabilometric technique for evaluation of lower limb instabilities. *American Journal of Sports Medicine, 17*, 118–122.

Garn, S. N., & Newton, R. A. (1988). Kinesthetic awareness in subjects with multiple ankle sprains. *Physical Therapy, 68*, 1667–1671.

Goodwin, G. M., McCloskey, D. I., & Matthews, P. B. C. (1972). The persistence of appreciable kinesthesia after paralysing joint afferents but preserving muscle afferents. *Brain Research, 37*, 326–329.

Grabiner, M. D., Lundin, T. M., & Feuerbach, J. W. (1993). Converting Chattecx Balance System vertical reaction force measurements to center of pressure excursion measurements. *Physical Therapy, 73*, 316–319.

Guskiewicz, K. M., & Perrin, D. H. (1996a). Effect of orthotics on postural sway following inversion ankle sprain. *Journal of Orthopaedic and Sports Physical Therapy, 23*, 326–331.

Guskiewicz, K. M., & Perrin, D. H. (1996b). Research and clinical applications of assessing balance. *Journal of Sport Rehabilitation, 5*, 45–63.

Horak, F. B., Nashner, L. M., & Diener, H. C. (1990). Postural strategies associated with somatosensory and vestibular loss. *Experimental Brain Research, 82*, 167–177.

Knapik, J. J., Wright, J. E., Mawdsley, R. H., & Braun, J. (1983a). Isometric, isotonic, and isokinetic torque variations in four muscle groups through a range of joint motion. *Physical Therapy, 63*, 938–947.

Knapik, J. J., Wright, J. E., Mawdsley, R. H., & Braun, J. M. (1983b). Isokinetic, isometric, and isotonic strength relationships. *Archives of Physical Medicine and Rehabilitation, 64*, 77–80.

Knuttgen, H. G., & Komi, P. V. (1992). Basic definitions for exercise. In P. V. Komi (Ed.), *Strength and power in sport.* Oxford: Blackwell Scientific Publications.

Lentell, G., Baas, B., Lopez, D., McGuire, L., Sarrels, M., & Snyder, P. (1995). The contributions of proprioceptive deficits, muscle function, and anatomic laxity to functional instability of the ankle. *Journal of Orthopaedic and Sports Physical Therapy, 21*, 206–215.

Lentell, G. L., Katzman, L. L., & Walters, M. R. (1990). The relationship between muscle function and ankle stability. *Journal of Orthopaedic and Sports Physical Therapy, 11*, 605–611.

Lephart, S. M., Kocher, M. S., Fu, F. H., Borsa, P. A., & Harner, C. D. (1992). Proprioception following anterior cruciate ligament reconstruction. *Journal of Sport Rehabilitation, 1*, 188–196.

Lephart, S. M., Warner, J. J. P., Borsa, P. A., & Fu, F. F. (1994). Proprioception of the shoulder joint in healthy, unstable, and surgically repaired shoulders. *Journal of Shoulder and Elbow Surgery, 3*, 371–380.

Macefield, G., Gandevia, S. C., & Burke, D. (1990). Perceptual responses to microstimulation of single afferents innervating joints, muscles, and skin of the human hand. *Journal of Physiology, 429*, 113–129.

Moffroid, M. T., & Whipple, R. H. (1970). Specificity of speed exercise. *Physical Therapy, 50*, 1692–1700.

Norkin, C. C., & White, D. J. (2003). *A guide to goniometery.* (2nd ed.). Philadelphia: F.A. Davis.

Pearson, D. R., & Costill, D. L. (1988). The effects of constant external resistance exercise and isokinetic exercise training on work-induced hypertrophy. *Journal of Applied Sport Science Research, 2*, 39–41.

Perrin, D. H. (1993). *Isokinetic exercise and assessment.* Champaign, IL: Human Kinetics.

Refshauge, K. M., & Fitzpatrick, R. C. (1995). Perception of movement at the human ankle: Effects of leg position. *Journal of Physiology, 488*, 243–248.

Rozzi, S. L., Lephart, S. M., Sterner, R., & Kuligowski, L. (1999). Balance training for persons with functionally unstable ankles. *Journal of Orthopaedic and Sports Physical Therapy, 29*, 478–486.

Ryan, L. (1994). Mechanical stability, muscle strength, and proprioception in the functionally unstable ankle. *Australian Physiotherapy, 40*, 41–47.

Schmitz, R. J., & Arnold, B. L. (1998). Intertester and intratester reliability of the Biodex Stability System. *Journal of Sport Rehabilitation, 7*, 95–101.

Tropp, H., Ekstrand, J., & Gillquist, J. (1984). Stabilometry in functional instability of the ankle and its value in predicting injury. *Medicine & Science in Sports & Exercise, 16*, 64–66.

Tropp, H., & Odenrick, P. (1988). Postural control in single-limb stance. *Journal of Orthopaedic Research, 6*, 833–839.

Tropp, H., Odenrick, P., & Gillquist, J. (1985). Stabilometry recordings in functional and mechanical instability of the ankle joint. *International Journal of Sports Medicine, 6*, 180–182.

Bibliography

Dvir, Z. (2004). *Isokinetics: Muscle testing, interpretation, and clinical applications* (2nd ed.). Edinburgh: Churchill Livingstone.

Enoka, R. M. (1994). *Neuromechanical basis of kinesiology* (2nd ed.). Champaign, IL: Human Kinetics.

Perrin, D. H. (1993). *Isokinetic exercise and assessment.* Champaign, IL: Human Kinetics.

Chapter 9

Reliability and Validity

Objectives

After reading this chapter, you will:

- Understand the differences among the types of reliability.
- Understand the differences among the types of validity.
- Know the components of an observed score.
- Be able to calculate an intraclass correlation (ICC) coefficient and the standard error of the measure.
- Understand the relationship between the different ICC forms and the Pearson correlation.
- Understand intertester and intratester reliability.

Questions

While reading this chapter, think about answers to the following questions:

1. When should I do reliability testing?
2. What conditions (assumptions) are necessary for reliability testing?
3. How high should a reliability/validity coefficient be?
4. Which ICC formula should I use?
5. Why don't I see more tests of the validity of measures?
6. What is the relationship between reliability and validity?
7. What does a standard error of measurement have to do with reliability?
8. Why are there different types of reliability and validity?

General Introduction to Reliability and Validity

The two major criteria for judging the quality of the measures you use are reliability and validity. Your aim is to have measures that have very little error (reliability) and that produce scores that are valid for your purposes. In this chapter we will explore various assessments of reliability and validity that can be used in athletic training research.

Reliability can be defined as "the extent to which a measurement remains constant as it is repeated under conditions taken to be constant" (Kaplan, 1964). In classical measurement, reliability has to do with error of measurement relative to "true" scores on the measure. Validity traditionally has dealt with the degree to which there is evidence that a measure actually measures what it purports to measure. For example, is joint reposition sense really a measure of proprioception?

 # Reliability

The Concept of Reliability

Classical measurement theory suggests that any measure is composed of a "true" score and error. The true score is a theoretical value that represents an error-free measure. For example, you can imagine that any patient or athlete has a true value for shoulder external rotation range of motion that is determined by the individual's anatomy and physiology at the shoulder. However, measurement theory suggests that you cannot actually measure the true external rotation without error. Thus, your measure of the individual's external rotation, i.e., the observed score, is a combination of the true score plus error. While the ideal is to have measures that are error free, two kinds of error can creep into our measures: random error and systematic error. Random errors are a function of random inconsistencies in the application of your measure or random inconsistencies in the subjects' responses on the measure. A subject's inconsistent performance may result from fatigue or from random shifts in motivation. Systematic error is a function of a defective measure or a misapplication of the measure. If an instrument has not been calibrated appropriately, the same error can repeatedly occur. A gas gauge on a car may consistently be off by 1 gallon. Isokinetic peak torque might always be off by 5 Nm. You, as the tester, might produce errors because you don't follow the testing protocols. Two athletic trainers might get different goniometer readings because one lacks the testing competence of the other.

If you repeatedly measure a subject's shoulder range of motion, your expectation is that the repeated scores will be about the same. You want differences between the repeated scores to be only random differences. You would not expect that the score would be exactly the same each time. If there are large differences from one time to the next, you should worry about the reliability of your measure. If there is no difference or very little difference between the scores, you can worry less about the reliability of the measure.

Effects of Unreliable Measures

Unreliable measures will produce inaccurate estimates of variables. In the athletic training room, you might have athletes externally rotate their shoulders as far as they can. You might then guesstimate how far they rotated their shoulders and conclude that an athlete has "very little flexibility." Certainly this qualitative measure of range of motion would be less reliable than a goniometric measure.

Unreliable measures can also lead to inappropriate conclusions in research. Inaccurate estimates of a variable (e.g., range of motion) will result in less powerful statistical tests. Less powerful tests may lead you to conclude that variables that you study are unrelated or that the treatments you implement are ineffective.

Test-Retest Reliability (Stability)

In athletic training research, test-retest reliabilities might be done for different purposes. They may be used to calculate equipment reliabilities, intertester reliabilities, and intratester reliabilities. Although the exact same calculations might be done in each case, the interpretations would be different. Equipment reliability refers to the consistency of the equipment's measures from one time to the next. You can test the consistency of an isokinetic dynamometer by assessing known weights two (or more) times in a row. If the reliability estimate is low, it is clear that something is wrong with the equipment. Interpretation of the other "types" of reliability is not so simple. Intertester reliability (i.e., the consistency of two different testers at taking the same measure) may vary with the skill of the judges or testers, inconsistencies in test procedures, or changes in the variable being assessed. Intratester reliability (i.e., the same tester's consistency at taking the same measure) may vary with inconsistency of the tester as well as changes in the variable being assessed. Intratester reliability tends to be higher for the kinds of data collection in which athletic trainers are typically engaged, and, as such, data collection by one tester is the approach of choice. Unfortunately, it is often impractical for one tester to collect all of the data for a research project, and it thus becomes necessary for more than one tester to collect the data. The testers should extensively practice the data collection procedures to ensure that intertester reliability will be acceptable.

Using the Interclass Correlation Coefficient (Pearson r) to Assess Reliability

The most common method of assessing reliability in athletic training research is to test (or judge) subjects more than once and assess the consistency (or stability) of the subjects' scores from one time to the next. An example is presented in Display 9–1. Range of motion has been assessed using a goniometer on the same shoulder two times for 10 subjects. If ROM scores have no error, you would expect that each subject would have the same score each time. Since these are 10 different subjects, you would also expect that the 10 subjects would exhibit different ROM. Finally, you would expect that the average score of the 10 subjects would be the same from one time to the next. In sum, if there is no error in our ROM measure, you would expect that the only variation in ROM scores would be between the subjects.

Range of Motion Tests for 10 Subjects

Subject	Trial 1	Trial 2
1	X_{1a}	X_{1b}
2		
3		
4		
5		
6		
7		
8		
9		
10	X_{10a}	X_{10b}

This is the basic model for assessing reliability. The actual reliability calculation is performed either through Pearson correlation coefficients (r) or intraclass correlations (ICCs). In the social sciences, psychometricians (specialists who design psychological tests) and others who develop and study measures of cognitive and affective tests usually calculate stability with a Pearson correlation coefficient (r). The formula for calculating the Pearson r is given in Chapter 15. Values of a Pearson r range from -1.0 to 1.0. A zero indicates no linear relationship, a 1.0 indicates a perfect positive linear relationship, and a −1.0 indicates a perfect negative linear relationship. A reliable measure would result in a high positive correlation between the scores from time one and time two. In other words, people who scored high the first time would tend to score high the second time, and people who scored low the first time would tend to score low the second time. A perfect positive correlation would mean that the order between people stayed exactly the same from one time to the next. A major difficulty with using the Pearson r is that it is not sensitive to changes across time as long as the subjects' scores stay in the same order.

In the Field

Marjie is conducting a study on hamstring flexibility after application of massage. To measure knee range of motion, she has decided to use an inclinometer rather than a standard goniometer. To do this she decides it is first necessary to assess the reliability of the inclinometer. However, she is uncertain whether to use the Pearson correlation or the ICC. As she lays out her research plan, she realizes that she is really interested in test-retest reliability. She knows that she could use the Pearson correlation to determine whether her subjects maintain their relative rank from one time to another. But she is equally interested in determining whether each subject's score remains the same from one trial to the next. Because of this, Marjie decides to look for another alternative.

Using the Intraclass Correlation Coefficient

Often athletic training researchers are concerned with score changes from one occasion to the next. You may want to be sure that your equipment remains calibrated, that an individual athletic trainer does not introduce errors from one occasion to the next, or that one of two or more testers do not produce more errors than the other testers. Unlike the Pearson r, the intraclass correlation (ICC) is sensitive to these changes.

Display 9–2 presents four alternative ICCs that have been suggested by Shrout and Fleiss (1979). Each has a different purpose. The first two (ICC 2,1 and ICC 2,k) are used when you want to make generalizations about reliability across different testers' occasions. Each assumes that the testers are a random sample taken from a theoretical population of testers. ICC 2,1 is used when all subjects are tested by the same testers, who are assumed to be a random sample of all possible testers. ICC 2,k includes the same assumption about testers, but the mean of k measures is used at each test time. The second two (ICC 3,1 and ICC 3,k) are used when you are not interested in making generalizations across testers (e.g., you are the only tester of interest and your measure will not be applied outside your study). ICC 3,1 is used when only one measure is taken at each test time, and ICC 3,k is used when the mean of k measures is used at each test time.

Each of the four ICCs in Display 9–2 is calculated using a subject by time repeated measures analysis of variance. A repeated measures analysis of variance (see Chapter 14) is used to partition the score variance into three types or "sources" of variance: variance between subjects, variance

Display 9-2

Formulae Used To Calculate the Common Forms of The Intraclass Correlation Coefficient (ICC).

$$ICC(2,1) = \frac{BMS - EMS}{BMS + (k-1)\,EMS + k(TMS - EMS)/n}$$

$$ICC(2,k) = \frac{BMS - EMS}{BMS + (TMS - EMS)/n}$$

$$ICC(3,1) = \frac{BMS - EMS}{BMS + (k-1)EMS}$$

$$ICC(3,k) = \frac{BMS - EMS}{BMS}$$

BMS = Between mean square
TMS = Trial mean square
EMS = Error mean square
n = Number of subjects
k = Number of trials

between occasions, and the interaction between subjects and tests (sometimes referred to as "error"). You will notice that each formula is a ratio or percentage of "true" score variance to "total" variance. Each has the same numerator. Error is subtracted from the between-subject variance to provide an estimate of true score variance. You will also note that each denominator is different. This is because the definition of total variance changes. In ICC 2,1 all three sources of variance (variance between subjects, variance between test occasions, and error variance) are included in the total. In ICC 2,k only variance between subjects and variance between test occasions are included in the total variance. In both ICC 3,1 and ICC 3,k the variance between occasions is not included in the total variance. Just as with the Pearson r (see Chapter 15), changes from occasion one to occasion two are not considered.

Possible Outcomes for the ICC

A look at some possible outcomes in reliability assessment and their effect on alternative reliability coefficients may help clarify these issues. Examples of four different possible outcomes are presented in Tables 9–1 through 9–4. For each example we have also calculated four different ICCs: ICC 2,1; ICC 2,k; ICC 3,1; and ICC 3,k. In Table 9–1, every subject has exactly the same ROM score on test 1 and test 2. There are no differences between subjects nor is there any difference between the scores on the two tests. This presents a dilemma. It might be that the measure is perfectly reliable. It also might be that the measure is not any good at all because it is unable to detect real differences in shoulder ROM between the subjects. You might never know for sure which is the case, but you would surely be skeptical of these results. Both the Pearson r and the ICCs are indeterminant (unable to be calculated).

Table 9–1 • **Correlation Coefficients When Subjects' Scores Are Identical**

Subject	Trial 1	Trial 2
1	52	52
2	52	52
3	52	52
4	52	52
5	52	52
6	52	52
7	52	52
8	52	52
9	52	52
10	52	52

$r = 0$
ICC 2,1 $= 0$
ICC 2,$k = 0$
ICC 3,1 $= 0$
ICC 3,$k = 0$

Table 9–2 • Correlation Coefficients When Subjects' Scores Are Repeated Across Trials

Subject	Trial 1	Trial 2
1	52	52
2	48	48
3	44	44
4	40	40
5	36	36
6	34	34
7	30	30
8	26	26
9	22	22
10	18	18

$r = 1$
ICC 2,1 = 1
ICC 2,k = 1
ICC 3,1 = 1
ICC 3,k = 1

The ideal case is presented in Table 9–2. There are ROM differences between subjects, and each subject has the same score on test one and test two. In addition, the mean for test one is the same as for test two. The only variation in ROM is between subjects. The Pearson r and the ICCs are each 1.0.

In Table 9–3, there are differences between subjects, but each subject has a score on test two that is 10 points higher than on test one. It appears that there has been some systematic change. How could this happen? Did

Table 9–3 • Correlation Coefficients When Subjects' Scores Are Increased by 10

Subject	Trial 1	Trial 2
1	52	62
2	48	58
3	44	54
4	40	50
5	36	46
6	34	44
7	30	40
8	26	36
9	22	32
10	18	28

$r = 1$
ICC 2,1 = 0.72
ICC 2,k = 0.83
ICC 3,1 = 1
ICC 3,k = 1

the subjects increase their ROM? Did you change your testing procedures? Did the goniometer become uncalibrated? The Pearson r is 1.0 but the ICC 2,1 is .72. The Pearson correlation remains high because the order of the subjects is the same for both tests. ICC 2,1 is lower because of the systematic difference in ROM across testings. The r is sensitive to the order of the subjects but not to the changes across testings. ICC 2,1 and ICC 2,k are sensitive both to the differences among subjects and to the changes from test 1 to test 2. Note that ICC 3,1 and ICC 3,k are each 1.0. This is because the change across time (TMS) is not included in the denominator. Just as with the Pearson r, ICC 3,1 and ICC 3,k are not sensitive to systematic changes.

In Table 9–4, there are differences among the subjects and each subject has had a change in ROM from test 1 to test 2, but half the subjects have increased their ROM and half the subjects have decreased their ROM. How could this happen? Is it due to subject changes – why would half decrease and half increase? Is it due to the test procedures or to having different testers? How could half of the goniometric measures increase on the second test and half decrease? We have seen this occur when obtaining goniometric measures of the left ankle and then of the right ankle. We suspected that it could have to do with the "handedness" of the tester in moving from one ankle to the other.

The effects of this on the ICCs is somewhat surprising and demonstrates the importance of plotting data when doing reliability testing. ICC 2,1 (.81) and ICC 2,k (.89) are actually higher than they were in Table 9–3. Remember that the systematic increase in scores in Table 9–3 from test 1 to test 2 depressed the values of ICC 2,1 and ICC 2,k. In Table 9–4, the systematic increase from test 1 to test 2 is canceled out, because half of them

Table 9–4 • Correlation Coefficients When Subjects' Scores Are Increased or Decreased by 10

Subject	Trial 1	Trial 2
1	52	62
2	48	58
3	44	54
4	40	50
5	36	46
6	34	24
7	30	20
8	26	16
9	22	12
10	19	8

$r = 0.965$
ICC 2,1 = 0.81
ICC 2,k = 0.9
ICC 3,1 = 0.8
ICC 3,k = 0.89

are decreasing. The average increase is almost zero. ICC 3,1 (.80) and ICC 3,k (.89) are both fairly high. We would have missed this pattern if we had not plotted the scores.

These four examples highlight very common issues with assessing the reliability of instruments. A "good" instrument must discriminate between subjects (see Table 9–1), not change from one time to the next (see Tables 9–2 and 9–3) and behave similarly for all subjects from one time to the next (see Table 9–4). When you conduct a reliability study, an inspection of these patterns can help you detect problems with your instrument. Systematic changes from test 1 to test 2 suggest changes in the subjects, the calibration of the instrument, or the testing procedures or testers. Changes from test 1 to test 2 like those in Table 9–4 suggest that different types of subjects are being tested differently, that different testers were used for different subjects, or possibly that a change occurred partway through the testing protocol or in the calibration of the instrument.

Mechanics of ICC Calculation

As suggested in the preceding section, to calculate an ICC you need slightly different statistical machinery. Specifically, rather than using the Pearson correlation you will use a repeated measures one-way analysis of variance (ANOVA; see Chapter 14). Figure 9–2 shows the printout created by data from Figure 9–1 using SPSS's repeated measures program. From this printout the ICC is calculated using the between mean square (BMS), the trial mean square (TMS), and the error mean square (EMS).

Once the components are obtained, they are simply put into the appropriate formula. You will note in the formulae two other values: n and k. The n is the number of subjects you tested for your reliability study. As

In the Field

Based on what Marjie now knows about ICCs, she decides that the ICC is a better option for her reliability study than the Pearson. Her new dilemma is to select the correct ICC formula. As part of her research plan, she has decided that she likes the inclinometer technique better than the standard goniometer, and she believes the other clinicians and researchers will like it as well. Because she now wants her reliability findings to generalize to all researchers and clinicians who might use an inclinometer for knee range of motion, she decides that either ICC 2,1 or ICC 2,k is the correct formula. Marjie must now decide between these formulas. Because average scores are more reliable than single scores, Marjie has decided to collect six measures and average the first three and the second three for her range of motion measure. She will then compare the average scores for her reliability study. Since she is using averages rather than single scores, Marjie selects ICC 2,k for her calculations.

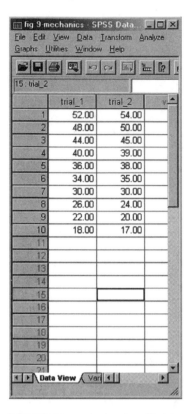

Figure 9–1 Data setup for a typical test-retest reliability assessment.

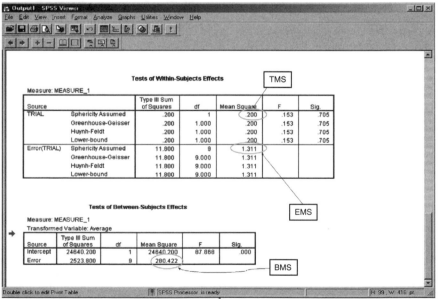

Figure 9–2 Statistical output for calculating ICCs. (EMS=error mean square, TMS=trial mean square, BMS=between mean square.)

indicated previously, k represents the number of scores averaged to create a trial. For example, you conduct a reliability study for ankle joint reposition sense. As part of this study you measure 20 subjects six times. Thus, you have six measures that constitute the six trials. In this case you would use formula (2,1), k would equal 6 (number of measures), and n would equal 20 (number of subjects). Alternatively, knowing that averages have less error than single scores, you decide to average the first three measures and average the last three measures. In this case the two averages constitute your trials. You would use formula (2,k). The k would equal 3 (for three scores averaged to produce each trial), and you would report the formula as (2,3). Finally, the n is still equal to 20.

Precision

The ICC is useful in telling you about the consistency of a measure. However, it does not provide information about the measure's precision. Although a measure may give consistent estimates of an individual's true score, this estimate will vary because of measurement error. Thus, it becomes useful to know how much a measure varies from random error. To do this, you can use the standard error of the measure (SEM). The formula for the SEM is:

$$SEM = S \sqrt{1 - ICC}$$

The S is the standard deviation of the scores from either trial 1 or trial 2. (Theoretically, the standard deviation is the same for both, so the selection of one or the other does not matter.) To understand this formula and the SEM, it is useful to look at it under two conditions. First, assume that you have perfect reliability (i.e., your ICC is 1). In this case, the portion under the square root becomes 0, and thus, the SEM equals zero. Put another way, when you have perfect reliability, there is no error to the score. In contrast, if your ICC equals 0 (i.e., completely unreliable measure), the square root becomes 1, producing an SEM that equals the standard deviation of the scores. In this case, all the variability in the scores is due to error. More realistically, assume that your ICC was equal to .75. Putting .75 into the equation produces a square root of .5. Multiplying this by the standard deviation reduces the standard deviation by $1/2$. In other words, $1/2$ of the variation in your measure is due to error. If your ICC was equal to .95, approximately 22 percent ($\sqrt{1 - .95} = .22$) of the standard deviation would be from error. Thus, as you can see, as the reliability increases, the SEM decreases.

Other Types of Reliability

Research in athletic training may include the measurement of complex variables that include different characteristics, or "items." A researcher may assess cognitive functioning of subjects who have suffered a head injury. The cognitive test may include a number of questions that subjects need to answer. An assessment of ankle instability may ask subjects to report their ankle instability during different functional tasks (e.g., walking on uneven surfaces or climbing up stairs). Measures of treatment compliance, patient satisfaction with treatments, or patients' perceptions of rehabilitation success would also call for the use of multiple assessment items.

Psychometricians warn against the use of test-retest reliability with cognitive, affective, or sociobehavioral measures. Since subjects change from day to day on these measures, it is difficult if not impossible to separate the reliability of the measure from real changes in the subjects. Psychometricians point out the potential of carryover effects of repeated testing and the tendency for subjects to respond in different ways because they are being measured. Subjects may try to please (or annoy) the researcher, they may respond differently because of the social context, or they may learn how to respond correctly. Lastly, and maybe most important, they may, in fact, have real changes on the measure between the time of the first and second test. One suggestion is to create parallel forms and another is to assess the internal consistency of the items within a single test.

Parallel Form Reliability

This method of assessing reliability is also sometimes called alternate form reliability or equivalence. The idea is that you want to have equivalent forms of the measure. You would want the two forms to measure the same thing so they could be used interchangeably. Two forms of the same measure would be developed. To develop a cognitive test of 20 items, you might develop 40 items and then randomly assign them to two forms. To test for reliability, a sample of subjects would then be tested with each form. The scores for the two forms would be compared. Typically this analysis would be done with a Pearson correlation coefficient (it could also be calculated with some form of an ICC). A high correlation between the scores on the two forms would indicate high reliability.

Internal Consistency

Internal consistency is the consistency of responses to different items in an instrument during a single administration of the instrument. This type of reliability assessment is appropriate for a test that has multiple items. Reliability assessment of this sort assesses the adequacy of the content sampling and/or the heterogeneity of the phenomenon being measured by the specific sample of items. For example, if you devise a survey with multiple questions on activities of daily living or quality of function, an internal consistency measure would determine whether the survey questions belong together as a set.

This measure of reliability is typically used with cognitive tests (e.g., IQ or reading achievement) or scales designed to assess personality character-istics or attitudes, but in athletic training, internal consistency analysis might be used for self-report measures of function or performance. A high reliability coefficient suggests consistency of responses within the measure. Since it is more likely that responses within a measure will be more consis-tent if all the items measure the same thing, internal consistency may assess the homogeneity or unidimensionality of the measure.

Split-Half Reliability and Internal Consistency

One way to assess consistency within a measure would be to split the test in half and see whether the scores from one half are consistent with those from the other half. Once scores have been derived from each half, a corre-lation is computed between the two half-scores. Since the test is now half as long, the Spearman-Brown prophecy formula is used to estimate the reli-ability for the total test.

As you can imagine, split-half reliability is dependent on how you divide up the halves. If the two halves are not equivalent in content because of difficulty or fatigue, for example, the reliability coefficient will be low-ered. Traditionally, the most common ways of splitting a test in half were first half versus second half, and odd versus even items. These are only two of many possible ways that a test could be split in half. You could ran-domly assign 20 items, for example, into two halves in many ways. As a result, Kuder and Richardson (1937) developed a method for simultane-ously assessing the internal consistency of all possible split halves. Their formulas were particularly appropriate for use with dichotomous (i.e., right/wrong) answers on cognitive tests. They developed five different for-mulas known as KR-2, KR-8, KR-14, KR-20, and KR-21. The five formulae make different assumptions about the data. As you might expect, the more assumptions made, the lower the reliability coefficient. This is because the data will be less likely to conform to the assumption and so some error is introduced. The KR-20 was used by the National Athletic Trainers' Association Board of Certification (NATABOC) to estimate reliability for the certification examination. They reported that "Internal consistency reliabil-ity estimates, using the KR-20 method, have been computed for the NATABOC examinations administered during 2000. The KR-20 calculation for each version of the written examination was .78 and .79, the four ver-sions of the practical examination ranged from .94 to .95, and the KR-20 estimate for both written simulation examinations was .89. These estimates suggest high reliability" (NATABOC, 1999).

Alternatively, Chronbach (1951) developed the alpha coefficient that has come to be known as Chronbach's alpha. Chronbach's alpha is the equivalent of the KR-20. It does not make the assumption of equal item dif-ficulty and thus it is useful with noncognitive measures (e.g., attitude scales or behavioral assessments).

Selection and Reporting of Reliability Coefficients

Since different reliability coefficients measure different kinds of things, you have to know which one a researcher is reporting and be clear which one you are reporting. The relevant reliability coefficient is the one that addresses the measurement concern that you have. Since cognitive and affective measures are more likely to be affected by learning and by the instability of the variable being studied, equivalence or internal consistency estimates might be more useful than would be test-retest estimates. In addition, internal consistency measures are only relevant when you have a measure that has multiple items (such as a survey), all of which purport to measure the same thing. Alternate form reliability or equivalence is relevant when you need to develop a different form to avoid testing effects.

When you report the value of a reliability coefficient, you also need to state which coefficient it is and the conditions under which it was taken. Other texts suggest specific values of reliability coefficients that are desirable. We hesitate to do this because we know that the standards for reliability coefficients vary by the nature of the variables being measured. Reliability of data produced by instruments (e.g., data from force plates) produce reliabilities in the .90s. If you don't reach this level, your measure (or your procedure) is not good enough. Measures that are affective (e.g., compliance) more typically have reliabilities in the .80s. These are probably satisfactory. A good researcher should be able to demonstrate reliability coefficients (or validity coefficients) that are as good or better than those produced by other researchers with the same instrument.

 Validity

As we mentioned earlier, instrument validity has to do with evidence either that the instrument actually measures what it purports to measure (e.g., postural stability) or that it is valid for some particular purpose (e.g., to screen injuries). The concept of validity is less intuitive and more complex than the concept of reliability. Demonstration of reliability simply calls for evidence of intratester or intertester consistency or consistency across forms or items of an instrument. There is no requirement that the instrument actually measures what it is supposed to measure. (You could have a weight scale that produces consistent measures but that doesn't measure weight at all.) You become more comfortable about the validity of the data if the instrument "looks right" (face or logical validity); if the operational measures demanded by the instrument contain elements that you believe are appropriate for measuring the phenomenon of interest (content validity); or if the scores produced by the instrument are related to other measures in ways that you believe they should be related (criterion validity or construct validity).

Establishing the validity of an instrument requires a number of steps. First, the target variable (e.g., postural stability) must be defined both conceptually (the ability to maintain your center of gravity within your base of support) and operationally (the standard deviation of the center of pressure measured on a force plate while standing quietly). Second, you must make a case that the elements (e.g., a set of functional performance tests or questions on a survey) of the instrument represent an operational definition of the target variable (see Chapter 6). Third, you must provide evidence that the scores resulting from the instrument do indeed measure the target variable or can be appropriate for some desired purpose. Scores from the instrument should behave like you think they should. They should be correlated with scores from other instruments that attempt to measure this variable. For example, if postural stability is measured by sway and postural stability is measured by the stork stand, then sway should be related to stork stand performance. If your purpose is to use postural stability as an indicator of functional ankle instability, then sway should allow you to distinguish unstable ankles from stable ones. Different strategies have been devised for each of these purposes.

Face and Content Validity

The simplest validity test is to inspect a measure or instrument and see if it looks like you think it should. This is referred to as face validity. While face validity is qualitative and not very sophisticated, it is the most commonly used method. When someone suggests that measures taken by having subjects stand on a force plate can indicate postural stability, you probably would say, "That sounds right." You wouldn't dismiss the measure out of hand. A more sophisticated, logical method would be for you to articulate the elements that ought to be included in a measure of postural stability and then check to see if they are included in the measure. This is fairly simple with measures taken from a force plate. There are two major measures: center of balance and sway. Sway scores indicate the deviations of movements away from the center of balance. That makes sense. Face or logical validity may be sufficient for a very concrete measure like clock time as an indicator of running speed.

Content validity is most useful for measures that include a number of discreet elements that are added together to form a measure. Recent measures of ankle instability, for example, include different aspects of functional ankle instability that, when added together, may constitute a better measure of degree of ankle instability than just asking subjects if they ever experience "giving way." Many psychological measures (e.g., self-esteem) and cognitive measures (e.g., a test of knowledge of how to assess ACL injuries) require an in-depth understanding of the concept to judge the adequacy of the content. Measuring an athletic trainer's knowledge of assessment of ACL injuries would require inclusion of questions about the

In the Field

> Craig is developing a questionnaire for assessing function after an ACL tear. His advisor has suggested that two things need to be done first: establish the face validity and the content validity of the questionnaire. Craig accomplishes the face validity easily. He reviews each of the questions to determine that each has some relationship to ACL symptoms. He finds the content validity part to be more problematic. His advisor suggests that he spend some time brainstorming different symptoms and their qualities (e.g., pain, when it occurs, how long does it last, does it throb; giving-way, when does it occur, how often do they experience it, does it interfere with sport activities/activities of daily living, and so on). After completing his list, he shares it with other athletic trainers to see if they would add or change anything on the list. Once his list is complete, he then compares it to his questionnaire to determine whether the questionnaire content is representative of his symptom list. In doing the comparison, Craig notices two or three symptoms that are not adequately represented and revises the questionnaire accordingly.

structure and movement of the knee as well as the causes and characteristics of an ACL. If these were not included in the assessment, you would probably judge it to not be a valid measure of knowledge of assessment of ACL injuries. The researcher must be able to articulate the desired content. If the researcher cannot do this, he or she cannot assess the content validity of the instrument. Makers of standardized tests develop "tables of specifications" that indicate the content to be covered and the number, type, and difficulty of items desired. Content validity is established by checking to be sure that the test items meet the table of specifications.

Criterion-Related Validity

Face and content validity are nonempirical (i.e., unmeasured) methods of assessing validity. There are a number of empirical (i.e., measured) ways to assess validity. One of these is referred to as criterion validity because some other measure is used as a criterion against which to judge the instrument. Scores produced by the instrument are compared with scores from another instrument (the criterion).

With physiological measures you might be able to compare measurements that you take with an outside standard. For example, you could place objects of known weight on a weighing scale and see if the scale reported the known weight. If it did, you would say that the scale gave us a valid measure of weight. If the reading on the scale were much lower or higher than that of the known weight, you would question the validity of the scale. While this is sometimes referred to as equipment reliability, it is better thought of as equipment validity.

Sometimes the criterion is thought of as a "gold standard," or the ultimate measure of the variable. For example, physician assessments of functional ankle instability might be considered to be a "gold standard" against which self-report measures of "giving way" might be compared. The expectation is that subjects who report "giving way" would be diagnosed by an orthopaedist as having functional ankle instability. Subjects who did not report giving way would not be diagnosed by the orthopaedist as having functional ankle instability. The use of an orthopaedist's diagnosis as the "gold standard" requires, of course, that the diagnosis be correct.

Another strategy would be to compare the scores of your instrument (e.g., the stork stand for balance) with another instrument that was designed to measure the same thing (e.g., postural sway on a force plate). You would expect the scores of the two measures to be correlated. If you didn't get similar results with the stork test and the force plate, you would be concerned with one or the other measure. Since these measures are taken at the same point in time, this type of criterion-related validity is referred to as concurrent validity.

Concurrent validity is often done to validate the choice of using a particular instrument instead of some other instrument. Is one measure as good as the other? Does it matter which one you use? You may wish to use one of the measures because it is less time consuming, less expensive, or less complicated. The stork stand can be done anywhere, and expensive equipment is not needed. In athletic training clinics, athletic trainers often use simple, inexpensive measures instead of sending patients to laboratories for extensive testing. Is that okay? Are skin-fold measures to estimate percent body fat "good enough" or should hydrostatic weighing be used? Do you get approximately the same scores? Why would weighing underwater be better or worse? Is it worth the cost to weigh everyone underwater? Are these measures interchangeable for a study of the effect of dieting on percent body fat? Could you use either measures from a KT-1000 or measures from a radiograph to assess laxity? Radiographs are expensive. If you could demonstrate that measures from the KT-1000 were as good as those from the radiograph or good enough for your purpose, you could probably test a lot more subjects and save a great deal of money.

Criterion-related validity may be used to demonstrate that scores from the instrument can be used to predict some other relevant criterion at a later point in time. This is referred to as predictive validity. Predictive validity is useful in making a case for using a measure to screen or classify subjects as well as to predict future behavior. You may want to use the instrument to screen athletes to predict future injuries.

Construct Validity

Many measures are designed to measure abstract constructs. Constructs are phenomena that are not directly measurable. Center of pressure is a specific measure. Postural stability is an abstract construct. Scores on a knowledge test are a specific measure. Knowledge is an abstract construct. Abstract concepts are not directly measurable. You develop indirect measures of them and then infer to the construct. To assess the validity of more abstract measures like proprioception or joint reposition sense calls for a sophisticated understanding of the nature and definition of the concept as well as an understanding (or at least sound hypotheses) of the role of the variable in physical activity. Many physiological measures and most cognitive, social, and psychological measures that are invented and used by researchers have no absolute standard against which they can be tested. As a result, researchers must build logical and conceptual frameworks based on the literature and their own expertise to contrive ways to determine whether the instrument is valid. The bottom line in terms of the starting point for validity assessment is a thorough understanding of the phenomenon. Without this it is difficult to decide on validation procedures.

The measure that you develop must include the appropriate elements (as you might demonstrate through content validity). The elements within the instrument must relate to each other in ways that you would expect them to relate. The scores on the instrument must relate to scores from other instruments in ways that you would expect them to relate. A single criterion would not be sufficient to establish construct validity. In validation research on a measure of postural stability, the researcher might hypothesize that subjects with lower sway scores (i.e., higher balance, more stability) would have fewer existing joint injuries, more sport experience, more flexibility, fewer injuries in an upcoming season, more ankle strength, and greater dancing ability. She might also hypothesize that sway scores would be unrelated to hair or eye color. The confirmation of these hypotheses would provide evidence that sway scores were indeed a measure of postural stability. This complex set of hypotheses may not be necessary in validating measures of postural stability. More abstract variables like self-confidence, desire to achieve, or aptitude as an athletic trainer may demand this approach. The measure of the athletic trainer's knowledge of ACL injuries was postulated to have four major dimensions (or factors): structure of the knee, movement of the knee, causes of ACL injuries, and characteristics of ACL injuries. In building the measure, you would insure that items were included to measure each of these factors. In trials of the instrument you would then do statistical analyses to see if the items in the four dimensions would form into correlated clusters or factors. To do this you might use a statistical technique called factor analysis (Tabachnick & Fidell, 2001).

As you can see, validity testing can be very complicated. When you use one measure to assess the adequacy of another measure, either measure could be at fault. The selection of the criterion variable becomes paramount. The criterion variable must have demonstrated reliability and validity. You must have a good rationale for choosing it. Is this really an alternative measure of the target variable? Is there a theoretical or empirical basis for choosing the criterion variable? Is there any evidence that the two variables should be related?

An Example of Validity Measures in Research

A researcher may be interested in testing the hypothesis that a concussion will result in reduced postural stability. The researcher might test the balance of subjects who have experienced a concussion and subjects who have not experienced a concussion. He wants to see if they differ in postural stability. Thus, the researcher needs a measure of postural stability. What is postural stability? How do you measure postural stability? How do you know that the measure actually measures postural stability? Subjects might be asked to stand on a force plate. Measures of "sway" might be derived by assessing the deviations of movement each subject makes around a "center of balance." Is that a good measure of postural stability? The more stable you are, the less you ought to move around your center of balance. That seems to make sense (face validity). If you had another measure (a criterion) of postural stability, you could have subjects take both measures during the same time period to see if they do about the same. You could ask the subjects both to perform the stork stand and to stand on the force plate. Your expectation would be that subjects who sway less on the force plate (who have smaller sway scores) would also be able to stand on one leg longer. If these two measures were in agreement, you would have evidence of concurrent validity. You could study the relationship of the force plate sway measures to measures of other variables that you think ought to be related to sway. Tropp and colleagues (1985) for example, found that individuals with greater perceived ankle instability had greater postural sway than individuals who perceived their ankles to be stable. You might also have more confidence in the validity of the force plate measure of sway if it was predictive of some functional outcome in the future. You might see whether subjects with more sway were more likely in the future to have injuries from falling down (predictive validity).

Which Type of Validity Do I Need?

As with different types of reliability, different types of validity are also more useful for different purposes. At one time your concern may be with having evidence that the measure is valid for measuring an abstract construct (construct validity). In other cases you might place more emphasis on predictive validity. Examples might be the use of physical characteristics (e.g., pronation) to predict injuries, psychological characteristics (e.g., autonomy) to predict compliance with rehabilitation, and cognitive characteristics (e.g., spatial ability) to predict academic success. You might place more emphasis on concurrent validity if you were testing out a measure that was potentially cheaper or more efficient than another measure.

Solutions to Common Problems

Although we commonly speak of instruments as "being reliable" or "being valid," we should really talk about the data, not the instruments, as being reliable or valid. The reliability or validity of data is also dependent on the characteristics of your subjects, the environment within which your measurement is taken, the exact procedures you used, and/or your skills in using the instrument. So you should be aware that even though other researchers have used a measure to produce scores that were reliable and valid, it does not ensure that the scores you get will be either reliable or valid.

Two conditions will artificially affect reliability estimates: real differences between subjects and real subject changes. If you conduct a reliability study of an instrument, two things are essential. First, be sure that you select subjects who are different on the target variable. If you are assessing joint reposition sense and the subjects are very similar to each other in joint reposition sense, the reliability coefficient will be lowered. This is not because your instrument is unreliable but because there is little subject variance. When you read about the reliability of an instrument, look at the standard deviation of the subjects tested. If it is very low, that may account for a low reliability coefficient. Second, when you take two measures, be sure that nothing has happened which would cause the subjects to change (e.g., fatigue). If, for some reason, they have changed, the reliability will be lower. Once again, this is not because your instrument is unreliable, but because the subjects have changed. When you read about the reliability of an instrument, look to see if the authors have described the testing conditions. Testing conditions may affect the reliability coefficient.

Summary

Reliability and validity of measures are fundamental to the research process. Reliability establishes the consistency of measures. Reliability can be conceptualized and measured in a variety of ways. In athletic training research, the most common type is stability and it is generally estimated using intraclass correlation coefficients. In contrast, the intent of validity is to establish whether a measure actually measures what it is purported to measure. As with reliability, validity can be conceptualized and measured in a variety of ways. The most common form in athletic training research is criterion validity. Regardless of whether you are doing reliability or validity assessment or both, as a researcher you should choose the form of reliability and validity that meets your specific purpose. Each method is designed for specific purposes, and your selected method should match your purpose.

Activities

1. Obtain an article that presents reliability information.
2. Identify the type of reliability and the method used to assess the reliability.
3. Obtain the measure you intend to use as part of your research and locate estimates of its reliability and validity.
4. Using the measure you intend to use in your research, outline a process for assessing its reliability. Be sure to include methods of intertester and intratester reliability, if appropriate.
5. Using the measure you intend to use in your research, outline a process for assessing its validity. Be sure to include face and/or content validity (if appropriate) and criterion validity.

References

Kaplan, A. (1964). *The conduct of inquiry: Methodology for behavioral science.* San Francisco: Chandler Pub. Co.

Kuder, G. F., & Richardson, M. W. (1937). The theory of the estimation of test reliability. *Psychometrika, 2,* 151–160.

NATABOC Test Development. (1999). Procedures used to develop the National Athletic Trainers' Association Board of Certification Examinations. Morrisville: Castle Worldwide.

Shrout, P. E., & Fleiss, J. L. (1979). Intraclasss correlations: Uses in assessing rater reliability. *Psychological Bulletin,* Tabachnick, B.G., & Fidell, L.S. (2001). *Using multivariate statistics.* Boston: Allyn and Bacon, 86, 420–428.

Tabachnick, B.G., & Fidell, L.S. (2001). *Using multivariate statistics.* Boston: Allyn & Bacon.

Tropp, H., Odenrick, P., & Gillquist, J. (1985). Stabilometry recordings in functional and mechanical instability of the ankle joint. *International Journal of Sports Medicine, 6,* 180–182.

Bibliography

Crocker, L., & Algina, J. (1986). Procedures for estimating reliability. In *Introduction to classical and modern test theory.* New York: Holt, Rinehart.

Fan, X., & Gansneder, B. M. (2004, August). *Assessing rater reliability: Intraclass correlations and generalizability theory.* Paper presented at the 28th International Congress of Psychology, Beijing, China.

Meyers, J. (1972). *Fundamentals of experimental design* (2nd ed.). Boston: Allyn & Bacon.

Denegar, C.R., & Ball, D. W. (1993). Assessing reliability and precision of measurement: An introduction to intraclass correlation and standard error of measurement. *Journal of Sport Rehabilitation, 2,* 35–42.

Chapter 10
Alternative Measures

Objectives

After reading this chapter, you will:

- Know when it is appropriate to use surveys for data collection.
- Learn rules for writing items.
- Know the difference between a closed- and open-ended item.
- Be aware of selected factors that may influence the reliability and validity of survey data.
- Understand the difference between nonprobability and probability sampling.
- Know the factors that influence the precision of population estimates.
- Understand issues related to getting responses from survey subjects.

Questions

While reading this chapter, think about answers to the following questions:

1. How could I use surveys for research in athletic training?
2. Can survey data be used to generalize to a population?
3. Are survey data reliable and valid?
4. What kinds of questions can I ask on a survey?
5. How do I write an item that is reliable and valid?
6. How do surveys compare to other self-report measures?

Introduction

The use of surveys and interviews in athletic training research has been increasing. This reflects an increased knowledge of methodologies from the social sciences and education. Psychologists and sociologists value these methods and use them routinely (over 90 percent of social science research is thought to be done with these methods). This increased use may also reflect a desire of athletic training researchers to focus on information that may best be collected directly from certified athletic trainers, athletes, students, and patients.

Researchers in athletic training are more familiar with concerns about the collection of physical data: adhering to specific protocols, appropriate calibration and use of machines (e.g., isokinetic dynamometers) or electronically produced data (e.g., EMG), processing and checking these data, and analyzing the data. They are skilled at ensuring that the data are appropriate for the research question, that the subjects can produce the data, and that the data are reliable and valid. Most athletic training researchers are much less familiar with the development or use of measures that request subjects to report their physical characteristics (e.g., ankle instability), their effort or pain, their behavior (e.g., adherence to a rehabilitation protocol) or their feelings/opinions (e.g., about the appropriateness of treatment). Since most of the published research in sports medicine/athletic training involves the assessment of physiological variables, the use of surveys represents a major shift.

In athletic training, surveys have a wide variety of potential uses. They might be used to determine values about curricular options or training needs. Surveys could be used to determine the characteristics that prospective employers would like to see in certified athletic trainers. Employer data might be used to make judgments about the kinds of courses that certified athletic trainers ought to take or that might be included in a masters or doctoral program. Surveys could be used to have athletes report their physical condition (e.g., ankle instability), injury history, and rehabilitation experiences or even to report the physical functions that they are able to perform.

Surveys of faculty and students could be used to evaluate the quality of a textbook or other instructional resource (e.g., videotape, web-based program, etc.). We may want to know if they like the text, find it readable, believe that it is at the right level of difficulty, has the right coverage, and so on. They can tell us how they feel if we ask them.

In the athletic training clinic surveys can be used to ask patients about how and when an injury (which we did not observe) occurred. We can ask them how much pain they have (which we cannot feel). We can ask them whether the injury limits performance of daily activities (which we are not present to observe). Almost any kind of information can be collected by survey. We can ask respondents what they know (cognitive), how they feel (affective), or what they do (behavioral). We can ask them about themselves, about other people (e.g., their coaches), and about other things (e.g., their schoolwork).

When Is It Appropriate to Use Surveys for Data Collection?

Survey data are one type of self-report data. Other examples of self-report methods include face-to-face and telephone interviews, focus groups, personality measures, and the use of visual analog scales (to report pain or effort). In each case subjects are asked to reveal something they know, feel,

In the Field

Rowena was interested in determining what kinds of characteristics employers were seeking in athletic trainers. She felt that this was an important question. She thought that if she knew the answer, she would be better prepared to help her students pursue careers in athletic training. She decided to develop a survey and use it to ask employers across the United States what these characteristics were. To do this, she had to develop the survey, identify the population of employers, decide who to sample, send the survey to the sample of employers, have the employers return the survey, and then make sense of the results. Rowena followed the principles presented in this chapter, which enabled her to publish her findings in the Journal of Athletic Training. As such, she was able to help athletic training educators across the country become better prepared to help their students pursue careers in the athletic training profession.

or can do. Self-report data are desirable when they are relevant for the research question being asked, when the respondent is the best source of the data, or when the most efficient way to collect the data is to ask a respondent.

Surveys are a way to collect self-report data in a systematic manner from each subject. They can be administered to large numbers of subjects relatively quickly and inexpensively. Since the researcher does not need to be present when a survey is completed, the impact of researchers' personal characteristics such as gender, dress, mannerisms, and voice are removed. Since surveys are written documents, they are best for respondents who have both the comfort and the skills to deal with written documents. Written surveys ought not to be used with nonliterate subjects or with subjects who do not know the language in which the survey is written. Ideal survey respondents would include adults, with a minimum of a high school education, who are literate and who are comfortable with written materials.

In general, surveys are susceptible to the weakness of any self-report data. Respondents may refuse to answer questions. They may not want to be honest about certain information (e.g., having an eating disorder). Often respondents are unable to answer specific questions. They may have forgotten the information. A respondent may not remember events that occurred last week, last month, or years ago. Respondents may not know why they do various things or even if they do them. (How many times did you scratch your head in the last 10 minutes?) Respondents may not have the information at all or have less precise information than you would like to collect (e.g., athletic trainers may not know how many unstable ankles they have treated the past 2 years). The researcher who uses surveys must try to develop the survey in a way that will minimize these weaknesses and maximize the collection of useful, reliable, and valid information.

Developing a Survey

The starting point of doing a survey is the same as it is for doing any research. Rather than beginning by writing questions to ask people, start by defining and refining your research question. In the beginning you may have some hunches about what the elements of the survey should be. You need to read the literature on the topic, develop an appropriate conceptual framework, and identify specific indicators to be used in the survey. Eventually, those indicators will be translated into specific items to be included on the survey (you may use someone else's items or need to develop your own). In surveys that have more than one part or aspect, each aspect of the survey needs to be approached the same way. Define the research question, use extant literature to help you define the concepts and identify potential measures, and translate these to survey items. If you don't do this, you will just have a bunch of questions to ask people. When you get the data, you will have a tendency to do mindless descriptive analyses that are not driven by a meaningful research question.

In an employer study about desirable hiring characteristics, you might start with a very simple framework suggesting that employers want to hire athletic trainers who have appropriate knowledge, experience, and skills. A search of the literature might reveal these are indeed the general kinds of characteristics that employers look for in hiring people. They want to know about prospective employees' formal training, their credentials, and their specific types of experience. Employers of athletic trainers may look for the same characteristics, only modified for athletic training. Thus athletic training credentials might include NATABOC certification in athletic training, teaching, CPR instruction, and National Strength and Conditioning Association certification.

Writing Survey Items

In writing survey items, the goal is to write items that all the respondents will interpret the same way, that respondents can respond to accurately, and that respondents are willing to answer (Dillman, 2000). Survey items are composed of a stem and a way for respondents to provide an answer. The stem is the question or statement. The mode for respondents to answer is called the response alternative(s).

There are two major types of survey items, open ended and closed ended. Open-ended items provide space for the respondents to answer in their own words. Closed-ended items provide specific answers from which respondents are asked to choose (see Display 10–1).

Open-ended and Closed-ended Items

In general, open-ended questions require respondents to formulate a personal response to the question and write their response in the space provided. An open-ended item may have an expected answer. If you ask someone, "What kind of car do you drive?" they can write down, "a Buick." If you ask an athletic trainer, "How many years have you been a certified athletic trainer?" she can write down the number of years. This type of open-ended question is easy for the respondent to answer, has limited clear answers, and can be analyzed easily by the researcher.

An open-ended item may have no expected answer and require the respondent to write out an answer ("Why did you become an athletic trainer?" or "What do you believe are the most satisfying things about being an athletic trainer?"). In the employer survey, we could have just asked employers one question, "What characteristics are most important to you in hiring athletic trainers?" An employer respondent would have to decide what kinds of characteristics to mention (e.g., knowledge, certification, academic preparation, and clinical experience) and then decide which ones to write down. The apparent advantage is that the respondents would write down the things that were most important to them, not just the things that the researcher thinks are important. On the other hand, the respondent might just put down a few things that come to mind instantly without much thought. Since the researcher is not present, probing or follow-up is impossible. This type of open-ended item is usually more difficult for the respondent to answer. The respondent has to reflect and formulate a response and then write it in whatever space is given. As a result, many respondents will not answer the question. Typically only about 20 to 30 percent or less of the respondents will answer this kind of open-ended question. Use of this kind of open-ended item also increases the task of the researcher. The answers have to be coded. They could be entered into a computer file as text. The text would then need to be analyzed to identify categories, themes, or metaphors. Because of the uncertainty of the meaning of the responses and because of the limited return, we advise against their use on mailed or web-based surveys. This type of question is much more suitable for face-to-face or telephone interviews. If you do use them, be sure that you really need the question and that you know how you want to use the information. The suggestions we make below about writing items are applicable to both open-ended and closed-ended items, but are primarily directed toward closed-ended items. Pilot test the items to make sure that you have not violated any of these suggestions.

Writing Item Stems

Item stems provide the content to which the respondent is to reply. In an eating disorder study, you might be interested in inappropriate behaviors associated with eating disorders such as vomiting, not swallowing food, and so on. If so, you should have developed a framework from the literature so that you know that you have included all of the relevant behaviors. Be sure you haven't left any out and you haven't included irrelevant behaviors. If two questions are implied, they need to be separated into two questions (see Display 10–2). Don't use jargon, technical terms, or acronyms unless you are sure the respondents will understand them. If respondents don't understand the question, they may refuse to answer or give a meaningless answer. Make sure the terms or phrases are correct (e.g., athletic trainer, not trainer). The respondent may refuse to respond because he thinks that since you did not use the right term, you are sloppy and/or not credible. Use language that is appropriate for the respondents. Avoid using complicated sentences or double negatives.

Writing Response Alternatives

Response alternatives are the response choices that you provide for the respondent. In closed-ended questions, respondents are asked to select from among the choices provided. They may range from a simple yes or no to complex expressions of opinions (see Display 10–3). You have probably seen a number of different types of response alternatives used with questions or statements. You might have seen a survey that asked respondents whether they agree or disagree with some statement and requested that they circle or check one of the words provided, such as "Strongly Agree," "Agree," and so on. You may have seen a graphic scale like the visual analog scale used to measure pain or effort. There are a number of basic types of response alternatives (see Display 10–3). The response alternatives may be ordered or unordered. Ordered response alternatives suggest an underlying continuum such as "Degree of Agreement" or "Degree of Compliance." The task for the respondent is to determine where he or she fits in that ordering. Unordered response alternatives are a list of categories that are presented in no particular order. Respondents must choose one of the categories that best represents their answer. To do this, the respondent has to make comparisons among the categories and then choose one.

The alternatives presented should be exhaustive (they should include all relevant answers). The alternatives should also be mutually exclusive (there should be no overlap between categories). Display 10–2 presents violations of this sort. Be sure that the alternatives you use are logically related to the stem. You may provide a verbal example of each category or just specify the end categories (e.g., Happy...............Sad). Sometimes only the end categories are defined because of the difficulty of inventing the right words to be used for each category. Questions with closed-ended alternatives are used for two major reasons: to increase the likelihood that responses will be comparable across respondents and to minimize the difficulty of the task required of respondents. If you use structured response alternatives, you assume that their meaning is widely shared, that respondents understand a given stimulus in roughly equivalent ways, and that, as a result, you can compare the responses across respondents.

Many surveys include middle responses as one of the possible response alternatives. The middle response is seen as providing the respondent the opportunity to indicate that they are neutral about the stem. Unfortunately,

Display 10-1 | **Types of Survey Items**

An open-ended question with no expected answer:
What do you like about being a certified athletic trainer?
An open-ended question with an expected answer:
How long have you been a certified athletic trainer?
A closed-ended question with ordered alternatives.
To what extent do you agree or disagree that all athletic trainers should be certified?
(Strongly Agree Agree Disagree Strongly Disagree)
A closed-ended question with unordered alternatives
Which of the following do you usually use? (Tape Orthotics Brace)

Display 10-2 | **Violations of Rules**

Each stem should include one and only one question:
"My rehabilitation has resulted in less pain and more flexibility" should be made into two statements:
"My rehabilitation has resulted in less pain"
"My rehabilitation has resulted in more flexibility"
Don't use jargon, technical terms, or acronyms:
NATA should be National Athletic Trainers' Association
CEU should be Continuing Education Unit
If you do spell out an acronym make sure it is correct:
NATA is not National Athlete Training Association
If items are stated as questions, write out the entire question:
Ask, "How old are you?" not "Age?"
Don't use double negatives:
"I don't believe that athletes aren't compliant with rehabilitation" could be restated as "Athletes aren't compliant with rehabilitation."
Avoid collectively exhaustive violation:

Please check your highest level of education:

☐ Elementary
☐ High School
☐ College

Avoid mutually exclusive violation:

Please check the length of time that you have dieted:

☐ 1–4 weeks
☐ 4–8 weeks
☐ 8–12 weeks
☐ More than 12 weeks

Display 10-3 | **Possible Response Alternatives**

2-point scales

Yes	No
Agree	Disagree
High School	College
Tape	Prosthesis

3-point scales

Yes	Don't Know	No
Agree	Neutral	Disagree
High School	2 yr College	4 yr College

4-point scales

Strongly Agree	Agree	Disagree	Strongly Disagree
Always	Often	Seldom	Never
Definitely Yes	Yes	No	Definitely No

5-point scales

Strongly Agree	Agree	Neutral	Disagree	Strongly Disagree
Always	Often	Fairly often	Seldom	Never
Definitely Yes	Yes	Unsure	No	Definitely No

End Point Only scales

Compliant ———————————	Not Compliant
Very Painful ———————————	Not At All Painful
Very Favorable ———————————	Very Unfavorable
Excellent ———————————	Poor
Extremely Satisfied ———————————	Extremely Dissatisfied
High Priority ———————————	Low Priority
Very Successful ———————————	Very Unsuccessful

Numerical scales

Lowest Quality (1) to Highest Quality (7)
Lowest Quality (1) to Highest Quality (10)
Lowest Quality (1) to Highest Quality (100)

Signed numerical scale

Lowest						Highest
-3	-2	-1	0	1	2	3

the meaning of the middle response is unclear. It could be that the respondent actually holds a neutral position about the attitude object. On the other hand, the respondent may not care about the object at all, not know anything about it, not hold an opinion about it, not want to take a stand, or not want to tell you. If the respondent is actually neutral, the midpoint is quite appropriate. When you are in doubt about the possible meaning, we suggest that you leave out the midpoint and present an even number (four or six) of closed-ended alternatives.

Many surveys also provide a space for respondents to indicate that they have "No Opinion" or that they "Don't know." We recommend that you include "Don't know" or "No opinion" only when you believe that these are viable and important responses. You should do this when you expect large numbers of "Don't know" "No opinion" responses or when you specifically want to know that response. In a study of curriculum content you might believe that many athletic trainers would not know "How many programs include a course in statistics?" or that they really had no opinion about whether athletic trainers should earn a Ph.D. In such cases you may want to include these options. For researchers who are attempting to develop scales ("Satisfaction in being an ATC"), "No opinion" and "Don't know" responses present a unique problem. Respondents who indicate either of these become missing data for those particular items.

Respondents are sometimes reluctant to select an extreme answer, especially in attitudinal items. If you pilot a question like, "How often do you demonstrate a stretching routine to an athlete for rehab?" with the answers "Always," "Sometimes," and "Never," you may find that few or no respondents say "Never." In order to identify respondents who use demonstrations more or less often you might change the end alternatives to "Almost always" and "Almost never."

To create items that have never been used before takes patience and the willingness to write items, try them out, and rewrite them again and again. Often it is possible to use or adapt items that have been previously used. If so, there may be information on the quality (e.g., reliability and validity) of the data that have been collected using these items. Another advantage of using previously used items is that it makes it possible to compare the data across different studies. If the same question has been asked in the same way in different studies, it is possible to directly compare the responses. We advise you to try to use extant items whenever possible. Just as you don't need to develop a new instrument to assess balance each time you do a study on balance — you use force plates that are commonly used by other researchers — you don't need to develop new questions each time you conduct a survey.

Reliability and Validity

As you learned in Chapter 9, the major criteria that we use to judge the quality of data are reliability and validity. We judge survey data by the same criteria. A survey is actually composed of a number of separate measures (items). Since a survey is not a unitary thing but a composition of items, we determine the reliability and/or validity of the items (or sets of items), not the survey as a whole. The reliability/validity will be different from one item to another. An item asking for respondent demographics (age or sex) may produce very reliable data, while an item requesting the average amount of third party reimbursement in a clinic might produce unreliable data. So reliability and validity coefficients need to be presented for separate items or for separate scales. That said, the issues of reliability and validity of survey data should be approached in the same way as data from other research instruments.

Reliability Estimates for Survey Data

You can estimate stability by administering the same items on two separate occasions to see if you get the same (or similar) responses on both occasions. Although the use of intraclass correlations (ICCs) to assess reliability is not unknown to survey researchers, they are more likely to use the Pearson r to assess either stability (test-retest reliability) or equivalence. A survey may include a set of items designed to measure a more complicated variable such as the social climate of an athletic training room, athletic trainers' interest in continuing education, or eating disorders. Reliability of these measures would be best done with estimates of internal consistency such as Kuder-Richardson coefficients or Chronbach's alpha.

Validity Estimates for Survey Data

As with reliability, the types of validity estimates presented in Chapter 9 (face, content, criterion, and construct) are appropriate for survey data. Survey researchers tend to use the Pearson r to estimate each of these various types of validity. They might attempt to validate an eating disorder scale by the correlation of the scale score with observed eating disorder behaviors. They might use a correlation to see if the scale scores correlated with physician diagnoses. Some survey data might be judged to be valid if they accurately reflect "reality." For example, if we ask respondents to indicate the number of continuing education units (CEUs) they have completed, we would like the number reported to be the actual number of CEUs they have completed. Other survey data that consist of attitudes or belief might be considered to be valid if they accurately measure the actual beliefs of the respondent. These beliefs may have little to do with "reality." If you ask athletic trainers to indicate the kinds of professional preparation they need, their responses may have nothing to do with their "real" educational needs (an analysis of competencies might be a better way to identify actual educational needs). But we will consider the scores valid if they accurately reflect the athletic trainers' beliefs. Since there are few "gold standards" for much of survey data, survey researchers are more likely to rely on face validity (the items appear to be appropriate) or content validity (the items include the characteristics implied by the definition of the construct, such as ankle instability or job satisfaction).

Factors That Affect the Reliability and Validity of Survey Data

Reliability and validity of survey data may be affected by the quality of the survey including the presentation (e.g., paper or Internet, for example), format, and directions. They are also affected by the nature of the data. Reliability coefficients for items such as demographic characteristics, family background, and high school achievements are typically high (.90 to 1.0). Reliability coefficients above .90 have been reported for academic aspirations and career plans, while those for attitudes, opinions, life goals, future behavior estimates, and parental attributes tend to be lower, ranging from .50 to .80. Reliabilities for scales presented within surveys tend to be higher than for individual items. Even affective scales can achieve internal consistency coefficients in the .80s and .90s.

Data about present events are more reliable than those about past or future events. Data that are about one's self are more reliable than those about other persons. Data about important events or factors are more reliable than those about unimportant events or factors. Data that are factual are more reliable than data that are affective. Reliability is affected by the number of items in a scale and the number of response alternatives presented. Scales with more items and items with more response alternatives tend to be more reliable. Reliability and validity may at times be related to respondent characteristics. For example, students who do better in school report their grades more reliably and validly than those who do worse in school. The fact that reliability coefficients vary with the nature of the data being collected should sharpen the difference between instrument/machine reliability and the reliability of data filtered through the perspective of individual persons. Individuals provide more reliable information about some things than others under some conditions and not other conditions. In addition, their perceptions and feelings change from one time to the next. As a result, reliability measures that are dependent on consistency over time (stability coefficients) or across alternate forms (equivalence) will be lower than the consistency of physical measures like balance or force production. How people feel about things fluctuates from one time to the next. These changes are not measurement errors. They are real changes. But they result in lower reliability coefficients. This is why survey researchers are more likely to use alpha coefficients or the Pearson r to measure reliability and why they might use relative standards for reliability depending on the kind of information collected.

In sum, respondents produce more reliable data on information that is concrete, specific, relevant, more significant, and more recent. They provide more reliable data when they understand the words used in the survey and the meaning of questions. They provide more reliable data when they understand the context and time frame within which they are supposed to respond. They also provide more reliable data when they care about the topic and when they are not afraid to respond.

These factors lead us to a number of specific strategies for increasing the reliability and validity of the data. Be sure that you have written the items well (follow the guidelines presented earlier). Be sure that they are clear, at the right level of complexity, and answerable. Pilot test the items to check these points. Whenever possible, use items that have been used by others and have known reliability or validity. Increase the number of response alternatives. Within limits (up to 4 or 6), increases in the number of response alternatives will improve reliability. Since the use of multiple items to measure variables increases reliability, increase the number of items. The aim should be to develop scales by summing the scores from each item. Anything that will mislead the responder will reduce reliability. So make sure that the directions for responding are clear, that the directions for going through the survey are clear, and that the format and printing make the survey easy to read and easy to follow. All of these things will help to increase the reliability of the data.

Using Surveys to Generalize to a Population

The use of surveys is often connected with the desire to make generalizations about some target population. This is not a necessary use of a survey. A survey could be used to get responses from just one individual of interest. You could ask an incoming athlete to complete a survey regarding what she likes to eat, whether she would like to have a roommate, and so on, in order to understand the athlete's likes and dislikes. You might not care in the slightest about what other athletes like and dislike. You could give your modalities class a survey to determine their prior knowledge of modalities so that you could decide how much time to spend in class on each modality. You might only be interested in that class, not the population of students who take modality classes. However, in many cases, a survey is conducted in order to draw conclusions about a target population. To generalize from a sample to a population you have to identify the population, draw a sample from the population, and then collect the data from that sample.

Researchers use a variety of ways to acquire samples that do not involve random sampling (i.e., nonprobability sampling). These samples are often easier to get and in some cases may have particular characteristics in which the researcher is interested. The disadvantage is there is no way to know for sure whether the sample is representative of the target population. Sometimes the process is judgmental and purposive. Most of the experimental studies in athletic training acquire subjects purposively. Subjects are not randomly sampled. They are chosen because they fit certain age, fitness, or injury characteristics. Sometimes quota sampling is used. Specific numbers of subjects are sampled to fit the distribution of that characteristic in the population. A researcher might decide that 25 males and 25 females are needed. The researcher would simply survey available respondents until data were collected from 25 males and 25 females. Sometimes a snowballing technique is used to identify subjects. Using this process, the researcher would identify one or more subjects to survey. Those subjects would identify other subjects that would be surveyed. For example, a researcher may want to survey athletic trainers who are very knowledgeable about ACL injuries. One subject is identified and that subject suggests other athletic trainers who ought to be surveyed. Data from these samples cannot be directly generalized to a population.

Identifying the Population and Sampling Frame

The first step is to identify the target population. To whom do you want to generalize? Do you want to generalize to all certified athletic trainers in the world, the United States, a region of the United States, a state, region of the state, or a school district? Let's assume that you want to generalize to all of the certified athletic trainers in the United States. You would need a list of every certified athletic trainer in the United States. Can you get such a list? You might be able to get a list of the athletic trainers who are members of the NATA in a given year. The list represents your sampling frame. Is the list complete? Does everyone join the NATA? Does the list include people who used to be members? It won't include people who become members the day after you get the list. It won't include athletic trainers who haven't paid their dues. There will be some gap between the target population and the population from which you actually sample. You will need to decide if the gap is too big. What if the list included only high school athletic trainers and not college athletic trainers? You would have to get a new list, redefine your population, or give up.

If you decide that the list is appropriate, you will then draw a probability sample of athletic trainers from the list. In probability sampling, all of the members of the population have an equal chance of being sampled, resulting in a sample that is representative of the population. The most common procedure is to draw a simple random sample from the population. Sometimes a table of random numbers is used. These tables are particularly useful with small populations. The population size is specified, a sample size is also specified, and elements of the population are numbered. Numbers are then selected from the table of random numbers. Elements of the population whose numbers correspond to the random numbers selected are designated to be the sample. Procedures to select random samples are available on most statistical computer packages and on spreadsheets. Stratified random sampling is a variation of simple random sampling. Strata are subcategories of a variable. The strata for sex are male/female. Clinics might be stratified by the size of the population served (small, medium, or large). The purpose is to increase the representativeness of the sample by sampling subsets that are quite different from another (heterogeneous) but that are made up homogeneous elements. The variable "sex" is often used for stratification, since sex is correlated with many variables we are interested in such as experience and strength. The population would be divided into males and females. Then a random sample of males would be drawn and another random sample of females would be drawn. A third possibility would be to do systematic sampling. From a list of population elements, every second, third, or fourth element would be sampled. Systematic sampling is useful with finite populations and will result in a random sample as long as the sampling frame doesn't include some systematic ordering that would introduce a systematic error. For example, the platoon leader in an army platoon is a lieutenant. Typically there are 36 enlisted soldiers in a platoon. If we sampled every 37th person, we could, by accident, have a sample of only lieutenants. Sometimes, when strict random sampling cannot be done, the researcher may identify naturally occurring clusters from which to sample. A cluster is not a subset of some variable. It is a grouping that has occurred for some other reason. Apartment houses are clusters that have a number of people in them. A state is a cluster. Clinics are clusters. We might sample a number of clinics (a cluster) and then draw a random sample from within the clinics. The disadvantage of cluster samples is that the initial clusters may not be representative of the target population. It may be possible to overcome this by randomly sampling clusters and then randomly sampling subjects within the cluster.

Precision of Sample Estimates

Sample data are used to estimate population characteristics. We might use sample data to estimate the average number of CEUs held by ATCs. We could use sample data to estimate the percentage of ATCs who have more than 50 CEUs. Let's assume that in our national study we want to estimate the percentage of ATCs who have taken a course in survey research. The precision of our estimate will depend on three things: the variability in the population, the size of the population, and the size of the sample. The formula for the error of estimate, also called the standard error, is given in Display 10–4. You will see these three elements (population variability, sample size [n] and population size [N] in the formula.

Notice the calculation $1 - n/N$ in the formula. It is a correction for pop-

Display 10-4	**Calculation of Standard Error (SE)**

$$SE = \sqrt{\frac{s^2}{n}\left(1 - \frac{n}{N}\right)}$$

SE = Error rate
s^2 = Variance
N = Population size
n = Sample size

ulation size. When the sample size is large relative to the population size, the standard error is reduced substantially (If $N = 500$ and $n = 400$, $1-400/500 = 1-.8 = .20$). A population of 500 is a "small" or finite population. A population of 200,000,000 is a "large" or infinite population. As you can see the correction is not very relevant when you have an infinite population. You have little control over the population size. But you should recognize that estimates to small populations are "easier" than estimates to large ones. They do not require as large a sample to get very good estimates.

The population variance also affects the precision of estimates from a sample. You can intuitively see that if a population consists of 95 percent males and 5 percent females (variance $= .0475$) it will be easier to estimate the percentage of males in the population than it would if the population consists of 50 percent males and 50 percent females (variance $= .25$). If you plug these two variances in the formula, you see that it has a dramatic effect on the standard error. You have little control over the variance in the population. But you should recognize that estimates to populations with low variance (homogeneous populations) are "easier" than estimates to populations with high variance (heterogeneous populations). Homogeneous populations do not require as large a sample to get very good estimates.

The third element in the formula is the sample size, or n. As the sample size goes up, the standard error will go down. You have a great deal of control over sample size.

Sample size affects the precision of the generalizations that can be made. Given that a representative sample of subjects has been drawn and they have returned the surveys, larger samples provide more precise generalization from the sample to the population from which it was drawn. If the sample is not representative of the target population, the size of the sample matters little in terms of generalization. For example, if you have surveys from patients with ACL injuries from contact injuries, your results will not generalize to patients with ACL injuries from noncontact injuries regardless of the sample size. Generalizations will be limited to patients with ACL injuries from contact injuries. A more obvious example may help. A researcher is about to draw a sample of 50 athletes at the University of Virginia. He is advised that the study would be more generalizable (meaning to other universities) if he had 500 athletes. It would not. It would still only generalize to the University of Virginia.

An Example

Let's consider an example of a study to determine whether ATCs have taken a survey research course. We know that N is 6500. We know that n is 500. We don't know the population variance. The variance for a proportion (s^2p) is equal to the percent who say yes (Y) times the percent who say no ($1 - Y$). Since 20 percent of our sample said yes, our sample variance is .16 (.20 times .80). The population variance for proportions is at its maximum when the population has a 50–50 split. It would be .50 times .50 = .25. Let's use this worst-case possibility and plug it into the formula. The resulting standard error is .024, or 2.4 percent. Our best estimate is that the percentage of ATCs who have had a course in survey research is 20 percent +/− 2.4 percent. (This represents a 68 percent confidence interval.) Survey research typically provides error rates with a 95 percent confidence interval, which is approximately 2 standard errors. In this case, our estimate is that the percentage of ATCs with a course in survey research is 20 percent +/− 4.8 percent. We are 95 percent confident that the true percent lies between 15.2 percent and 24.8 percent. If we had a larger sample, the error would be smaller. For a sample of 1200, it would be .0144, or 1.4 percent. At the 95 percent confidence level, it would be 2.8%

Standard errors for proportions for samples drawn from finite and infinite populations are given in Figure 10–1 to 10–3. Each graph presents the reduction of error with an increase in sample size (from $n = 100$ to $n = 1200$). As you can see, the standard error decreases as the sample size gets larger. Figure 10-1 shows the standard error for a proportion or percentage when the population percentage is 50. The dashed line displays error reduction with increases in sample size ($n = 1$ to $n = 1200$) for an infinite population and the dotted line shows error reduction for a finite population ($N = 1200$).

For an infinite population, the reduction in standard error decreases (i.e., the line is flattening) at around $n = 1200$. This is why pollsters do not usually draw samples larger than 1200. With $n = 1200$, the standard error for a proportion is approximately $1\frac{1}{2}$ percent. At two standard errors (approximately 3 percent), the researcher can be more than 95 percent confident that the population percent is between −3 percent and +3 percent of the observed sample percent.

Here is another example. Assume that you asked a random sample of 1200 ATCs if they had a master's degree, and 61 percent said yes. Your best single estimate would be that 61 percent of ATCs have a master's degree.

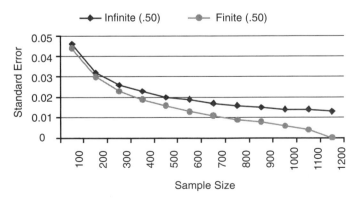

Figure 10–1 Sampling error as a function of population size and sample size when population percentage equals .50.

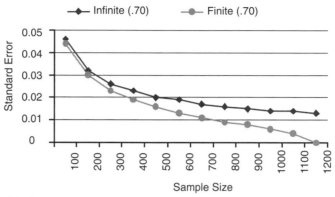

Figure 10–2 Sampling error as a function of population size and sample size when population percentage equals .70.

You could be 95 percent confident that the population percentage falls between 58 percent and 64 percent. With infinite populations, the sample represents a very small percentage of the population. With finite populations, a sample may represent a major percentage of the population. As a result, much smaller samples can produce results with the same or even smaller error. A sample of 600 from a population of 1200 is 50 percent of the population. If 61 percent of the 600 indicated that they had a master's degree, you could be 95 percent confident that the true percentage fell within about the same limits (58.2 to 63.8 percent).

Figure 10-2 shows the reduction in standard error for both finite and infinite populations when the population percentage is 70. This population is more "homogeneous" than the population whose percentage is 50. Note that the standard error is smaller for the more homogeneous population. It is easier to estimate population values when the population is homogeneous.

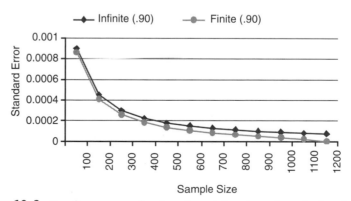

Figure 10–3 Sampling error as a function of population size and sample size when population percentage equals .90.

Determining the Sample Size Needed

A formula for estimating the size of sample needed is presented in Display 10–5. While this formula may be somewhat intimidating, a closer look at it reveals the principles that we have discussed previously. The size of the sample you need depends on the size of the population, the homogeneity of the population, and how precise you want your population estimates to be. Using this formula with our population of 6000, a population percentage split of .50 and .50, and with a desired error rate of $+/-$ 3 percent (95 percent confidence), the desired sample size is 1034:

$$ns = \frac{(6000)\,(.5)\,(.5)}{(6000-1)\left(\frac{.03}{1.96}\right)^2 + (.5)\,(.5)}$$

Response Rates

It is not sufficient to draw a representative sample. You must also receive a representative sample. If the researcher wants to generalize to a specific population, it is essential that the sample that was drawn and the sample that is received are the same. Unless this is the case, the researcher cannot be confident that the sample is representative of that population. He or she would have to assume that there was not some systematic bias linked to not responding. Anyone who has read about mailed surveys or has attempted to conduct them knows that it is unreasonable to expect a 100 percent response rate, so we need some guidelines for making decisions about incomplete samples. It might help us to answer the following questions: What is a response rate? What is a *good* response rate? What kinds of response rates do survey researchers achieve? What is the effect of different response rates? What factors influence response rates? What are the characteristics of respondents/nonrespondents?

Display 10-5   **Calculation of Sample Size**

$$ns = \frac{(Np)\,(p)\,(1-p)}{(Np-1)\left(\frac{B}{C}\right)^2 + [(p)\,(1-p)]}$$

ns = Desired sample size
Np = Size of population
p = Proportion of the population expected to choose 1 of 2 response categories
B = Desired amount of sampling error (e.g., 3%)
C = z associated with confidence level (often $z.95$)

Calculation of Response Rate

Response rates refer to the proportion of completed surveys returned. You will find different ways to calculate response rates. Two alternative calculations are provided in Display 10–6. They differ in terms of what is meant by "completed" and by who is included in the calculation. Response rate is calculated by dividing the number of completed returns by the total number of people who were eligible. If the survey was sent to 1200 persons and 825 returned completed surveys, the response rate would be 825/1200, or 68.75 percent. Completion rate adjusts the denominator of this formula to take account of the fact that some respondents may not be reachable because their address is incorrect, they have moved, they are deceased, and other factors. If 50 of the 1200 persons were deemed unreachable, the completion rate would be 825/1150, or 72 percent. If these factors are random occurrences, it makes sense to drop these persons from the return rate. If, on the other hand, respondents have moved because they are unable to get along with other staff members, the returned sample may have an inherent bias.

The Effect of Different Response Rates

If the nonrespondents would have responded similarly to the respondents, the researcher could treat not responding as a random and therefore somewhat irrelevant phenomenon. But nonrespondents could be radically different from respondents. Nonrespondents pose a problem for the researcher because the researcher cannot be certain that the returned sample is representative of the population of interest, since not all cases are accounted for. While it is possible that the nonrespondents are just random drops, it is also likely that they did not respond for a particular reason. They may not be interested in the topic. They could be very negative and not want to respond. They could be very positive and think that it is unnecessary to respond. If so, the returned sample has some degree of bias. If the proportion of nonrespondents is small, there may be little bias. If the proportion of nonrespondents is large and the respondents are very different from the

Display 10-6   **Calculation of Response Rate**

Response rate: C/E

   $C=$ Number completed
   $E=$ Number eligible

Completion Rate:

$$\frac{\text{Number completed}}{\text{Number sent } - \text{ (noneligible } + \text{ nondeliverable)}}$$

respondents, the "actual" results could be drastically different from those achieved.

Unfortunately, we seldom know anything about nonrespondents. As a result, survey researchers often assume that they are the same as the respondents. This could be a very bad assumption. Low response rates combined with respondent bias can have a dramatic effect on population estimates. Consider this example. A researcher wants to know whether a workshop on issues related to ankle instability should be given at the NATA Clinical Symposium. She draws a random sample of 1000 athletic trainers from a national list of athletic trainers. Of this sample, 100 athletic trainers respond. Her response rate is 100/1200, or 10.0 percent, a particularly poor response rate. Of the respondents, 75 percent indicate that they want a workshop on ankle instability. First, let's assume that the 100 respondents are indeed a random sample of the population (this also assumes that nonrespondents were random). The researcher's error rate will be higher than it would have been with a larger sample, but she can generalize to the original population. Her best single estimate is that 75 percent of the population would want the workshop. Now let's assume that the nonrespondents were not random. In fact, let's assume that none of the nonrespondents believe that there should be a workshop on ankle instability. If so, the best single population estimate would be that only 7.5 percent of the population (75 of 1000) would like to have a workshop on ankle instability. The combined effect of low response rate and biased returns is dramatic. She would probably decide not to have the workshop.

Although we never know for sure whether the nonrespondents are different from the respondents, we can develop some "what if" scenarios to see what kind of effect response bias might have on population estimates. We have presented a number of these in Figure 10–4. As you look at Figure 10–4, assume the same survey described above. A researcher has sent a single question instrument to a random sample of 1000 certified athletic trainers. She has asked each person the following question: "Should there be a workshop on the treatment of ankle instability at the NATA Clinical Symposium?" The possible answers are yes or no.

We have presented five different scenarios in Figure 10–4. The impact on survey results of two factors, the percentage return and the degree to which the nonrespondents agree with the respondents, is plotted. In every case, 95 percent of the respondents indicate yes, when asked whether athletic trainers should be certified. The top line represents the best case scenario. All of the nonrespondents (100%) agree with the respondents. In that case, even a 10 percent return would be fine. The bottom line represents the worst-case scenario. None of the nonrespondents (0%) agree with the respondents. If 10 percent of the sample returns the survey and none of the nonrespondents agree with the respondents, the results actually reverse, changing from 95 percent yes to only 5 percent yes. You can see that in the worst-case scenario, the results are very discrepant unless the response rate is close to 100 percent.

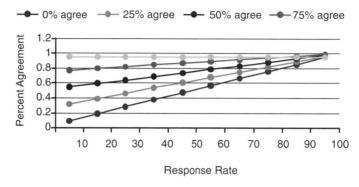

Figure 10–4   The effect of response bias and response rate on estimates of population values.

What Is a Good Response Rate?

As suggested above, the best result is a 100 percent response. You can also see that the adequacy of a response rate is highly dependent on the nature of the nonrespondents. If respondents and nonrespondents are not different from one another, a 20 or 30 percent response rate might be adequate. The problem is that the distribution of nonrespondents is almost never known. You can see from Figure 10–4 that response rates below 40 to 60 percent could result in extremely biased samples. The results from this figure suggest that a good response rate would be in the 65 to 75 percent range. This is the point at which the effect of having biased nonrespondents is diminished. Another way to arrive at a standard for response rates would be to look at response rates that survey researchers typically get.

Babbie (1990), on the basis of many years of experience, has suggested that a return of 50 percent is adequate, a return of 60 percent is good, and a return rate of 70 percent or more is very good. Dillman (2000), on the other hand, believes that return rates above 70 or 80 percent can and should be achieved. We could search through the literature and see what kinds of return rates have been achieved. Fortunately, a number of meta-analyses have been done on survey response rates and on factors influencing them (see, for example, Fox et al., 1988; Heberlin & Baumgartner, 1978; Yammarino et al., 1991). Heberlin and Baumgartner (1978) report a range of returns from 20 to 80 percent. Initial return rates have been reported from 28 percent to 68 percent (Babbie, 1973). Heberlin and Baumgartner (1978) reported an average return rate of 48 percent from the initial mailing.

Factors that Influence Response Rates

There are a number of factors that influence response rate. The major factors that have been empirically demonstrated to be related to response rate are whether respondents receive a notice that a survey will be sent to them before the actual mailing of the survey, the number of follow-ups made by the researcher, the perceived salience or importance of the topic, and the provision of incentives. You might expect that length of the survey would have a direct influence on response rates, but the effect of length appears to be dependent on the salience of the topic for the target population. Surveys that the target population believes are important might attain fairly high response rates even though they are quite long. In spite of this finding, we suggest that you limit the length of surveys, probably to four to six pages (60 to 100 items). Although there has been little empirical research on the effect of the general quality and presentation of a survey on response rate, our experience suggests that these are very important. People tend to throw away trashy looking mail.

Increasing Salience (Letters to Respondents). Because of the fact that you cannot converse with the respondent face to face, the letters you write to the respondents take on great significance. As well as describing the study and explaining what the respondent needs to do in order to complete the survey, a major purpose of the cover letter is to convince the respondent to respond. You need to convince the respondent that the issue is an important issue in general, that it is personally important to the respondent, and that it is critical that the respondent responds. Educated respondents such as ATCs will understand the logic of random samples and the necessity of getting complete returns from everyone in the sample. When you pilot the instrument, ask pilot subjects why they would return or not return the survey. Use these as points to be made in letters to the respondents.

Notification and Follow-ups. The initial instrument should have included a letter to the respondent describing the purpose of the survey and the importance of both the topic and the respondent. It should also give directions for returning the survey. This letter would include the use of the "motivators" that you identified in the pilot study. A few days after the survey is sent, you should begin a series of follow-ups. The first follow-up is a post card. The post card should be sent so that it will arrive 3 to 5 days after the respondent has received the instrument. The post card reminds the respondents that they had received a survey, asks them to please complete it and return it, and provides a way to get a new instrument if needed. About 1 week later (10 to 12 days after the initial delivery), you should send a longer letter that restates the purpose of the study and the importance of the topic and of the responder. After another 1 to 1.5 weeks (17 to 25 days after the initial delivery), you should send another letter and a new copy of the survey to those who still have not responded. We suggest that you keep track of respondents. Inform them that this is simply for the purpose of doing follow-ups and that the tracking mechanisms will be destroyed when the survey is returned (see Display 10–7 for a Checklist for Reviewing Surveys).

Alternative Survey Methods

Interviews

Researchers might choose to collect the data through a face-to-face interview rather than through a mailed survey. There are a number of potential advantages in doing surveys in this way. You can control the conditions under which they survey is completed. Since you are with the respondent,

Display 10-7	**A Checklist for Reviewing Surveys**

1. **Was a survey appropriate for this study?**
   - ☐ Were self-report data appropriate?
   - ☐ Did the survey fit the research question?
   - ☐ Was a copy of the survey included?
2. **Did the survey appear to:**
   - ☐ Be attractive?
   - ☐ Be of reasonable length?
   - ☐ Have clear directions?
   - ☐ Have appropriately worded questions?
   - ☐ Have appropriate response alternatives?
3. **Were survey variables/scales substantiated by other**
   - ☐ Research?
   - ☐ Theory?
4. **Has the survey been used before?**
   - ☐ Yes. If yes:
     - ☐ Did the researcher include reliability/validity estimates from that research?
     - ☐ Was the research with a similar population?
     - ☐ Are the current results similar to those found before?
5. **Reliability/Validity**
   - ☐ Were coefficients provided?
   - ☐ What type of reliability?
     - ☐ From previous research?
     - ☐ Done by the authors?
       - ☐ Were they adequate?
6. **Sampling**
   - ☐ Is the intended population identified?
   - ☐ Is the sampling frame identified?
   - ☐ Does the sampling frame include the right elements?
   - ☐ Is the sample a:
     - ☐ probability sample?
     - ☐ nonprobability sample?
   - ☐ Was generalization appropriate?
7. **Data Collection Procedures**
   - ☐ Were there timely follow-ups?
   - ☐ Were the letters to respondents motivating?

(Continued on following page)

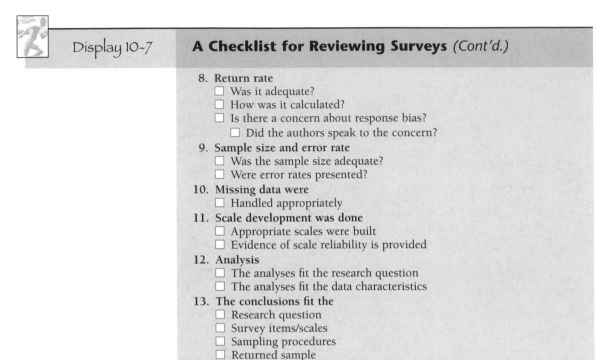

Display 10-7   **A Checklist for Reviewing Surveys** *(Cont'd.)*

8. **Return rate**
   - ☐ Was it adequate?
   - ☐ How was it calculated?
   - ☐ Is there a concern about response bias?
     - ☐ Did the authors speak to the concern?
9. **Sample size and error rate**
   - ☐ Was the sample size adequate?
   - ☐ Were error rates presented?
10. **Missing data were**
    - ☐ Handled appropriately
11. **Scale development was done**
    - ☐ Appropriate scales were built
    - ☐ Evidence of scale reliability is provided
12. **Analysis**
    - ☐ The analyses fit the research question
    - ☐ The analyses fit the data characteristics
13. **The conclusions fit the**
    - ☐ Research question
    - ☐ Survey items/scales
    - ☐ Sampling procedures
    - ☐ Returned sample

you can ensure that the respondent is paying attention, has no distractions, understands the directions, and, of course, is actually the person who completes the survey. The fact that you are face to face with the respondent also increases some risks. The physical and emotional characteristics as well as the skills of the interviewer can either enhance or reduce the quality of the data. A skillful interviewer can draw out a respondent, exploring issues in more depth than might be possible with a mailed survey. An unskilled interviewer may not know how do this. A researcher who is biased may prod the respondent into responses that he or she would not have made otherwise. The mere presence of the interviewer may increase the likelihood of a more positive (or more negative) response. Finally, the amount of time the researcher needs to spend getting data from each respondent dramatically increases. As a result, researchers who use interviews often resort to interviewing small samples that are purposively chosen. This, of course, limits both generalizabilty and accuracy.

The Telephone Survey

The telephone survey is a kind of hybrid between the mailed survey and the face-to-face interview. Given both the person and technical resources, it is a way to combine the advantages of both approaches. Most people have phones. You can probably get phone listings, particularly if the target population is athletic trainers, coaches, or athletes. This will make it possible to draw appropriate samples (or, with some very small populations, to survey the entire population). Data can be collected relatively quickly. The phone interviewer can be given structured questions and be trained to ask them with appropriate cadence and inflection. The phone interviewer can record the data instantly either on paper or electronically. It is possible to interact with potential respondents to answer questions they may have and to personalize the encouragement to respond. The phone interviewer can do follow-up questioning to probe open-ended responses.

Email and Web Surveys

Increasingly, researchers are using both email and the Internet to do surveys. Each of these makes conducting follow-ups much easier and less costly. Increases in the number of follow-ups by email and Internet do not add appreciably to the cost. The timing of follow-ups can be extremely flexible. It is possible to interact with potential respondents to answer questions they may have and to personalize the incentives to respond. Formatting is limited in email surveys, but in web-based surveys there are many formatting alternatives. Alternative formats can be present but unseen by the respondent. Skip patterns can be imbedded in the survey so that a particular response moves a respondent to skip to another set of questions. Similarly, subsets of questions can be built in that are germane only to a specific subset of respondents (e.g., athletic trainers who are in clinics). Special instructions for particular items can be presented with pop-up or drop-down boxes at the moment the respondent starts the question. These are almost impossible to do with a mailed paper-based survey without increasing the length substantially. Potential respondents can be informed of a Website and given a password (a PIN number) that only they can use. This ensures that no one else will complete their survey. The password and the survey responses can be separated. As a result, the follow-ups can be done to the respondent, and researcher cannot connect the respondent to her data. Earlier in this chapter, we suggested that open-ended questions on paper surveys were difficult for respondents, and resulted in poor response rates, and poor quality of data. The Web survey may increase both the amount and quality of open-ended responses, since respondents can type their responses in open-ended boxes.

A major issue with the use of either email or web-based surveys is the degree to which the target population has access to computers. High school athletic trainers may have less access to computers at their high school than athletic trainers in a college. This, of course, can reduce return and result in response bias, which will limit the generalizability of the results.

 ## Data Analysis

Extensive treatment of the analysis of survey data is beyond the scope of this chapter, but we would like to remind you of a few points. You need to think about data analysis during the construction of the survey, not afterwards. Surveys should be developed to answer research questions and they should be analyzed to answer those questions. Decisions about the use of specific statistics for analysis of surveys must be made on the basis of the same principles that decisions about the analysis of any data need to be made. Analysis should be consistent with the research questions of the study. While simple descriptive statistics can be informative, they are often taken to mean more than they do. If, for example, the researcher has hypothesized that the use of alternative modalities is associated with the type of educational preparation athletic trainers have had, it is not sufficient to present frequency data on the use of alternative modalities and frequency data on levels of educational preparation and then imply that the two are connected. The researcher should directly test that hypothesis using some statistical technique (e.g., Pearson r or chi square).

Since much of the data collected through surveys is qualitative, decisions about the nature of the data are more problematic than with other measures in athletic training research. Concerns about the nature of the data are minimized somewhat by the development of continuous scales (e.g., a single "satisfaction" item versus a satisfaction scale). Categorical (nominal) independent variables can be dealt with by the use of dummy coding, effect coding, or orthogonal coding, just as might be done with analysis of variance/multiple regression analyses. Categorical dependent variables can be analyzed with logistic regression.

We strongly urge you to develop subscales within surveys. The appropriate use of multiple items to measure a phenomenon will increase the reliability and validity of the measure. Reliability and validity work should precede the collection of survey data, but sometimes the final development of subscales is done with the actual data. Internal consistency analysis may be done to do final selection of items for analysis and for the calculation of reliability coefficients (e.g., Chronbach's alpha). Because so many individual pieces of data are collected in a single survey, a number of additional research questions may emerge after the data are collected. National data sets, such as might be collected by NATA, can be used by researchers to invent research questions that may not even have been thought of by the survey developers.

 ## Respondent Subjectivity

Many researchers in athletic training seem to be unsure about the use of surveys and other methods that collect self-report data as research tools. The data are treated as subjective and therefore untrustworthy. This is somewhat ironic, since the bulk of information available in athletic training rooms is self-reported and qualitative. Athletes are routinely questioned about their injuries, their fitness, and their rehabilitation success or failures. Athletic trainers use this information to help them make clinical judgments. If this information is useful for clinical judgments, it ought to have many uses in research.

Institutional Review Board (IRB) Approval of the Study

As with other forms of athletic training research, if you hope or intend to disseminate the findings of your survey research, it will be necessary for you to obtain permission for your study from your institution's review board for the protection of human subjects. In some cases, the study may be exempted from needing to obtain informed consent from the respondents, but this exemption must be granted by your IRB.

Summary

Surveys are a way to systematically collect data from individuals about what they know, how they feel, or how they behave. Appropriate writing of survey items can result in data that are reliable and valid. Surveys can be used with only a few individuals or with representative samples from populations. When samples are drawn correctly, the results can generalize to that population. The correctness and precision of population estimates is dependent on appropriate sampling, getting an adequate return rate, the size of the population, the variability of the population, and the size of the sample. Survey data, and other types of self-report data, can provide insights about athletes and athletic training that cannot be provided by physiological data alone. We have provided you with a checklist that you can use in evaluating your own survey or in evaluating a published study using a survey (Gansneder, 2002).

Activities

1. Using a table of random numbers, draw a random sample of 25.
2. Calculate the standard error for each of the following:
   In percentages for a sample of 500
      From an infinite population with population percentage of .50
      From an infinite population with population percentage of .70
      From an finite population with population percentage of .50
      From an finite population with population percentage of .70
   In means for a sample of 500
      From an infinite population with population with *mean* = 28, *standard deviation* = 2
      From an infinite population with population with *mean* = 50, *standard deviation* = 4
      From a finite population with population with *mean* = 28, *standard deviation* = 2
      From a finite population with population with *mean* = 50, *standard deviation* = 4
3. Identify three research questions that could be answered using surveys.
4. Write questions to determine each of the following Write each question as an open-ended question and as a closed-ended question

  a. Age, sex, and years as a certified athletic trainer
  b. Usage by athletic trainers of alternative modalities for rehabilitation
  c. Athletes' compliance with rehabilitation protocols
  d. Athletic trainers' belief in the value of completing a Ph.D.
  e. Number of hours athletic trainers work each week
5. Develop a sampling plan to draw a sample of athletic trainers in your state.

References

Babbie, E. R. (1990). *Survey research methods.* Belmont, C.A.: Wadsworth Publishing Company, Inc.

Dillman, D. A. (1978). *Mail and telephone surveys: The total design method.* New York: John Wiley and Sons.

Dillman, D. A. (2000). *Mail and telephone surveys: The tailored design method.* New York: John Wiley and Sons.

Fox, R. J., Crask, M. R., & Kim, J. (1988). Mail survey response rate: A meta-analysis of selected techniques for inducing response. *Public Opinion Quarterly, 52,* 467–491.

Gansneder, B.M. (2002, June). Issues in the use of surveys in athletic training/sports medicine research, *Journal of Athletic Training.* Dallas, TX: NATA workshop.

Heberlin, T. A., & Baumgartner, R. (1978). Factors affecting response rates to mailed questionnaires: A quantitative analysis of the published literature. *American Sociological Review, 43,* 447–462.

Yammarino, F. J., Skinner, S. J., & Childers, T. L. (1991). Understanding mail survey response behavior: A meta-analysis. *Public Opinion Quarterly, 55,* 613–639.

Bibliography

Kviz, F. J. (1977). Toward a standard definition of response rate. *Public Opinion Quarterly, 41,* 265–267.

Pitney, W.A., & Parker, J. (2002). Qualitative research applications in athletic training. *Journal of Athletic Training, 37,* S168–173.

Turocy, P. S. (2002). Survey research in athletic training: The scientific method of development and implementation. *Journal of Athletic Training, 37,* S174–179.

Chapter 11

Formulating and Writing the Methods

Objectives

After reading this chapter, you will:

- Understand the key aspects to developing a sound methodology for your study.
- Understand the essential sections for writing the methods.
- Know how to describe the selection and characteristics of the subjects used in the study.
- Realize the importance of obtaining appropriate institutional review board approval for the use of human subjects.
- Be able to accurately explain the instrumentation used for data collection.
- Appreciate the importance of controlling the data collection environment.
- Understand the importance of pilot testing the methods before beginning actual data collection.
- Know how to clearly explain what was examined and what was done to answer the questions.
- Be able to clearly present the statistical procedures used to analyze the data.

Questions

While reading this chapter, think about answers to the following questions:

1. How much detail needs to be included in describing the methods?
2. Under what circumstances is it necessary to obtain institutional review board approval to use subjects?
3. What if the research setting doesn't have an institutional review board for the use of human subjects?
4. When is it necessary to establish the reliability and validity of the instrumentation you will use for your study?
5. Can the statistical procedures be determined after collection of the data?

Formulating the Methods

This chapter will explain the keys to developing a sound methodology for your study. The main elements of a methods section of a manuscript will also be presented. The keys to a sound methodology are developing an appropriate research design, obtaining approval for the use of human subjects, pilot testing, establishing the reliability and validity of the instrumentation that will be used for data collection, and analysis of the data using correct statistical techniques. The methods section of a manuscript should be written in enough detail that someone could replicate the study by simply reading this section of your paper. The main topics of the methods section include subjects, instrumentation, procedures, and statistical analysis.

Research Designs

In Chapter 7, you learned about the designs commonly used in athletic training research. It is essential that your research design is appropriate to answer the questions put forth in your problem statement and hypotheses. The incorrect application of a research design is one of the fatal flaws that lead to rejection of manuscripts submitted to scholarly journals. For example, once the study is completed, if you didn't randomly assign subjects to treatment and control groups, you can't go back and do this during the process of revising the manuscript. If you should have counterbalanced treatment interventions and you did not do so, it is also too late once the data collection is completed.

Subjects

Selection

The purpose of your study should determine the characteristics of the subjects you choose to study. One good way to think about subject selection is to consider the population to which you hope to generalize your findings. Consider the following example. Assessment of mild head injury has been studied extensively in high school and college athletes, using a whole host of assessment instruments such as the Standardized Assessment of Concussion (SAC), Balance Error Scoring System (BESS), and others. We know that hundreds of thousands of children participate in youth sports programs across the country and are susceptible to sustaining mild head injury. Yet very little research has examined the utility of these assessment instruments for children. A study to determine the reliability and validity of using the SAC and BESS in youth sports would require the inclusion of subjects from this age group in order to generalize findings to the broader population of youth sport participants.

Sometimes it is acceptable to use subjects from a sample of convenience for your study. If, for example, you are interested in determining the rela-

In the Field

> *Jenny is collecting data on subjects with multiple ankle sprains and wants to compare their ability to reposition their ankle (i.e., reposition sense) to the ability of individuals with no ankle sprains. She is aware that the typical characteristics reported are height, weight, and age, but she wonders if other characteristics should be reported. Since she is interested in generalizing her findings to individuals with repeated sprains, she adds the average number and range of sprains reported by the injured subjects. In consulting with her advisor, she also decides to report the severity of the initial sprain and how much time individuals were restricted from returning to sport participation or work.*

tionship between female sex-specific hormones and knee joint laxity across the menstrual cycle, you might draw your subjects from a population of normal menstruating college-age females. If, however, you are interested in generalizing your findings to female athletes at high risk for injury to the anterior cruciate ligament, you would need to recruit subjects who participate in sports like basketball and soccer.

Should you include males, females, or both in your study? Our recommendation is that unless the purpose of your study is gender specific (e.g., effect of prophylactic knee bracing in football players), both sexes should be included. In 1987, the National Institutes of Health (NIH), the largest health research funding agency in the world, spent only 13 percent of its budget on women's health. Since that time NIH has placed greater emphasis on the inclusion of females (and ethnic minority populations for that matter) in federally funded research protocols. Indeed, proposals for funded research to the NIH must now include females or provide clear evidence for why the exclusion of females is appropriate.

Number of Subjects

Perhaps the most frequently asked question by students during the development of research proposals is "How many subjects do I need?" One way to think about this question is to consider what the norm is in the published literature. A more scientific approach would be to calculate an a priori statistical power analysis (Cohen, 1988).

Institutional Review Board Approval

The purpose of the institutional review board (IRB) process is to protect individuals' rights in research and assure that the risks of the research are compatible with the expected benefits. As a general rule, any research conducted with the intent to disseminate the findings of the research through presentations or publications requires the review and approval of an Institutional Review Board for the Protection of Human Subjects. Most reputable journals will not review and accept manuscripts submitted for publication if the study has not been reviewed and approved by an IRB.

Another common question of new researchers is "Do I need IRB approval for pilot testing?" Our best answer is the same general rule: if the intent of the research is to disseminate the findings, then IRB review and approval should be sought and obtained. In some cases, research can be "exempted" from the process of obtaining consent to participate, but that exemption must be granted by the Institutional Review Board for the Protection of Human Subjects.

It is possible that you might find yourself wanting to conduct a research project while you are in a work setting (e.g., sports medicine clinic or industrial workplace) that does not have an Institutional Review Board for the Protection of Human Subjects. The best solution might be for you to find a faculty member at a local college or university with whom you could collaborate. In this case, the study could be reviewed and approved by the institution of the collaborating faculty member. If there are no colleges or universities in the immediate area, local and regional hospitals often have institutional review boards. Perhaps you could identify a physician or other health care professional at the hospital who might be interested in collaborating with you on the research project.

In the Field

Alan is developing a technique for assessing hip proprioception. As a first step he has decided to conduct a reliability study. Although the process is noninvasive and has minimal risk, according to university and federal policy, he decides to submit it to the IRB at his institution. Eventually it is approved and Alan proceeds with his study. In contrast, Melanie is at a similar point with a survey on job satisfaction. But Melanie determines that because her study is only a reliability pilot and her data contain no information about personally sensitive or criminal behavior, under her university's policy, the study would be exempt from IRB protections. Because of these considerations she decides to not submit it to her IRB. Alan and Melanie each recruit 30 subjects equally distributed between males and females. Both find that their instruments have good reliability. Additionally, both discover that men and women respond differently. Because of these unexpected findings, both decide to submit their data in manuscript form for publication. After a couple of revisions Alan's manuscript is accepted for publication. However, Melanie's manuscript is rejected after the initial submission. In consulting with the journal's editor, Melanie is told that because her study had not been reviewed by the IRB, it did not qualify for publication. Melanie counters by stating that under her institution's policy, her research is exempt. The editor responds that while that may be, only the IRB, not the researcher, can make the exemption determination and that she must submit confirmation from her IRB that the project met the exemption criteria. Melanie subsequently contacts her IRB to request an exemption, but is sternly advised that the IRB does not grant exemptions (or approvals) retroactively.

The IRB process is an extremely important aspect of developing your methods, and you should not engage in any data collection until you have met the standards and followed the protocol of your institution's IRB. The approval of your study by the IRB is not a given. In making a decision, the committee will carefully assess the risk-benefit ratio of the proposal. Please keep in mind that the process of IRB review and approval can be a lengthy one and as such you should plan accordingly.

Appropriate procedures for the study of human subjects are discussed at length in Chapter 20. You should review this discussion and become very familiar with the requirements of your institution's Institutional Review Board for the Protection of Human Subjects.

Recruitment

The recruitment of your subjects is one of the most difficult aspects of conducting a research project. It is important that you be realistic in the likelihood you will find and recruit the kind of subjects you wish to study. For example, if you want to study shoulder proprioception in baseball players, you need to ascertain early if the baseball coach is willing to make his athletes available to study before proceeding too far with your research proposal. If you are interested in studying the effects of a particular cryotherapy intervention on edema in acute ankle sprained subjects, you should review the historical incidence of this kind of injury in your prospective study population to determine if it is adequate. In general, the type of research being performed will influence how easy it is to recruit subjects. Studies perceived by your subjects as important, easy, or painless (literally and figuratively) or studies using healthy populations will be easier from which to recruit.

It may be acceptable to provide an incentive for subjects to participate in your study, such as a monetary payment. However, you should not coerce or threaten subjects to participate, and all subjects have the right to withdraw at any time without threat of reprisal or penalty. Your institution's IRB

In the Field

Aimee is interested in studying ACL injuries in women. Specifically, she is interested in comparing the speed of recovery between men and women. To do this she consults with her orthopedist to confirm that she may have access to his patients. Her orthopedist states that he probably sees 20 to 30 per year. Aimee feels confident that this should yield an adequate number for her study. However, at the end of one year, she has been able to recruit only 9 subjects. In reviewing patient records she discovers that actually 14 new ACL patients were treated but only 9 volunteered. She also discovered that the annual average was not 20 to 30 for the clinic, but 16. In retrospect, Aimee realizes that just because subjects are treated doesn't mean they will volunteer for research. She also begins to suspect that because clinicians see the same patients repeatedly, they tend to overestimate their actual number of patients.

will have specific policies for incentives, and you should follow those policies. However, typical guidelines are as follows. Incentives should be proportional to effort required by your subjects. Extremely lucrative incentives are considered coercive. Incentives may be prorated and should be prorated for multistage studies. In multistage studies, your subjects should be reimbursed in a prorated fashion for those portions of the study for which they enroll. This includes reimbursement regardless of whether they complete that stage of the study or the whole study. Finally, instructors cannot require students to participate in research studies. However, your institution may allow instructors to require a research experience. In this case, the instructor would have to offer at least two options: participation as a research subject or completion of an alternative project. The alternative project should make no greater demand on the student than serving as a research subject. In our experience this is usually measured in time required to complete each activity, but your institution may define it differently.

Recruiting subjects can be done in a variety of ways. Flyers are often effective if posted in areas frequented by potential subjects. Subjects might also be recruited through your team physicians or local physician groups. Our experience shows that classified ads in student newspapers can also be effective. The support of coaches may be helpful in the recruitment of subjects from the athletic population. Finally, recruitment of subjects for some research protocols, especially those using invasive procedures, will be more successful when compensation is provided for participation.

Instrumentation

For purposes of this discussion, instrumentation is broadly defined as a device, test method, survey, or some other apparatus you will use to collect data. Examples include an isokinetic device to measure strength, an agility test to measure functional performance, or a questionnaire to determine the perceived outcome of a treatment intervention. It is imperative that your instrument measures what it is intended to measure (validity) and is consistent and reproducible in its measurement (reliability) (see Chapter 9). You can establish its reliability in one of several ways.

If the reliability of the instrument you are using has been documented in the published literature, it may be acceptable for you to simply provide that reference in support of your use of the device or test. This assumes that you are using the same instrument and following exactly the same protocol from which its reliability was established. If your instrument varies from previous protocols, or is a novel test, it will be important to establish its reliability. One way to establish the test-retest reliability of instrument is to randomly select a subset of subjects from your study to return for a repeat test session. This approach is not without risk, since you might determine posthoc that your measurement was indeed not very reliable. A safer approach would be to determine the reliability of the test a priori through an independent protocol using subjects similar to those who will ultimately participate in your study. In any event, if you hope to publish the findings of your study, you must be able to defend the reliability and validity of your measurement instrument.

Pilot Testing

Perhaps the single best piece of advice we can provide in this book is to pilot test, pilot test, and pilot test your methods! Pilot testing is essentially rehearsing the data collection procedures you will use in your study. Invariably there will be unknowns and kinks in the data collection process that can only be uncovered through the actual testing of human subjects. If you fail to pilot test, it is likely that the first several subjects you test for your study will ultimately become pilot test subjects. This can adversely affect certain aspects of your design (e.g., random assignment or counterbalancing) as well as presenting a greater challenge in subject recruitment.

Writing the Methods

The methods section of a manuscript should be organized into subsections, which can vary depending on the authors' guide to which the paper will be submitted. For purposes of this discussion, the following sections will be used: subjects, instrumentation, procedures, and statistical analysis.

Subjects

The number and characteristics of the subjects should be clearly and concisely described and presented in the text. In cases where more complex descriptive demographics are relevant, reference may be made to this information in the text (Display 11–1) or in a table (Table 11–1). An indication that the study was reviewed and approved by an Institutional Review Board for the Protection of Human Subjects and that consent was obtained for participation by the subjects should also be included.

Instrumentation

This section describes the instrument, apparatus, or tests used to collect the data. The device should be presented in enough detail that one could use this information to order the instrument. For example, the brand name and model should be listed, along with the city and state of the manufacturer of the equipment. It is also appropriate to address the reliability of the instrument here, either by providing a reference from the published literature or by explaining the process by which reliability was established in the

Display 11-1 | **Subjects**

Thirty-two uninjured high school student-athletes (age = 16.94 ± 1.56 years, grade = 11 ± 1.19, body mass = 72.47 ± 10.93 kg, height = 177.09 ± 8.78 cm) volunteered to participate in this study. Subjects were randomly assigned to either the control (n = 16) or practice (n = 16) group. All subjects participated in either recreational or interscholastic athletics on the soccer, lacrosse, track, cheerleading, tennis, basketball, or baseball teams. Subjects were excluded if they had sustained an MHI or a lower extremity injury in the last 6 months or suffered from any visual, vestibular, or balance disorders. All subjects read and signed an informed consent form approved by the university's human investigations committee, which also approved the study. The parents of all minors also read and signed an informed consent form before their children participated.

From: Valorich, T.C., Perrin, D.H., & Gansneder, B. M. (2003). Repeat administration elicits a practice effect with the balance error scoring system but not with the standardized assessment of concussion in high school athletes. Journal of Athletic Training, 38, 51–56.

author's laboratory. The model of any computer interfacing and the manner by which data are to be processed should also be included.

If the instrument is novel and one that would be unfamiliar to the reader, it would also be appropriate to depict the device in a figure containing a photograph or drawing of the instrument. (We will explain the use of

Table 11–1 • **Group Demographics**

Variable	Mean ± SD	Range
Height (cm)	163.7 ± 6.1	152.0–174.5
Weight (kg)	65.2 ± 11.5	45.4–88.8
BMI (wt/ht^2)	24.4 ± 3.5	18.4–30.0
AGE (yr)	23.0 ± 3.5	19.6–30.5
Cycle Length (day)	27.8 ± 2.4	24–36
Day of Ovulation	13.9 ± 2.7	9–20
Day of 1st E2 Peak (Ovulation)	15.0 ± 3.8	8–25
Day of 2nd E2 Peak (Luteal)	21.9 ± 3.1	15–27
Day of Progesterone Rise (>2 ng/mL)	17.4 ± 3.5	11–27
Day of Progesterone Peak	21.6 ± 3.1	15–27
E2 at Menses (pg/mL)	53.4 ± 10.2	33.4–81.6
Peak Estrogen (1st Peak) (pg/mL)	189.7 ± 53.4	85.6–295.0
Peak Estrogen (2nd Peak) (pg/mL)	143.9 ± 48.7	48.2–258.3
Peak Progesterone (ng/mL)	14.3 ± 5.8	3.6–26.8
Peak Testosterone (ng/mL)	68.9 ± 16.7	37.0–115.0
Maximum Laxity Change (mm)	3.2 ± 1.1	1.5–5.3

Source: From Shulz, S.J., Kirk, S. E., Johnson, M., Sander, T.C., & Perrin, D.H. (2004). Relationship between sex hormones and anterior knee laxity across the menstrual cycle. Medicine & Science in Sports & Exercise, 36, 1165–1174.

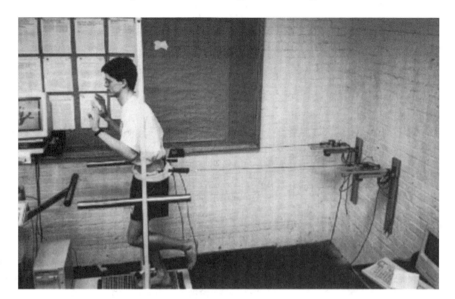

Figure 11–1 Device designed to assess neuromuscular response characteristics at the knee following a functional perturbation. (From: Shultz, S. J., Perrin, D. H., Adams, J. M., Arnold, B. L., Gansneder, B. M., Granata, K. P. (2000). Assessment of neuromuscular response characteristics at the knee following a functional perturbation. *Journal of Electromyography and Kinesiology*, 10, 159–170.)

tables, figures, and appendices in Chapter 16.) For example, Figure 11–1 is a photograph of a device designed to assess neuromuscular response characteristics at the knee following a functional perturbation. This was the original presentation of this device in the published literature, and it established the reliability and validity of this perturbation system. Thus, it would be appropriate for authors to present a figure of this novel instrument and to cite this publication in the methods section of publications using this device.

In Chapter 8, you learned about measurement in athletic training research, including common laboratory measures and the importance of calibration. It would be appropriate to include the manner by which the instrumentation was calibrated and the units of measurement that will ultimately be used for analysis of the data. The majority of sports medicine journals require that units of measurement be recorded as SI units (International System of Units). Table 11–2 presents the seven base units that refer to seven basic quantities of measurement. For a complete listing of SI-derived units, prefixes, and conversions, consult The International System of Units or a reference such as the *American Medical Association Manual of Style*.

Procedures

The procedures section should be presented in enough detail that a reasonably well-informed researcher could replicate the data collection procedures used in your study. The design of the study should be presented and the dependent measures identified. The protocol of the study should be explained, including what was done to cause a change (the independent

Table 11–2 • **SI Base Units**

Quantity	Base Unit Name	SI Unit Symbol
Length	meter	m
Mass	kilogram	kg
Time	second	s
Electric current	ampere	A
Thermodynamic temperature	Kelvin	k
Luminous intensity	candela	cd
Amount of substance	mole	mol

Source: American Medical Association. (1998). *American medical association manual of style: A guide for authors and editors* (9th ed.) Philadelphia: Lippincott Williams & Wilkins.

variables) and what was measured to assess any changes resulting from the treatment or intervention (the dependent variables). The number of times subjects reported to the laboratory, the manner by which instructions were explained, the number of practice or warm-up trials allowed and the rest intervals provided are among the details that should be included.

Statistical Analyses

The methods section should end with a clear and concise presentation of the statistical procedures employed to analyze the data. The statistical procedures that are used should be determined early in the development of the research project and should be designed to answer the research hypotheses and problem statement. Display 11.2 summarizes what the reader should learn from reading your methods section.

Summary

The methods of your study should be carefully developed and based on what is known and not known from the published literature. The methods section of your manuscript should be concisely written, yet in enough detail that an informed reader could replicate your study.

Activities

1. Review your institution's IRB guidelines for review procedures for submitting a research protocol, deadlines for submission, and the review schedule.
2. Complete the researcher training program required by your institution's IRB.
3. Create a data collection sheet specific to your research project.

Display 11-2

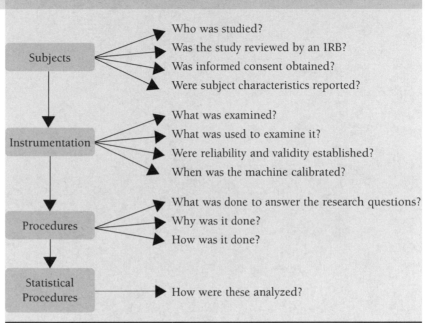

Flow Chart for Constructing the Study Methods

Subjects
- Who was studied?
- Was the study reviewed by an IRB?
- Was informed consent obtained?
- Were subject characteristics reported?

Instrumentation
- What was examined?
- What was used to examine it?
- Were reliability and validity established?
- When was the machine calibrated?

Procedures
- What was done to answer the research questions?
- Why was it done?
- How was it done?

Statistical Procedures
- How were these analyzed?

References

Cohen, J. (1988). *Statistical power analysis for the behavioral sciences* (2nd ed.). Hillsdale, NJ: Lawrence Erlbaum Associates.

Cohen, J. (1988). The t test for means, Statistical power analysis for the behavioral science (2nd ed.). Hillsdale, NJ: Lawrence Erlbaum Associates.

Iverson, C., Flanagin, A., & Fontanarosa, P. B. (Eds.). (1998). *American Medical Association manual of style* (9th ed.). Baltimore: Williams & Wilkins.

Bibliography

The International System of Units (SI). (1991). *Special Publication 330.* Washington, DC: US Department of Commerce, National Institute of Standards and Technology (NIST).

Part IV

Statistical Measurements

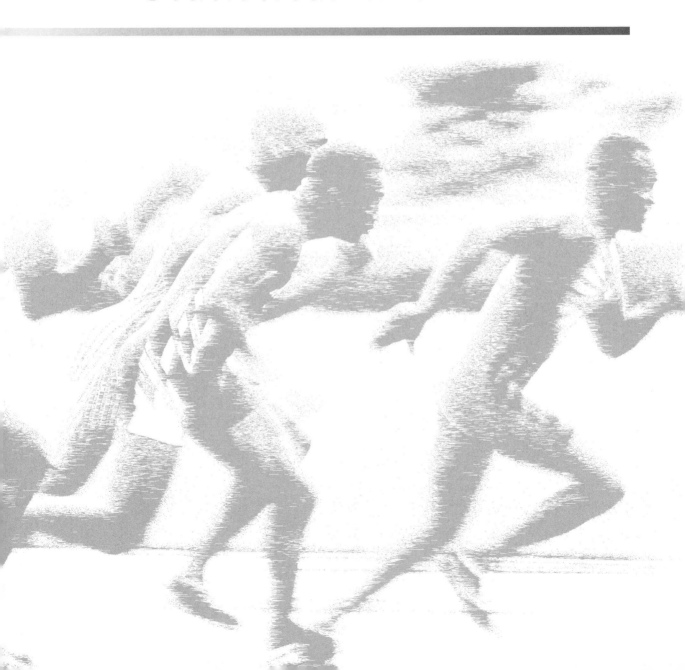

Chapter 12

Statistical Decision Making

Objectives

After reading this chapter, you will:
- Describe the z distribution.
- Explain the difference between the t and z distributions.
- Define a null hypothesis and an alternative hypothesis.
- Correctly select between an independent and dependent (or correlated) t test.
- Define alpha and p values.
- Read a statistical output for the t test.
- Define statistical power.

Questions

While reading this chapter, think about answers to the following questions:
1. Why do I perform statistical tests?
2. When do I use random sampling versus random assignment?
3. What is the difference between an independent t test and a dependent t test?
4. What is the difference between a correlated t test and a dependent t test?
5. When should I use alpha, and when should I use p values?
6. Why is statistical power important?
7. How do I increase statistical power?
8. If it is statistically significant, is it clinically significant?
9. What is a statistical error?

Introduction

To properly understand statistical testing, it is important to understand that statistical tests are simply tools used in hypothesis testing. You should also understand that hypothesis testing is a process of logic, not just mathematics, and that statistical tests and statistical distributions are based on mathematical assumptions about random variables and random distributions. You will apply these mathematics to real situations and real data. It's easy to confuse the mathematics of statistical tests with the logic of hypothesis testing and subsequently believe that statistical tests are the answer to all concerns about your experiment.

Thus, as you proceed through this chapter, keep in mind that the process of statistical decision making is one of logic and that statistics are used to *confirm* the logic. As you learn about statistics, do not forget the principles that you learned about research design (Chapter 7). Making conclusions about whether treatments work is primarily a function of the research design and not of the statistics you use. The statistics help you to decide whether differences or relationships are random. While this may be a necessary condition for making causal conclusions, it is not sufficient. Causal conclusions can only be made if you can rule out alternative causes through your research design. To decide that a difference is "real" and not due to chance does not mean that a treatment worked. Since this text is not intended to be a statistics text, we have tried to emphasize the *logic* behind the use of statistics, not their mathematics or their formulae.

 ## Statistical Definitions

Before beginning a detailed discussion of statistical testing, a brief introduction to some statistical terms and their formulae would be appropriate (Display 12–1). Three key terms will be important throughout the text: mean, variance, and standard deviation. The mean (or average) is a measure of central tendency, whereas the standard deviation and variance are measures of dispersion of scores about the mean. The mean is represented by the following formula:

$$\bar{X} = \frac{\Sigma X}{n} \quad (12\text{–}1)$$

where ΣX is the sum of the scores and n is the number of subjects in the group. You probably have a very good, practical sense of the value of the mean. However, it should be emphasized that the mean is a measure of central tendency, indicating the central point about which the subjects' scores vary.

The second important statistical term is the variance, which is calculated as:

$$s^2 = \frac{\Sigma (X - \bar{X})^2}{n - 1} \quad (12\text{–}2)$$

Where the numerator is the sum of the squared deviations of subjects' scores, i.e., X, from the mean, and n is the number of subjects. Variance is a measure of score spread. The larger the variance, the larger the spread of the scores. Note that this spread is based on a score's distance from the mean. Compare the variance formula to the mean formula. You'll notice that both numerators contain a sum of scores (sum of the subjects' scores for the mean and the sum of the squared differences for variance). You will also note that the denominators of both contain n. This isn't a coincidence. In actuality, the variance is a mean. It is the average of the squared differences. Squared deviations from the mean will be smaller than squared deviations from any other possible value (e.g., the median). This is known as the method of least squares. Each of the statistical tests presented (i.e., t test, F test, and Pearson r) are based on this least squares principle.

Closely related to the variance is the standard deviation. Its formula is:

$$s = \sqrt{\frac{\sum (X - \overline{X})^2}{n - 1}} \quad (12\text{–}3)$$

Compare this formula to the variance formula. You should notice that the only difference is the square root. In other words the standard deviation is the square root of the variance and is another measure of deviation from the mean. As you will find in Chapters 13 and 14, variance is very useful. However, it isn't very intuitively useful. For example, if you measured a group's height in meters and got the average (2 meters) and then calculated the variance (0.04 m^2), the variance of the height would be in meters squared. In this case, it would appear that you calculated an area that is not a meaningful description of height variation. By converting the variance to a standard deviation (0.2 m), the units convert to a unit that makes intuitive sense and provides a more meaningful measure.

Populations and Samples

In addition to the basic statistical definitions, an understanding of populations, samples, random selection, and random assignment is necessary. A population represents a whole group that you might be interested in. For example, you might be interested in ACL injuries in women or you might be interested in ACL injuries in women basketball players. Both of these represent populations and each could be broadened or narrowed. Obviously, populations are quite large and, as such, are more difficult to measure. Thus, rather than measuring whole populations, we can randomly select individuals from these populations. The purpose of random selection is to derive a representative sample of the population. From this representative sample, inferences about the whole population (e.g., how many women receive ACL injuries annually) can be drawn.

In athletic training research, random selection is rarely done. Rather, we start with an available sample and then randomly assign individuals of the sample to a control or experimental group. By giving one of the groups a treatment (e.g., static stretching), you are in effect trying to change that group's population. If the stretching is effective, members of the stretch group are no longer part of the original population but instead belong to a

Display 12-1

Statistical Definitions

Term	Definition
Mean	Average
Variance	Dispersion of scores from the mean in units of squared deviations
Standard deviation	Dispersion of scores from the mean in units of the original measure
Population	The entire group of which you are interested (Typically too large to be studied, e.g., all college baseball players)
Sample	A representative subgroup of individuals from a population (Typically selected at random)
Random selection	The selection of a sample by a predetermined, random process
Random assignment	Assignment of individuals within a sample to either the control group or the experimental research group by a predetermined, random process

new population, one that stretches. At first glance this may seem odd. If a treatment changes the population, how do we study the population of interest? In fact, we don't. In the case of experiments, we study the phenomenon of the treatment and are not interested in the population. If the population is of interest, random selection from the population—rather than random assignment of the sample—is necessary.

The Normal (*z*) Distribution and the *z* Test

To understand how statistical tests work, it may help to start with an explanation of some basic statistical distributions. The most fundamental distribution is the normal (or *z*) distribution (Fig. 12–1). If you measured the hamstring flexibility of everybody across the United States, the range of flexibilities and the number of people with those flexibilities would proba-

In the Field

Nicole is interested in studying the impact of rotator cuff stretching on rotator cuff impingement in baseball pitchers. She realizes that she cannot study the entire population of collegiate baseball pitchers. Because she only has access to her college's baseball team, she also realizes she cannot randomly select from the population. Instead she makes the assumption (see Chapter 6) that her baseball team is a representative sample of the population and randomly assigns the pitchers to a stretching and no-stretching group.

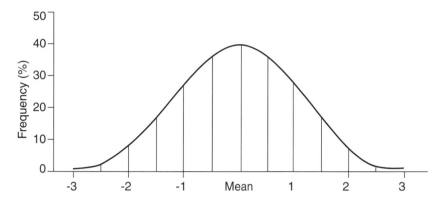

Figure 12–1   The normal (z) curve.

bly be normally distributed. The curve that describes this distribution is known as the standard normal distribution or the z distribution. In the middle of the normal curve is the mean (i.e., average) flexibility of the population. The curve is highest at the mean because the greatest number of people will have the average flexibility (or at least be very close to the average flexibility). You will also notice that to the left and right of the mean is the location of the first standard deviation (marked as +1 and –1 standard deviation). In this case, the positive and negative only indicate on which side of the mean the standard deviation is, i.e., it indicates direction not size. An important feature of the normal curve is that 68 percent of the measures (i.e., hamstring flexibility) will always be between +1 and –1 standard deviation. Furthermore, 95 percent of the flexibility scores are in the area of the curve between +1.96 and –1.96 standard deviations. This is an important feature of the normal curve because if a data set is normal, you know how often a given range of values occurs. As you will see, this principle is an essential feature of statistical tests.

You should understand that this exact distribution is not a unique or necessary feature of hamstring flexibility. But it is a necessary feature of the normal or z distribution and data sets that are normally distributed. A companion to the z distribution is a statistical test known as the z test. The z test can be used to test whether a sample or samples are drawn from a known population. To use the z test, the researcher must know the population standard deviation and know or estimate the population mean. The formula for the z test is presented below. Note the use of Greek symbols for the mean (μ) and the standard deviation (σ) in the formula:

$$z = \frac{\mu - \bar{x}}{\sqrt{\dfrac{\sigma^2}{n}}} \quad (12\text{–}4)$$

where:

$\bar{x}$ = mean
μ = population mean
σ^2 = population variance
n = sample size

This should alert you to the fact that the use of the z test requires knowledge of the population mean and standard deviation.

Student's *t* Distribution

Although the normal distribution and the z test are fundamental to statistical testing and important to your understanding of statistics, the z test is rarely used in research in athletic training. This is because its use requires specific knowledge about the population. Instead of using the z distribution, other distributions such as the t distribution and the F distribution are used. Conceptually, the t distribution is the easiest, so we will start with it.

The t distribution and the t test were derived in 1908 by William Sealey Gosset, who was employed by the Guinness brewery in Dublin, Ireland. The t distribution, like the z distribution, is a mathematically derived distribution. Gossett was faced with the task of trying to determine the quality of a vat of beer. He needed to make decisions about the population (the vat) from a sample (or samples) of beer drawn from the vat. Since the z test required knowledge of the population mean and standard deviation, it was not usable. Gossett figured out that he could estimate the population standard deviation. He also figured out that the resulting distribution was dependent on the size of the samples drawn. It was different for every different sample size. Instead of there just being one distribution, as is the case with the z distribution, there is an "infinity" of distributions. Thus, the shape of the t distribution is dependent on sample size. He called the test the student's t test and the distribution the t distribution. (This was because the Guinness brewery would not allow their employees to use their own names in a publication.) Unlike the z distribution, it is a distribution of outcomes occurring from repeated sampling from unknown populations. Also unlike the z distribution, there is not a single t distribution but a multitude of them (more about that later).

Gosset developed a t test for single samples drawn from an unknown (or theoretical) population and another t test for drawing pairs of samples (independent or dependent) from an unknown population. He realized that even when two samples come from the same population, the means of those samples would probably be different from each because they are samples. This is also called "sampling error." But how big would this difference be? Most of the time it would be fairly small. But some of the time the difference could be quite large just due to the vagaries of sampling or "by chance." The *t* distribution provides the distribution of these differences. When we use small samples, we will tend to get a larger proportion of big differences between the sample means just by chance. The result is that with small samples, the *t* distribution does not look like the *z* distribution. In general, it is flatter and wider. On the other hand, with larger and larger samples, the *t* distribution approximates the *z* distribution.

But if sample means are always going to be different from each other, how could you ever decide that was because they really came from different populations (e.g., a population that receives some treatment and one that does not)? Gosset's logic was as follows. It is possible to draw two samples from the same population and find that the difference between their means is quite large. But this rarely happens by chance. If that probability is small, say only 5 percent or less of the time, one might be willing to believe that the difference is "real" (not a chance difference). Gosset's distribution, the *t* distribution, provides those probabilities for samples of various sizes. This is, in general, the logic behind the use of all statistical tests. We apply mathematical distributions of what happens randomly, or by chance, to actual occurrences that we observe in the conduct of our research.

Imagine that you have drawn a random sample from some "population." You can calculate the mean of the sample. Now, place this original sample back into the population, draw a second random sample and calculate a new sample mean. If you repeat this process 100 times (or more, if you want) you will get 100 different means. None of them will be exactly the same. These differences are a direct result of the sampling process and are referred to as sampling error. If you have done this with large samples, the sample means will be normally distributed about the overall or grand mean (i.e., the mean of the 100 means, which is a very good estimate of the population mean). This feature is referred to as the central limit theorem, and it works to your advantage by converting non-normal sample distributions to normal distributions. The standard deviation of these means is known as the standard error of the mean. (You will frequently find references to standard errors in statistics textbooks and journal articles. When you see references to standard errors, you should think of them as standard deviations of statistical distributions. The term *standard deviation* should be reserved to identify the standard deviation of the population or a sample of the population.) Knowing the shape of this curve is important because it describes how often the means of random samples occur. For example, if the distribution is normal, the means of the 100 random samples that are between +1 and –1 standard errors from the grand mean occur 68 percent of the time by chance and means that are between +2 and –2 standard errors occur approximately 95 percent of the time by chance. When sample sizes are smaller, the distribution will not be normal. It is, of course, vital to know the shape of those distributions for the same reasons.

Statistical Decision Making (Hypothesis Testing)

Let's consider a hypothetical experiment. For this experiment you want to determine whether a specific stretching protocol is useful in increasing quadriceps flexibility as measured by knee range of motion. To accomplish this, you randomly assign half the subjects to a treatment group that gets the stretch, and half to a control group that receives no stretch. Based on this design, you have three potential hypotheses (Display 12–2). Your first is the null hypothesis (identified as H_0) and states that the range of motion of the treatment group after stretch will not be different from (or will be equal to) that of the control group. Your second, or alternative hypothesis (identified as H_{A1}), is that the treatment group will have greater range of motion than the control group. Your third hypothesis (also an alternate hypothesis and identified as H_{A2}) is that the experimental group will have less range of motion than the control group. This last hypothesis is often neglected, ignored, or forgotten by researchers, but it is always implied as part of hypothesis testing and is important to statistical decision making.

Why Use Statistical Decision Making?

Statistics are used to help make decisions regarding differences between groups. In the stretch experiment, this means the differences between the control and stretch groups. By looking at the means in Table 12–1, you don't need a statistical test to tell you that the stretch group has more range of motion than the control group. If you were only interested in knowing whether these two groups are different, using the means would be acceptable. However, generally you are not interested in whether groups are different from each other. You want to know whether the two groups came from different populations, in this case, a population that doesn't stretch.

Display 12-2

Hypotheses for the Stretch Experiment	
Hypothesis Type	**Definition**
Null (H_0)	Range of motion will not be different for the stretch and no-stretch (control) groups.
Alternative 1 (H_{A1})	The stretch group will have greater knee flexion than the control group.
Alternative 2 (H_{A2})	The stretch group will have less knee flexion that the control group

Table 12–1 • **Stretch Experiment Data**

	Control	Stretch
	95.51	95.75
	96.05	101.64
	94.68	95.98
	106.69	110.49
	97.75	95.85
	104.95	108.9
	98.38	98.41
	106.62	105.67
	102.85	108.25
	103.06	106.07
	90.97	93.04
	109.6	114.18
	98.03	102.14
	100.46	99.97
	96.37	99.28
	106.29	107.47
	102.37	101.36
	103.22	102.45
	96.45	99.96
	93.88	96.31
	105.79	112.34
	103.73	109.56
	104.9	110.48
	96.25	103.06
	95.16	102.17
	99.06	98.29
	108.44	109.67
	97.06	96.78
	99.48	97
	100.89	104.78
	102.32	108.76
	99.77	106.97
	109.13	115.76
	90.2	91.11
	102.25	99.77
	100.69	104.65
	107.59	108.6
	95.16	102.37
	105.09	111.52
	97.24	94.89

Mean	100.61		103.29	
Standard deviation	5.01		6.20	
Independent t test		Dependent t test		
t value	2.128	t value	5.439	
p value	0.037	p value	0.000003	
		Correlation between control and stretch groups	0.867	

The Independent t Test

One way to test your hypothesis is to use the *t* test and, in this case, the independent *t* test. The formula for it is:

$$t = \frac{\overline{X_E} - \overline{X_C}}{S_{\overline{X_E} - \overline{X_C}}} \quad or \quad \frac{\text{Difference between the means}}{\text{Standard error of the difference of the means}} \quad (12\text{--}5)$$

$$\text{Where } S_{\overline{X_E} - \overline{X_C}} = \sqrt{S_C^2 \Big/ n_C + S_E^2 \Big/ n_E} \quad (12\text{--}6)$$

It is appropriate for comparing two groups of different subjects. To understand how the *t* test can be used for statistical decision making, let's go back to our example. Referring to the information in Table 12–1, you will see that the difference in the means of the control and experimental group is 2.68°. The easiest way to calculate the value for the *t* test is to employ a computer package such as SPSS (SPSS Inc., Chicago, IL). By inputting the data into the computer, SPSS can calculate a *t* value and its probability (or *p* value). In this particular case, the *p* value is approximately .04. This means that a difference this big or bigger between the means (i.e., 2.68°) could occur 4 times in 100 by chance when the null hypothesis (that there is no real difference between the range of motion of the stretch group and the control group) is true.

Researchers commonly use *p* values that are equal to or less than .05 (5 times in 100) as a standard for rejecting the null hypothesis. Since *p* = .04 is less than *p* = .05, you would reject the null hypothesis and select one of your two alternative hypotheses. Logically, this is the equivalent of believing that you have identified a nonrandom difference. You do not know whether the difference was due to the treatment itself, only that the likelihood that it occurred by chance was low. Choosing the correct alternative hypothesis simply requires selecting the one that matches your results.

You should notice that we did not say that you accept the alternative hypothesis. Instead we said you reject the null hypothesis. This is because you did not test the alternative hypotheses. You tested the probability that the null hypothesis is true and decided that it probably was not true. You rejected the null hypothesis even though it would be true 4 times in 100. Thus, you can never truly reject the null hypothesis with certainty, because it is always possible (although improbable) that the null is true.

The Correlated t Test

An alternative approach to your experiment could have been to use only one group and measure them once before the stretching treatment and once after. By doing this, you could test differences in ROM from pre- to posttreatment. Using the data from Table 12–1, assume that the control data represents a pretest (i.e., a measure before stretching) and the experimental data represents a post-test taken after stretching. Thus, instead of two groups, you now have one group measured twice. With repeated measures designs, the dependent or correlated t test is used. The correlated t test is the same test as the independent t test, except that it is "adjusted" for the relationship between the pretest and post-test data. It has the same formula as the independent t test except that the denominator has an extra term (the extra term is the adjustment):

$$t = \frac{\overline{X}_E - \overline{X}_C}{\sqrt{\underbrace{S_C^2\big/n_C + S_E^2\big/n_E - \left(2r \cdot S_C^2\big/n_C \cdot S_E^2\big/n_E\right)}}} \quad (12\text{–}7)$$

Adjustment to denominator

Whenever you collect measures on subjects twice, it is almost always true that the first set of scores will be correlated with the second set of scores. For example, using our experiment, if you find a person's ROM at pretest is the largest in the group, it is very likely this person will have the greatest ROM at post-test. Conversely, the person with the least ROM at pretest will is very likely to have the least ROM at post-test. Using this kind of information for the whole group, you can establish the relationship between the pretest and post-test scores for the whole group. This relationship is measured by the correlation statistic r (see Chapter 15 for a detailed explanation of r). This correlation is used to adjust the independent t test to produce the correlated (or dependent) t test. The effect of adjusting this term is to increase the size of the t. Using the data in Table 12–1 and treating it as a repeated measures design, you will see that the t increases from 2.13 to 5.44 and the p value changes from .04 to .000003. The correlated t test is more sensitive to the difference between the means. One effect of this is that smaller differences are more likely to lead to rejection of the null hypothesis. However, you should understand that the correlated t test has this effect only when subject scores are related.

Reading the Statistical Output

Figure 12–2 (see page 190) is a partial SPSS output for the independent t test for the stretch experiment. The full output has been excluded because additional information is printed that is not essential to the statistical analysis. In the upper panel, you can see that the means, standard deviations, standard errors of the means, and number of subjects (N) in each group (control and stretch) are reported. When examining the output, always check the value of N to make sure it is correct. This is a good quick check to make sure you have analyzed the correct data. The second panel is the

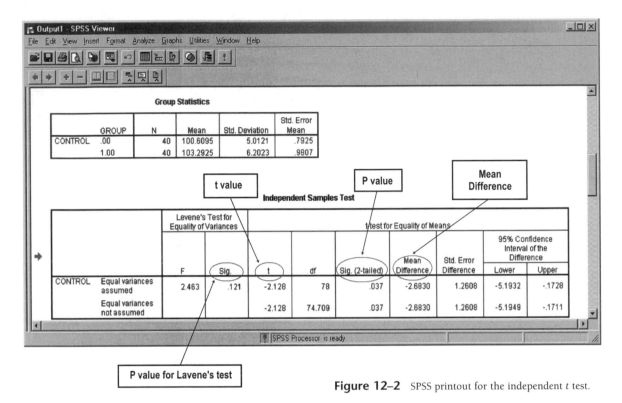

Figure 12–2   SPSS printout for the independent *t* test.

results from the independent *t* test. The fourth column is the actual *t* value. The sixth column, labeled "sig." (two-tailed), is the *p* value (the two-tailed test is the most common form of *t* tests; see our subsequent section on Statistical Power), and the seventh column is the difference between the means. You will also note that there are two rows labeled "equal variances assumed" and "equal variances not assumed." One of the assumptions of the *t* test is that the variances of each group are not statistically different. The SPSS output will include a test of equality of variances (Levene's test). If this test indicates that the variances are equal ($p \geq .05$), the top row contains the information you need. However, if the group variances are different from each other, use the bottom row. As you can see in this example, as is often the case, there is no difference in the *t* and *p* values between the rows.

Figure 12–3 contains the output for the dependent *t* test and is labeled "paired samples," which is another name for the correlated or dependent *t* test. As you can see, the top of the output is identical to the independent *t* test output. In the second panel, the third column contains the correlation (*r*), which measures the relationship between the pretest and post-test scores. The column labeled "sig." is the *p* value for the correlation, not the *t* test. The last two panels contain the dependent *t* test results. In the bot-

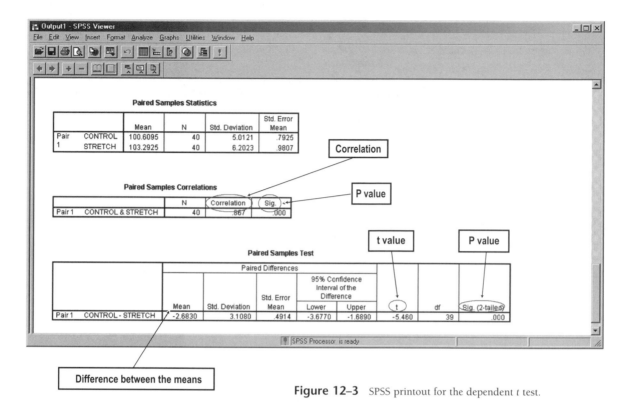

Figure 12–3 SPSS printout for the dependent *t* test.

tom panel, the second column contains the difference between the means. The third column contains the standard deviation for all the scores, the sixth column has the *t*, and the last two columns contain the degrees of freedom and the *p* value, respectively.

The Alpha and p Levels

We previously described the use of the *p* value, the probability with which the *t* could occur by chance. The *p* value applies to other statistics such as the *F* test and the Pearson correlation (*r*). You may also see alpha levels reported. Alpha levels are *p* values that are set prior to the experiment. Traditionally, alpha levels have been an integral part of the decision-making process. Researchers would specify these values before the experiment to indicate the risk they were willing to take in making a wrong decision to reject the null. For example, in the above experiment we used the *p* values after the study was completed. Alternatively, we could have set the alpha level at .05 and rejected the null hypothesis if the *p* value was any value less than .05. When using alpha levels, you do not need to report the actual *p* value.

Which method you use will depend on the journal in which you intend

In the Field

Eric is trying to decide whether to use alpha levels or p values. He has already decided that he will use .05 as the cutoff value, but recognizes that it would be just as easy to report the actual p values. To solve the problem, he consults the author's guide of several journals of interest. Based on this there is no clear answer, since some report the alpha and others report p. In preparing the first draft of his manuscript, he decides to include the actual p value. This way, the exact values are presented but can be easily deleted if he needs to report only the alpha level. Otherwise, by initially only including the alpha, he would later have to make several insertions of p values.

to publish. The *Journal of Athletic Training* uses the American Medical Association's guidelines (Iverson et al., 1998), which require *p* values. The preference for alpha levels or *p* values reflects a different decision strategy. Many researchers mistakenly believe that smaller *p* values mean the result is more important. This may explain why *p* values are preferred. It is important to understand that smaller *p* values do not indicate the importance of the finding. Rather, they only indicate that there is a smaller probability that the finding could have occurred by chance.

Researchers generally prefer *p* values and alpha levels to be at least equal to or below .05. How this is decided also reflects the researcher's decision strategy and a desire to minimize incorrectly rejecting the null hypothesis. However, you can apply a couple of rules of thumb. First, what is the alpha level other researchers have used? You can determine this by reviewing the articles in your literature review. You will probably find a pattern or convention that is used by previous researchers. Second, if no convention exists, then your decision is a judgment call. If you want to be very conservative, select the .01 level, but keep in mind that differences will be more likely to at .05 than at .01.

Statistical Power, Statistical Significance, and Clinical Significance

By now you should realize that the purpose of hypothesis testing is to detect differences, typically between (or among) group means. But what are your chances of finding a statistically "significant" difference? Obviously you do not want to develop a research project that will not find differences. This would be a waste of time and resources. Thus, you will find it useful to determine your chances of success before beginning the experiment.

Statistical Power

The *p* value indicates the probability of rejecting the null hypothesis when it is true. It is the probability of concluding that differences are due to chance when in fact they are due to chance. What we would really like to

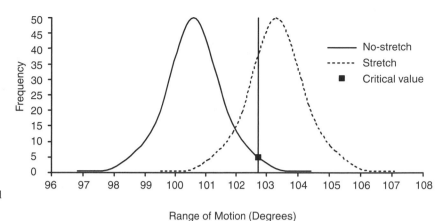

Figure 12–4 No-stretch and stretch group distributions of the differences of the means.

know is the probability of rejecting the null hypothesis when it is false. This is known as statistical power. Figure 12–4 illustrates the basic concept behind statistical power. You will notice that the figure contains two hypothetical normal (bell-shaped) curves. Each curve represents a sampling distribution of many means. Assume that we have taken repeated samples and calculated the mean for each sample. Using the stretching experiment, the left curve represents a sampling distribution of many means for the no-stretch condition of our experiment. Conversely, the right curve represents the means of samples that receive the stretching treatment. Thus, the left and right curves represent the null and alternative hypotheses, respectively. The mean of the no-stretch curve is 100.5°. Notice that even when the null is true, different samples (represented by different points along the curve) will have different mean ROMs. This entire distribution is a chance distribution. Thus we can determine the probability of any difference occurring by chance. A small percentage of the samples have means that are very different from the population mean of 100.5°. These discrepancies are due to chance (or sampling error). We have added a line above which only 5 percent of the means fall that represents the upper end of the .05 significance point. In other words, flexibility mean scores to the left of the line occur 97.5 percent of the time by chance, whereas flexibility scores to the right of the line only occur 5 percent of the time by chance.

You will remember that if the difference between the means could occur less than 5 percent of the time by chance, you would declare that that there was a real difference between the stretch and no-stretch groups. If that is the case, then you are making the assumption that the right curve correctly represents the stretch population.

From these curves you can determine the statistical power of your experiment. Specifically, the area of the stretch curve to the right of the .05 line represents the power of your statistical test. The more of the stretch curve that is to the right (or beyond) of the .05 line, the greater the chance you will find a difference. It should be obvious to you that the further the curves are apart, the more statistical power you will have. The distance between the stretch and no-stretch curves represents the treatment's effect size, the offset that is produced by the treatment. If the treatment had no effect, the stretch curve would completely overlap the no-stretch curve, and the two curves would be indistinguishable from each other. Thus, as the effect size increases, the two curves overlap less. In planning experiments, it is important to be sure that you are using an effective treatment, since this will increase your effect size and thus your statistical power.

Statistical power is also affected by sample size and the alpha level. For example, if you change the alpha level from .05 to .01, this would move the significance point further to the right and reduce the amount of the stretch curve to the right of the line (Fig. 12–5A). Conversely, increasing the number of subjects in the groups increases power by narrowing the two curves. As the curves narrow, they overlap less, and more of the stretch curve is to the right of the significance point (Fig. 12–5B).

Statistical power is also affected by whether tests are one-tailed (i.e., directional) or two-tailed (nondirectional). The example given in Figure 12–4 is a one-tailed test. In other words, the 5 percent rejection area was placed on one side of the curve. If the test had been two-tailed, the 5 percent area would have divided in half (i.e., 2.5 percent) and each half distributed to either tail of the distribution (Fig. 12–5C). As you can see from the figure, this results in less of the stretch curve being to the right of the critical point and a reduction in statistical power.

Two other factors that increase power are correlated measures and measurement reliability. As illustrated with the correlated t test example above, when your measures are correlated, the same difference between the means in the data will produce a larger t value. Similarly, the more reliable your measure, the more powerful your statistical test. As discussed in Chapter 9, low measurement reliability results in more measurement error, and error can be thought of as the background noise in your measure. Obviously, if you can reduce the background noise (i.e., error), then you have a greater chance of finding a difference (i.e., more power).

Statistical versus Clinical Significance

Unfortunately, statistical significance and statistical power cannot tell you whether your results are important. Statistical decision making is a process of logic, and the statistics are only tools to help you make logical choices. Likewise, whether the difference you found is important or not does not depend on the statistical finding. One factor it depends on is your judgment. You will recall that in the stretching study the two groups differed by 2.68°. Thus, the treatment produced an increase in knee range of motion of approximately 3°. And you will recall that this difference was statistically significant. But is this difference important? If you believe, or if other research has shown, that this 3° increase reduces quadriceps strains, then it

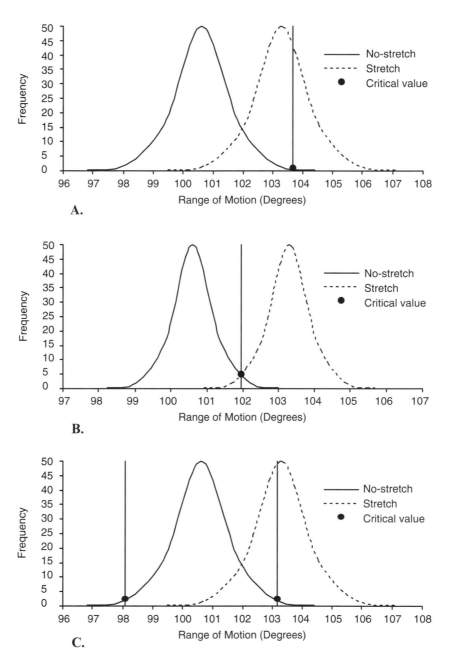

Figure 12–5 (A) Statistical power is diminished by changing the alpha from .05 to .01 (B) Increasing the number of subjects narrows the curves' widths, decreasing the overlap and increasing the statistical power. (C) A two-tailed test divides the alpha level into two sections, reducing the statistical power.

is important. This coincides with Cohen's (1988) definition of effect size. He defines effect size as:

$$\text{Effect size} = \frac{\text{Difference of knee ROM}}{\text{Control group ROM standard deviation}} \quad (12\text{--}8)$$

Cohen suggests that an effect size of .30 is low, an effect size of .50 is moderate, and an effect size of .80 is high. He also suggests that an effect size of .80 is visible to the naked eye. So an effect size of .80 should be obvious to a clinician. Knowing what difference are or are not important is one of the major challenges that you will face as a researcher.

Statistical Errors

Researchers want to demonstrate that the null hypothesis is not true. If you believe that there is only a small chance that the null hypothesis is true (e.g., less than 5 times in 100), you reject the null hypothesis. If other causes can be ruled out, this may mean that the treatment worked. But what if the treatment did not work and your significant results are due to chance? Using the stretching experiment example, the independent t test had a p value equal to .04, meaning that the findings of the experiment could occur by chance 4 percent of the time. What if that is exactly what happened and the results were due to chance and not the treatment? Obviously your decision to reject the null hypothesis would be wrong. That is, you rejected the null hypothesis when it was true. This is called a type I statistical error. Generally, we want to reduce our type I error, and we do this by keeping our alpha values low. How do you know that you made a type I error? You never do for sure, but replicating a study will increase your confidence. If you get the same results more than once from several different experiments, then you can be more certain that your results are due to the treatment and not chance.

Conversely, it is also possible that you will not reject the null hypothesis when the alternative hypothesis is true. In other words, you would declare the treatment did not work when it did. This is called a type II error. In general, researchers prefer to make this error than a type I error. It is believed that it is scientifically "safer" to miss a real difference than to declare a difference when none exists. Finally, it is important to understand that these two errors are inversely related to each other. In other words, as you reduce your chances of making a type I error, you increase your chances of making a type II error, and vice versa.

Solutions to Common Problems

Several problems are common in using statistics in athletic training research. The most common problem with statistical testing is selecting the alpha or *p* value. Should you use .05 or .01? There is no clear answer to this question. In athletic training research, either value is acceptable, and we usually use .05 as the criterion. A second problem is increasing statistical power. This can be achieved by making sure that your treatment is as potent as possible, that you measure a precisely as possible, and that you have enough subjects. The latter factor is the easiest for you to control. Although it creates more work, we encourage you not to be skimpy with your number of subjects. Probably the most difficult problem to solve is determining how big of a difference for which you should look. There is no clear answer to this. You might be guided by results from pilot testing and the results of other studies.

Summary

The purpose of hypothesis testing is to provide a logical method by which to make research decisions. The statistical tests that you use are tools to help you make those decisions. Specifically, they help you determine whether your results occurred by chance. Statistical tests help you go beyond the specific group differences and make inferences to hypothetical or real populations.

Activities

1. Find research studies that used the independent *t* test and the dependent *t* test. Summarize the studies and why each test was used.
2. Take the data given in Table 12–1, enter it into SPSS and run the independent *t* analysis.
3. Use the same data and run the dependent *t* analysis.

References

Cohen, J. (1988). *Statistical power analysis for the behavioral sciences* (2nd ed.). Hillsdale, NJ: Lawrence Erlbaum Associates.
Iverson, C., Flanagin, A., & Fontanarosa, P.B. (Eds.). (1998). *American Medical Association manual of style* (9th ed.). Baltimore: Williams & Wilkins.

Bibliography

Myers, J., & Well, A. (1991). *Research design and statistical analysis*. New York: Harper-CollinsPublishers.
Runyon, R.P., & Haber, A. (1991). *Fundamentals of behavioral statistics*. New York: McGraw-Hill, Inc.

Analysis of Variance

Objectives

After reading this chapter, you will:
- Be able to design a one-way analysis of variance.
- Be able to design a factorial analysis of variance.
- Know how to interpret an *F* table.
- Be familiar with different methods of post hoc testing.
- Know how to interpret post hoc tests.

Questions

While reading this chapter, think about answers to the following questions:
1. What is the difference between the *t* test and the *F* test?
2. Can I use the *t* test to compare multiple groups?
3. Can I test for how two different variables interact with each other?
4. How do I structure the data for two independent variables?
5. What is a mean square?
6. Why are there different post hoc tests?
7. Which post hoc test is best?

Between Subjects Designs: Analysis of Variance

In Chapter 12 we introduced selected statistical concepts you need to know when you conduct or read research. We also introduced a statistical test known as the *t* test. The *t* test is used in studies to compare the means of two sets of data. Sometimes a comparison is made of the means of two groups (independent *t* test), e.g., between a group that receives compression after an ankle sprain and one that does not; these are often referred to as "between subjects" designs. And sometimes a single group is measured twice and the means from the two times are compared (dependent *t* test), e.g., testing balance before and after wearing orthotics; these are often called "within subjects" designs. In the next two chapters, we will deal with the use of the analysis of variance (ANOVA) to analyze data from between subjects and within subjects studies. This chapter deals with between subjects designs (the independent t test equivalent), and Chapter 14 deals with within subjects designs (the dependent t test equivalent). Between subjects designs are particularly useful when you are concerned about learning or carryover effects (e.g., fatigue) or when you want to minimize the task to be completed. They are also useful when the independent variable cannot be manipulated (e.g., occurrence of an ACL injury or gender).

Limitations of the t Test

The use of the t test is associated with relatively simple research questions—questions about two groups. For example, what is the effect of stretching on flexibility? Is joint reposition sense different at 30° degrees than at 90°? Is ankle mobility different with a brace than without? Clearly, these are very limited research questions.

The t test model is too simple to be used to simultaneously contrast a number of different variations of an intervention. For instance, if you wanted to study which ways of stabilizing the knee (e.g., a neoprene sleeve, a functional brace, taping) are more effective than one another or than not bracing at all (i.e., a control), the t test could not be used to compare the multiple methods of stabilization. The t test is also too simple to simultaneously look at the effect of more than one independent variable. For instance, if you wanted to examine the effect of different variations of bracing (independent variable one = type of bracing) for knees that vary in terms of the severity of the injury (independent variable two = severity of the injury), the t test could not be used to make all of these comparisons *simultaneously*

We commonly make statements like, "Athletes would have better range of motion if they stretched." We assert that stretching would improve range of motion; but certainly individual athletes differ in the amount of ROM they have. Thus, you might propose that ROM is a function of stretching and individual differences. It should be fairly obvious that if you want to test this proposition alone, then it is absolutely necessary to be able to rule out any other factors that might affect range of motion, e.g. tissue warming from a hot pack.

You would have to devise a study (see Display 13–1) in which the only sources of variation in measures of ROM would be stretching and uncontrolled individual differences (including measurement error). This implies that you can control who gets the treatment, when they get the treatment, and the exact nature of the treatment. (As you will remember, these are the procedures of experimentation.) To do this, you would take some number of subjects and randomly assign them to different groups. One group would

Display 13-1	**Research: ROM Is a Function of Stretching and Individual Differences**

Research question:	Is ROM a function of stretching?
Dependent variable:	Knee range of motion
Independent variable:	Stretching
Statistical test:	Control group + static stretching = *t* test

complete a stretching protocol (e.g., static stretching) and the other would not (the control group). Random assignment removes systematic differences (such as only the less flexible people being assigned to the treatment group) between the groups. When they were finished, you would measure the ROM of all subjects and compare range of motion of the two groups using a *t* test. But you could not add a third group (e.g., PNF stretching) and compare the groups with the *t* test. This leaves you hanging—you have a valid question and a well-designed study, but no way to reach a conclusion.

ANOVA

Fortunately, R.A. Fisher, a statistician working in the field of agriculture, developed a technique called the analysis of variance (ANOVA) that allows you to make many comparisons simultaneously. The basic logic of ANOVA is that, under certain conditions, you can analyze an observed behavior by breaking it down into the components that produced it.

Fisher introduced us to a new way of thinking that includes partitioning variations in the behavior. Specifically, behavior is partitioned into the factor or factors that may have produced the differences between the groups and into randomized and uncontrolled factors (these include individual differences and measurement error).

Going back to our ROM research from the previous section, you wish to determine whether or not the control and stretch groups are different from each other. But you need a way of thinking about the components that make up any individual's score. If all of the individuals were identical and drawn from a population of identical persons, then all of the knee ROM scores would be the same and they would each be equal to the mean of the population. However, you have treated each group of individuals differently and thus you would expect that any individual's score would be equal to the population mean (average knee ROM) plus whatever effect the treatment (stretching) had. This effect of the treatment is defined as the deviation of the treatment mean from the population mean. But individuals will differ from one another even if they are treated equally. We call this error (*e*). Error is the deviation of individuals' scores around each treatment population's mean. In other words, your knee ROM or any other person's rarely matches the population's mean knee ROM. The difference between your knee ROM and the mean population knee ROM is the error.

We have begun to talk about a score as being a function of two types or sources of variability. One type is due to variability of treatment means around the mean for all treatments—the grand mean. The other is due to the variability of individual scores around a treatment mean. If we could subdivide, or partition, the total amount of variation of a set of scores into these two components, we might find a way to test the relative influence of the two components on the total amount of variability. In simpler terms, we might find a way to determine the proportion of the variability of individuals' scores that is an effect of belonging to a treatment group. The model for the design above suggests that ROM is a function of whether you stretch or not and error (ROM = Stretching + Error). An alternative model would suggest that stretching had nothing to do with ROM (ROM = Error).

This is the basic logic of the analysis of variance. We need a little machinery to turn this logic into statistical analysis. The basic formulae for the *t* test and the *F* test used in the analysis of variance are presented below:

$$t = \frac{\overline{X}_E - \overline{X}_C}{S_{\overline{X}_E - \overline{X}_C}} \quad \text{or} \quad \frac{\text{Difference of the means}}{\text{Standard error of the difference of the means}} \quad (13\text{--}1)$$

$$F = \frac{n\sum_j (\overline{Y}_j - \overline{Y}_{.})^2 / (a-1)}{\sum_i \sum_j (\overline{Y}_{ij} - \overline{Y}_{.j})^2 / a(n-1)} \quad (13\text{--}2)$$

As you recall, the *t* test is a ratio of the difference between a pair of means and an estimate of the "average" difference in pairs of means under the null hypothesis. Fisher created a ratio that was not limited to two means but could be applied to any number of means. Instead of comparing the means directly (as in the *t* test), he formed a new ratio that had the variance between group means (any number of means) as the numerator and the variance of the scores within the groups as the denominator (Formula 13–3).

$$F = \frac{\text{Variance between 2 or more group means}}{\text{Variance within groups}} \quad (13\text{--}3)$$

Not only did he create a statistic that was appropriate for any number of means, he also mathematically portioned the variance of the scores into two parts (variance between groups and variance within groups). These two parts correspond to the model above: ROM = Stretching + Error.

You can build a fairly complete picture of this process by developing an ANOVA summary table. This table documents the calculation of the variance components as well as the calculation of the *F* test (Table 13–1). The first column identifies the Sources of Variance. These "sources" should

Table13–1 • ANOVA Summary Table

Source of Variance	Degrees of Freedom (df)	Sum of Squares (ss)	Mean Square (ms)	F
Stretching (between groups)	1	143.97	143.97	4.53
Error (within groups)	78	2479.98	31.80	

reflect your research model. In this case it is that ROM = Stretching + Error. Two sources are given in the first column of the table: Stretching and Error. These are often referred to as "Between Groups" (Stretch) and "Within Groups" (Error). You will remember that a variance is equal to the sum of the squared deviations of scores around a mean divided by degrees of freedom. The degrees of freedom (df), the sum of the squared deviations (ss), and the variance or mean of the squares (ms) are in columns two, three, and four of the table. The value of the F test is given in the fifth column. Note that in this particular case, it is a ratio of the between group variance over the within group variance.

The simple logic for this is that if the variance between the stretch and no-stretch groups is no more than the variance within the groups (individual differences), you would probably conclude that a stretching protocol does not add anything to ROM over and above individual differences. The statistical logic has to do with the expected values of these variances. The expected value of the between group variance includes both the "effect" of the stretching protocol and "error," while the expected value of the within group variance includes only error.

Expected value of the between group variance =   Error + Stretching

Expected value of the within group variance =   Error

Note that if there is no effect of the stretching protocol, then stretch = 0 and this ratio reduces to error/error. In other words, when the null hypothesis is true, there is no statistical difference between the stretching protocol groups in ROM. ROM is apparently just a function of individual differences.

The One-Way Analysis with Two Groups

The one-way analysis is used to test multiple groups on only one factor. In the example above, the factor was stretching with two groups (or levels), stretch and no stretch. In contrast, let's assume you decide to study the effect of ankle fatigue on single leg balance (Display 13–2). Fatigue is the factor with two groups, fatigue and no fatigue. To do this you randomly assign people to the groups. The first group will not receive the treatment and will serve as the control group. Subjects in the second group have their ankle fatigued on an isokinetic dynamometer. More specifically, the fatigue group performs repetitive isokinetic inversion and eversion contractions until the peak torque of the evertors falls below 50 percent of the peak torque of the first three contractions. Following fatigue, postural sway is measured using a force plate. The data for this are shown in Figure 13–1. The first column (fatigue) is the grouping variable. Zero indicates the no-fatigue group and 1 indicates the fatigue group. This is how the computer program will recognize which balance scores belong to each group. There is no specific rule for coding the groups. However, it often is logical to label

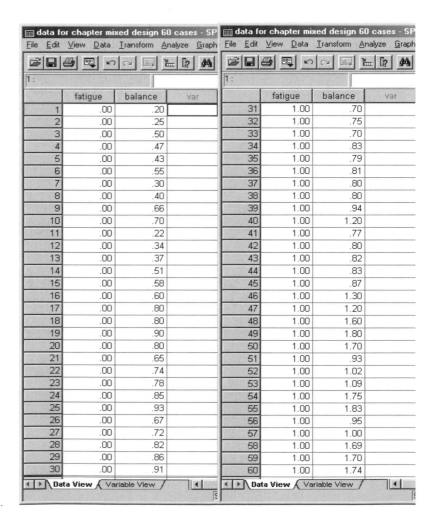

Figure 13–1 Data structured for the one-way ANOVA.

the control group with the lowest code (i.e., 0). The second column (balance) is the individual's postural sway score. Look at the scores. Does every subject have a score? The scores range from .20 to 1.74. Do the scores look reasonable to you, given what you know about measuring postural sway? Once you "eyeball" the data to make sure it looks correct, you should also look at the "Descriptives" analysis included with the ANOVA (see description below). This will report the means and standard deviations. This should help you detect scores that are excessively high or low (otherwise know as outliers). If you detect outliers, you should double-check the individual score to ensure that it is correct. Sometimes outliers are real scores, but most of the time they are data entry errors.

The F Table

Figure 13–2 provides the results from using the General Linear Model Analysis of Variance program from SPSS (Statistical Package for the Social

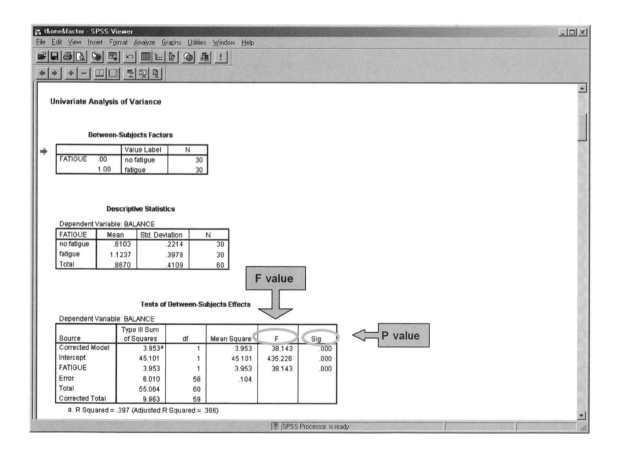

Figure 13–2 SPSS output for the two-group one-way ANOVA.

Display 13-2 | **Research: The Effect of Ankle Fatigue on Single-Leg Balance**

Research question:	Does ankle fatigue have an effect on single-leg balance?
Dependent variable:	Postural sway
Independent variable:	Fatigue with two levels (fatigue and no fatigue)
Statistical tests:	One independent variable with 2 groups = t test or one-way ANOVA

Sciences). There are three subtables in this figure. The first subtable, "Between-Subjects Factors," gives the name of the independent variable (or factor) in the first column, the levels (called value labels) in the second column, and the number of subjects (N) in each of the groups in the third column. The second subtable, "Descriptive Statistics," provides the sway means and standard deviations for each of the subgroups and for the total group of subjects. Look at the means. Is one higher than the other? Is the difference between the means what you thought it would be? Look at the standard deviations. Are they small or large relative to the means? Are the standard deviations of the two groups similar? The third subtable, "Tests of Between-Subjects Effects," is the analysis of variance summary table that we described previously and showed in Table 13–1.

You will notice that the tests of between-subject effects include some additional information not mentioned above. Let's look at the information that is most relevant to our discussion. The subtable contains six columns. The first lists the sources of variance—Fatigue and Error. In your model, these are the only factors that account for score variance. The second is the Sum of Squares. The third is the Degrees of Freedom (labeled "df"). The fourth is the Mean Square or variance for each factor. The fifth and sixth column are the F value and p value (labeled Sig. for significance), respectively. Of these six columns, you will report only three of them in a journal article: F, df, and Sig.

You will also note that the table includes six rows. For your purposes, you should focus on the rows labeled Fatigue and Error. Scan across the row labeled Fatigue until you get to the F value. It is 38.143. As explained above, this F is a ratio of the between groups variance over the within groups variance (labeled error), or 3.953/.104. The between groups variance is 38 times as big as the within group variance.

The printout gives the chance probability of this F as .000. (It would appear that there is no probability at all of obtaining an F value of this size, or bigger, when the null hypothesis is true. This is wrong.) This value has been rounded by SPSS. You should read it as $p < .001$ and when you report it in a paper or article, you should report it as $p < .001$. (You should note that SPSS truncates p values at three decimal places. If the fourth decimal is

.0005 - .0009, it will round p to .001 and report p as .001. If the fourth decimal is .00049 or smaller, it will round down and truncate p to .000. Thus, $p = .000$ implies the true p value was $< .0005$.) You will also need to report the degrees of freedom associated with the F test. You will report the degrees of freedom for both the numerator (between groups) and the denominator (within groups). Just as there are an infinite number of t distributions (one for each sample size or degrees of freedom), there are an infinite number of F distributions. Each F distribution is dependent on the number of groups (numerator) and the number of subjects within the groups (denominator). In this case, the degrees of freedom for groups is 1 (number of groups minus 1). The degrees of freedom for subjects within groups are 58. Each of these is found in the table under the column labeled df. In an article you would report this particular result as $(F = 38.14, df = 1,58, p < .001)$. Since the chance probability of the F is less than .05, you would reject the null hypothesis. You would also state that average sway was greater in the group that had been fatigued than in the group that had not been fatigued. Since this is a randomized experiment, you have evidence to conclude that fatigue has an effect on balance (at least as measured by sway).

The Relationship between F and t

In this first example, we have compared two groups. You probably recognize that this is exactly what we did with the t test in Chapter 12. So what is the difference? In the two-group design there is no difference in the results provided by the t test and ANOVA. Figure 13–3 has the results from the t test calculated on this exact same data set as we used for the ANOVA. Comparing the ANOVA results to the t test results you should notice at least three things. First, the degrees of freedom for the t test and the error term of the ANOVA are identical. Second, the square of the t value (i.e., –6.176) equals 38.143, which is the F value for fatigue. Finally, the p value for the t test and F test are also identical.

To emphasize, in the two-group design the t test and the F test produce the same results. They are different methods of obtaining the exact same result. You could use them interchangeably. The important thing is that ANOVA and the F test provide a model and a mechanism for pursuing much more complex research questions. The analysis of variance for two groups can be extended to three or more groups. In addition it extends to include multiple independent variables (factors).

Before we introduce designs involving more than two groups or more than one independent variable, let's review a few concepts and terms with which you need to be familiar. These terms are also shown in Display 13–3. The two-group design we reviewed above is referred to as a completely randomized design, since subjects are randomly assigned to groups. Since there is only one independent variable (fatigue), it is also referred to as a one-way design. The independent variable is also often referred to as a factor. The

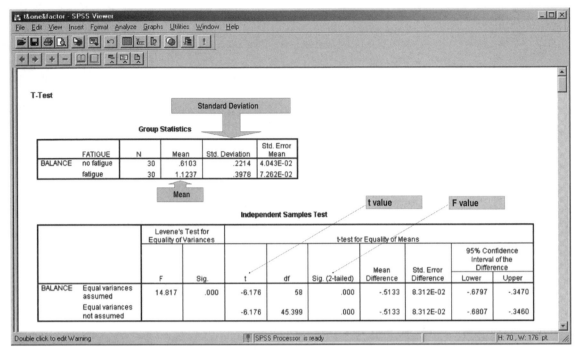

Figure 13–3 SPSS output for the *t* test using data from Figure 13–1.

independent variable in the example has only two conditions, or "levels." These are "fatigue" and "control." Theoretically, you could have any number of levels: you could have two or three or four alternative stretching methods, or you could include a placebo group as well as a control group.

Selection of levels should be theoretically justified and experimentally manageable. You could select the levels because they are the only levels in which you are interested. For example, in one experiment you might decide to study only static fatigue, while in another experiment you might want

Display 13-3

Vocabulary Review for Two-Group Designs

Completely randomized design	Design where subjects are randomly assigned to groups
One-way design	Study where there is only one independent variable
Factor	An independent variable
Level	The conditions for independent variables (factors)
Fixed factors	Factors that are the only levels of interest in a given study
Random factors	Factors that are randomly selected

to study both static and dynamic stretching. Regardless of the number of levels studied, if they are chosen because they are the only levels of interest, the independent variable is referred to as a fixed factor. When you complete your experiment, you can generalize only to the particular levels you studied.

In rare cases, the levels of a factor may be randomly selected. This factor would be called a random factor. For instance, it would be possible to randomly sample the angles at which isometric force measures are taken. Instead of taking force measures at 30°, 60°, and 90° of knee extension, the research could randomly sample some number (probably more than three) of angles from 0° to 90°. On completion of the experiment, the researcher could generalize the results across all angles.

The One-Way Analysis with Three Groups

The one-way analysis of variance can be used to compare three or more groups simultaneously. To illustrate the three-group design, let's design a study of the effect of visual reference on balance (Display 13–4). You believe that sway will increase with a restriction of visual reference. Although there are three groups, the general model remains the same. You expect that variance of the dependent measure is a function of only two things, the independent variable and error (Balance = Visual Condition + Error). Beginning with 60 subjects, we randomly assign them to one of three groups (20 subjects in each group):

1. With eyes open (control)
2. With eyes closed
3. With subjects wearing a conflict dome

The conflict dome is usually a Chinese lantern modified to fit on a person's head. Inside the lantern an "X" is placed directly in the person's field of vision for a reference. The individuals wearing the domes focus on the visual reference, which in this case sways with them. The purpose is to create an open-eyes condition without providing an external reference. This condition is considered to have a difficulty that is intermediate to the eyes-open and eyes-closed conditions. The data for this study are in Figure 13–4. The data file has two columns. The first column is labeled "balance" and contains each subject's sway measure. As before, you should inspect these data to see if the scores "look right" and if there are any obvious errors in the data. The second column is labeled "eyes." The numbers in this column represent group membership in the independent variable. Subjects in the control group have a 1 in this column, subjects in the conflict dome condition have a 2, and subjects in the eyes-closed condition have a 3. While you could use any numbers you want, we chose these numbers because we expect the most sway in the eyes-closed group (3) and the least sway in the eyes-open group (1).

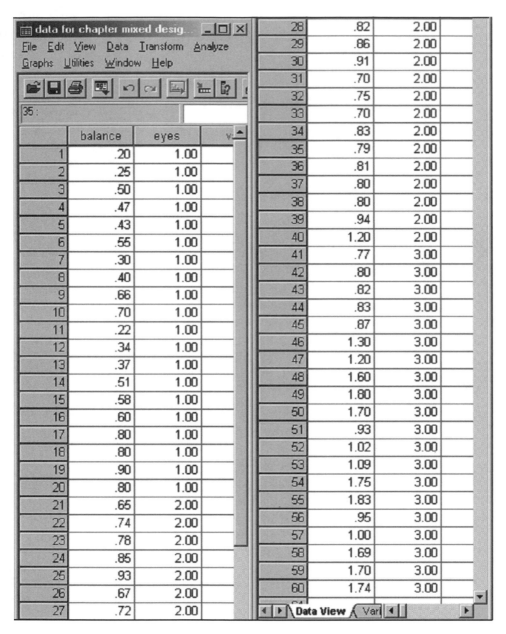

Figure 13–4 Data structured for the one-way ANOVA.

The F Table

The basic structure of the SPSS output for this analysis, Figure 13–5, is identical to that presented in Figure 13–2. There are three subtables. The first subtable, "Between-Subjects Factors," names the independent variable

Display 13-4

Research: The Effect of Visual Reference on Balance
Research question: Does visual reference have an effect on balance?
Dependent variable: Postural sway
Independent variable: Eyes condition (eyes open, conflict dome, eyes closed)
Statistical tests: One independent variable with more than two groups = One-way ANOVA

"Eyes," names the independent variable's groups (eyes open, conflict dome, eyes closed), and reports the number of subjects in each group (20). Be sure that these are what you meant them to be. The second subtable, "Descriptive Statistics," reports the means and standard deviations for the three groups. Note that the eyes-closed group has the highest mean and the eyes-open group has the lowest mean. Also note that the standard deviations of the three groups are quite similar. The third subtable, "Tests of Between-Subjects Effects," summarizes the ANOVA and provides the F test of interest.

As with the two-group case, the sources of variance, the sums of squares, degrees of freedom, mean squares, and Fs are given in the table. First, check each of these to see if they appear to be correct. One simple check is the degrees of freedom. The degrees of freedom on the "Eyes" row have changed from 1 to 2. Between-group degrees of freedom are always one less than the number of groups that you have. So for the two-group analysis it was 1 and for this analysis it is 2. The degrees of freedom for error (within group) have changed from 58 to 57. The calculation for this is:

df = (no. of groups)×(no. of subjects within each group -1) (13–4)

So df error = 3(20–1) = 57. The relevant F is calculated by dividing the variance for eyes (between-group variance) by the variance for error (within-group variance). The calculated F is in the Eyes row and it is 38.446. The between-group variance is more than 38 times as large as the within-group variance. As you can see from Figure 13–5, the F value is statistically significant with a p value reported as .000. As mentioned previously, you should report it as $< .001$. In an article, you would report it as $F = 38.45$, df, $= 2,57$, $p < .001$.

This F test provides what is known as an omnibus (all or overall) test. If the F test is not statistically significant, you would decide that you do not have enough evidence to conclude that these means are statistically different and you would discontinue your analyses. After a suitable mourning period, you would try to figure out what you did wrong and design a new study. Since this particular F is statistically significant, you would conclude that some pair of means (or pair combination) is statistically different from

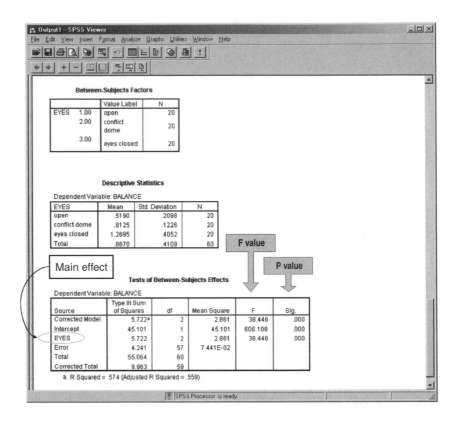

Figure 13–5 SPSS output for the three-group one-way ANOVA.

each other. But the *F* test does not tell which pair is statistically different. To find this out you must do additional tests. You need to directly compare the means. One alternative would be to use the *t* test to compare each of the possible pairs of means. You could, for example, calculate three *t* tests (eyes open versus conflict dome; eyes open versus eyes closed; conflict dome versus eyes closed). As we shall see shortly, the statistical probabilities for each of these three tests may not be appropriate for the set of three comparisons. As a result, statisticians have attempted to devise ways to hold the probability level constant across an entire set of comparisons. Sometimes these are referred to as multiple comparison tests or post hoc tests.

Post Hoc Tests

As we mentioned above, the statistical probabilities for multiple independent *t* tests after observing a statistically significant *F* may not be appropriate for the set of three comparisons. In Chapter 12, we introduced the notion of the type I error. Remember that statistical probability distributions provide us with the probability that the null is true. So when we reject the null hypothesis, there is always some probability that in fact the null is true. The alpha level is the probability of rejecting the null falsely that you, as the researcher, are willing to live with. One of the first decisions you make when using statistical tests has to do with the risk of rejecting the null hypothesis when it is actually true. It may be that this is why this kind of mistake is known as a type I error. The probabilities provided for the t distribution are probabilities derived for the case in which one t test is conducted, not two or three t tests. So when we make more than one comparison, these probabilities are not correct.

A simple example with coin tosses may help you understand. If you flip a coin, the probability of getting a head is .50. If you flip a coin a second time, the probability of getting a head on the second toss is also .50. But the probability of getting at least one head in the two tosses is .75 (How this is calculated is in Display 13–5.) Although the probability of getting a head on any single toss remains the same, the probability of getting at least one head continues to increase as the number of tosses in a "set" of tosses goes up. When the number of tosses in the set becomes quite large (say 10 or more), we can be fairly sure of having a head occur. But we are not usually interested in coin tosses in experiments. We are interested in things like the effect of alternative modalities on return to function. In our current example we are interested in different visual conditions. As we increase the number of comparisons in the set of comparisons to be made, we increase the probability of falsely rejecting the null hypothesis. Said simply, if we make lots of comparisons, we are almost certain to find one of them to be "statistically significant" when they really aren't.

Let's consider doing the three t tests for the current example. We might set an alpha level of .05 for each of the t tests. While this alpha level would be correct for each of the three tests, it would be incorrect for the *set* of three tests. The actual probability level for the set of three tests would be the sum of the alphas, .15. This is the probability of rejecting the null for at least one of the three comparisons. In other words, the probability of a Type I error for the set of three tests would not be .05 (which was our original alpha level), it would be .15. We would have accidentally increased our Type I error rate for this set of tests. As the number of comparison increases, the probability of a Type I error increases. Just like with the coin tosses, with large number of comparisons between means, it becomes very likely that at least one of them will be "statistically significant" when it really is not. A

Display 13-5	**Probability of Getting at Least One Head in Two Coin Tosses**			
		Coin Toss 1		
Coin Toss 2	Head = .5	Tail = .5		
Head = .5	Head × Head = .25	Head × Tail = .25	$3/_4$ = .75 or
Tail = .5	Tail × Head = .25	Tail × Tail = .25	.25 × 3 = .75

number of different post hoc tests have been devised (see multiple comparisons). Since the F test for visual condition was statistically significant, we decided to statistically compare the three pairs of means. The SPSS one-way analysis of variance program makes it possible to use a number of different post hoc tests. We used it to conduct a commonly used post hoc test devised by Tukey. The results of this test are given in Figure 13–6. As you can see, the post hoc table is organized into several columns. The first two columns identify the results of the comparisons among the three group means. The third column, Mean Difference, is the difference between the two respective group means. This can be useful in determining the size of the difference between groups. The next column is Standard Error of the difference between means (remember that this was the denominator of the t test). The probability values for each comparison are given in the column labeled Sig. The last two columns provide the upper and lower bounds of the 95 percent Confidence Interval.

The comparison between the eyes open and conflict dome means resulted in a p value of .003. Since our alpha level was .05, this comparison is significant. The comparison between the eyes open versus the eyes closed means resulted in a p value of .000 ($p < .001$). You conclude that these two means are statistically different and that sway is greater when the eyes are

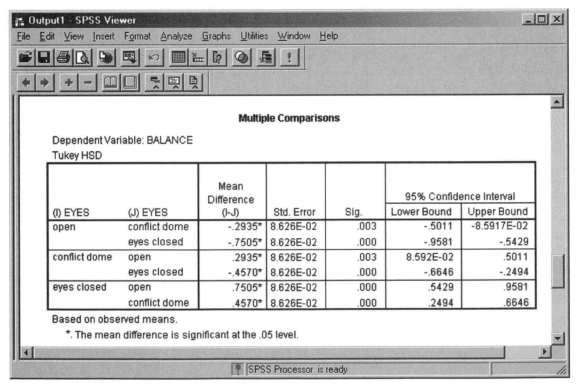

Figure 13–6 SPSS post hoc test output for the three-group one-way ANOVA.

closed than when they are open. (Do not be confused by the fact that the comparison between the conflict dome and eyes-open groups is repeated in this table.) The third relevant comparison is between the means for eyes closed and conflict dome. The *p* value is .000 Again this *p* value is less than .05, so you declare it to be statistically significant. Sway is greater with eyes closed than with the conflict dome on. You may conclude that the amount of sway with the eyes closed is greater than that with the conflict dome on, which is greater than that with eyes open.

The Factorial Analysis of Variance

Researchers in athletic training are often interested in studying the effects produced by two or more independent variables. Analysis of variance designs with multiple independent variables are referred to as factorial designs. To illustrate this, let's consider a study of the effect of fatigue and ankle instability on balance (Display 13–6). You believe that both fatigue and ankle instability may influence balance and that together there may be some kind of combined effect on balance. You suspect that fatigue will reduce balance. You also suspect that ankle instability will reduce balance. In addition, you expect that the presence of both ankle instability and fatigue will result in even poorer balance. We have presented an example of this in Figures 13–7 and 13–8. You recruit 60 subjects, 30 of whom have stable ankles and 30 of whom have unstable ankles. You randomly assign those with stable ankles to either a fatigue group or a nonfatigue group. Then you randomly assign those with unstable ankles to either a fatigue group or a nonfatigue group. The fatigue protocol described above is used. You now have four groups: (1) stable ankle with no fatigue, (2) stable ankle with fatigue, (3) unstable ankle with no fatigue, and (4) unstable ankle with fatigue. Each group has 15 subjects. From this four-fold table, you pose three research hypotheses. The first is that ankle instability will affect balance. The second is that fatigue will affect balance. The third is that there will be an "interactive" effect of ankle instability and fatigue on balance.

The data for this study are presented in Figure 13–7. There are 60 subjects. The first column, which is labeled "fatigue," is used to identify who is fatigued and who is not fatigued. Fatigued subjects are assigned a 1 and

Display 13-6

Research: Combined Effect of Fatigue and Ankle Stability on Balance

Research question:	Do fatigue and ankle instability affect balance?
Dependent variable:	Postural sway
Independent variables:	Fatigue (2 levels, fatigue and no fatigue) and ankle stability (2 levels, stable and unstable)
Statistical tests:	Multiple independent variables = Factorial ANOVA

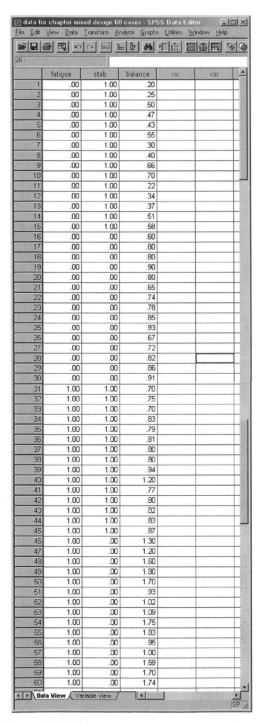

Figure 13–7   Data structured for the two-way ANOVA.

nonfatigued subjects are assigned a 0. The second column, labeled "stab," is used to identify subjects who have a stable ankle and those who have an unstable ankle. Those with a stable ankle are assigned a 1 and those with an unstable ankle have been assigned a 0. (Note that subjects with a stable ankle who have been fatigued have a 0 and a 1 in these two columns). The third column is labeled "balance." The sway scores for each individual subject are given in this column. Be sure that you inspect the data in each of these columns for potential errors.

There are three subtables in Figure 13–8. The first subtable, "Between-Subjects Factors," reports the number of subjects who have stable and unstable ankles (30 in each) and the number of subjects who have been fatigued and the number who have not been fatigued (30 in each). Descriptive statistics are given in the second subtable. Look carefully at this table. The sway means and standard deviations for each of the four groups are given. We can see a number of things in this table. Average sway scores (the value in the Mean column) are higher for the fatigued group than the not-fatigued group. Average sway scores are higher for the unstable ankle group than for the stable ankle group. The lowest average sway is for the subjects who have stable ankles and have not been fatigued. The highest average sway score is for the subjects who have unstable ankles and have been fatigued. These differences are what you might predict, but these differences may not be statistically significant. They may just be due to sampling error.

The F Table

A summary of the ANOVA is given in the third subtable, "Tests of Between-Subjects Effects," in Figure 13–8. Tests of the three hypotheses stated above can be found in this table. They are listed under "Source" (i.e., sources of variance) as stability (STAB), fatigue (FATIGUE), and (STAB*FATIGUE). Otherwise, the table is formatted exactly the same as the previous tables. By now you should be able to quickly find the F test and p value for each factor.

Main Effects

From the F table, you can see that the main effect for stability ($F = 78.145$, df $= 1,56$, $p < .0005$) and the main effect for fatigue ($F = 91.395$, df $= 1,56$, $p < .0005$) are statistically significant. Since both of these factors have only two levels (i.e., stable and unstable), no post_hoc test is necessary. We conclude that balance is worse for unstable ($\overline{X} = 1.1$) than stable ($\overline{X} = .63$) subjects and that balance is worse for fatigued ($\overline{X} = 1.12$) subjects than for subjects who have not been fatigued ($\overline{X} = .61$).

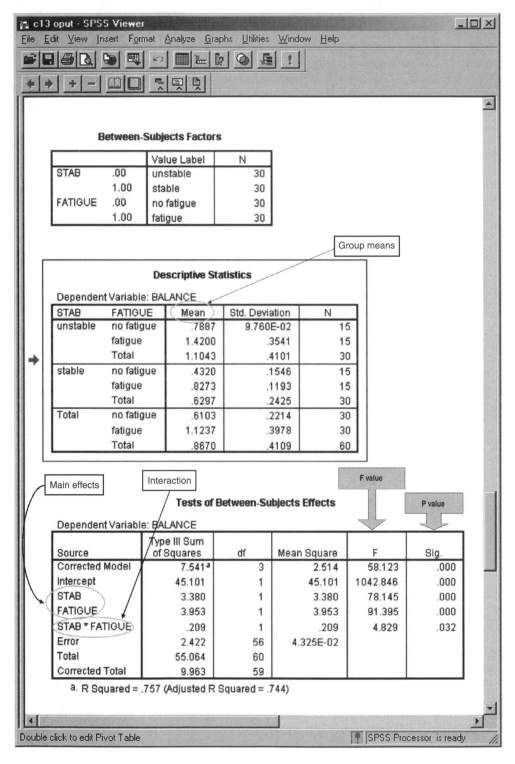

Figure 13–8 SPSS output for the two-way ANOVA.

Interactions

The third test is of the interaction. The F is statistically significant ($F = 4.83$, df $= 1.56$, p $= .032$). This indicates that the effect of fatigue on balance is different for stable subjects than it is for unstable subjects. The means for the four groups have been plotted in Figure 13–9. On visual inspection, you will note that the lines in the graph are not parallel. This is one simple way to detect the presence of an interaction. The pattern in the graph also suggests that fatigue has a bigger effect on unstable subjects than it does on stable subjects. However, we now have the same kind of problem that we had with three-group one-way ANOVA design. The F test does not indicate where the differences are. So we will conduct further (post hoc) tests. We have a number of different possibilities for post hoc testing. (See the Multiple Comparisons section.) The results of Tukey post hoc comparisons are presented in Table 13–2. There are six possible comparisons between means. Five of the six were statistically significant. The sway scores of subjects with unstable ankles in the no fatigue condition were not statistically different from the sway scores of subjects with stable ankles in the fatigued conditions. Table 13-2

Other Issues

More About Interactions

A significant interaction indicates that the effect of one independent variable is different over the levels of another independent variable. Interactions can take different forms. To illustrate this, assume you conduct an experiment on delayed-onset muscle soreness (DOMS). Specifically, you are interested in knowing whether ice applied after eccentric muscle contractions reduces pain as measured by a visual analog scale (VAS). You randomly

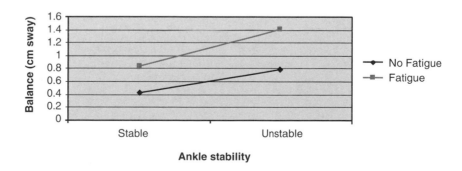

Figure 13–9 Graph of the interaction between ankle stability and fatigue.

Table 13–2 • **Critical Differences for the Tukey Post Hoc Test**

	Group Mean	Unstable, fatigued	Stable, fatigued	Unstable, no fatigue	Stable, no fatigue
		1.42	.8273	.7887	.4320
Unstable, fatigued	1.42		.593*	.631*	.988*
Stable, fatigued	.8273			.039	.395*
Unstable, no fatigue	.7887				.357*
Stable, no fatigue	.4320				

* $\overline{X}_1 - \overline{X}_2 \geq .222$ @ P=.05

assign subjects to either a control group or an ice treatment group. All of your subjects receive a DOMS manipulation. Because DOMS peaks between 48 and 96 hours, you decide to take pain measures at 24 hours, 48 hours, and 96 hours. Data for five possible outcomes are illustrated in Figure 13–10. In each of the five panels we have plotted the average pain scores for the control and DOMS groups at 24, 48, and 96 hours. Panels A and B illustrate a main effect but no significant interaction. The results in Panel A suggest a main effect for time. Pain increases from 24 to 96 hours at similar rates for both the control group and the group that receives ice. Ice doesn't seem to have any effect. Pain just gets worse across the three time intervals. The results in Panel B suggest a main effect for treatment factor (i.e., ice versus no ice). In this case no change occurs across time, but the ice group experiences less pain than the control group at each of the three time points.

Panels C and D represent two possible interactions. The results in Panel C suggest that while the pain after the first 24 hours for the control and ice group is similar, pain continues to increase across time for the control group but lessens for the ice group. Because of the fact that pain is not different at the first time period, conclusions about the impact of ice must be limited to the specific time periods. This pattern represents what sometimes is called a disordinal interaction. The results in Panel D suggest that pain is less for the ice group after the first 24 hours and even less as time goes on. There is less pain reported by the ice treatment group than the control group and the difference between the two groups gets even greater at later time periods. In this case it would be reasonable to talk about both a main effect for treatment and an interactive effect of the treatment and time. Sometimes this is referred to as an ordinal interaction. The results in Panel E suggest that there is no effect of the treatment, no effect of time, and no interactive effect of treatment and time on subjects' report of pain.

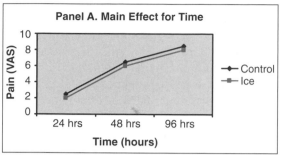

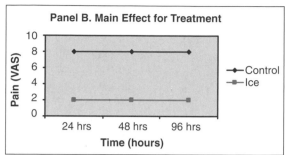

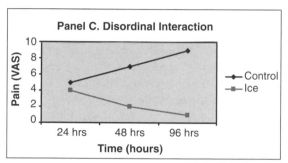

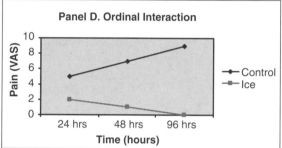

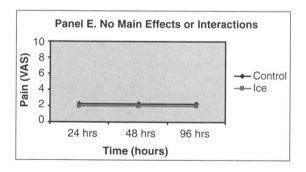

Figure 13–10 Graphical depiction of main effects and interactions.

Multiple Comparisons

When the researcher decides before conducting the research which comparisons are to be made, these are called a priori or planned comparisons. Planned comparisons are usually directly connected to specific research hypotheses that have been generated as a result of theory or previous research. As a result, they usually would not include all possible comparisons, which would provide a modicum of protection against type I errors. One choice would be to make only orthogonal contrasts. These are contrasts that are nonoverlapping (independent of one another), and the sum of the contrasts reflects the total variance. Since this is the case, no probability adjustment needs to be made for orthogonal contrasts. For example, Figure 13–11 illustrates a set of orthogonal contrasts among three groups (control, placebo, and ultrasound). For the orthogonal contrast to work, you must specify the contrasts in advance. In this case you hypothesized that the placebo and control group were not different (contrast 1). If this proves true, your plan would be to combine the placebo and control groups, and compare that new group to the ultrasound group (contrast 2). Nonorthogonal contrasts, on the other hand, are not independent of one another, and so the sum of nonorthogonal contrasts adds up to more than the total variance. Figure 13–11 also shows a nonorthogonal contrast. In this case, the placebo and control groups are compared to each other (contrast 1). Then the placebo and treatment groups are compared (contrast 2). In this case, the placebo group is used in both comparisons, making them related to each other or nonorthogonal. Dunnett devised a strategy that would contrast the mean of the control group with the mean of each experimental group. Comparisons would not be made between experimental groups. It is somewhat unfortunate that the use of planned contrasts has fallen into disfavor, since the concept of planned comparisons would seem to be consistent with thoughtful, purposive research.

On the other hand, it is often the case that researchers do not know exactly what tests they want do before they start the research. In addition, exploratory analyses can be an extremely valuable tool for a researcher involved in a continuing line of research. The desire to clarify results and the desire to do exploratory analyses has led to the use of a posteriori or post hoc testing. As the term suggests, post hoc testing is only done after

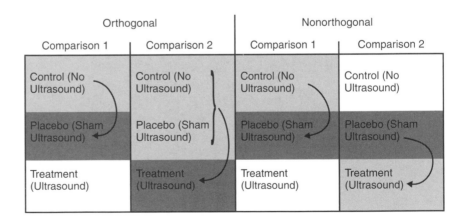

Figure 13–11 Orthogonal and nonorthogonal contrasts. In each column the light gray group is compared to the dark gray group. White groups are not included in the respective comparisons.

the occurrence of a statistically significant F. This provides an initial level of protection since further analysis is not done for a nonsignificant F.

A number of strategies have been devised to protect against an increase in type I errors. As you will see, a major difference among these strategies has to with how the research defines the set of comparisons to be made. As the number of comparisons within sets increases, the post hoc tests become more conservative, making it less likely to reject the null hypothesis. A researcher could theoretically define a set as all possible comparisons in the researcher's lifetime, all comparisons within a given line of research, all possible comparisons within a single experiment (experiment-wise), or all the comparisons with some conceptual or logical grouping (family-wise). It is the obligation of the researcher to make a case for the choice made.

The method of least significant difference (LSD) provides only the protection of the F. After a significant F, multiple t tests are performed. Since no probability adjustments are made, this strategy will result in more type I errors than other strategies. Two of the most common strategies are Tukey's honest significant difference (HSD) and the use of a Bonferroni correction. Tukey's test defines the set or family of comparisons as all the possible comparisons between some set of means. For example, in the ultrasound experiment described above there are three combinations:

1. Control + Placebo
2. Control + Ultrasound
3. Placebo + Ultrasound

The Tukey HSD error rate is held constant across the entire set of comparisons (in this case three, but it could be more). Simply put, the probability of one or more type I errors would be .05 for the whole family of comparisons. Using the Bonferroni correction, the researcher would divide the alpha level by the number of comparisons to be made. If you are going to make three comparisons, as in the ultrasound example, and your alpha level was .05, divide .05 by 3. The resulting probability .017 would be used as the new probability level for each comparison. Once again, this would maintain the alpha level for the family of tests at .05. If you made 20 comparisons with an initial alpha level of .05, each of the 20 comparisons would now be made with a probability level of .0025 (i.e., .05/20). You can see that if the number of comparisons is very large, the probability level becomes very small and thus conservative.

We would like to mention two more possibilities that we believe are appropriate for comparing means in athletic training research. Either could be used within a planned comparisons framework or post hoc comparisons framework, and either could be done using a Bonferroni correction. They are important for you because each of them is usually used *after* the occurrence of a statistically significant interaction. As you remember, a significant interaction indicates that the effect of one independent variable is different over the levels of another independent variable. In our example of a factorial design to study the effect of fatigue on the balance of subjects with stable and unstable ankles, we used Tukey post hoc tests to interpret the interaction. We did six different comparisons. We concluded that fatigue had a greater effect on subjects with unstable ankles than those with stable ankles. We could have demonstrated this effect with simple effects testing. With simple effects testing, we might have reached the same conclusion with only two comparisons: (1) a comparison of the sway scores of fatigued and nonfatigued subjects with stable ankles; and (2) a comparison of the sway of fatigued and nonfatigued subjects with unstable ankles. This would be a more powerful test, since with a Bonferroni correction (.05/2) we would use a probability of .025.

The last strategy we would like to mention is more complex but more targeted to what an interaction really is. This strategy would involve a complex contrast. The complex contrast that would be appropriate would be to compare the difference in sway scores of fatigued and nonfatigued subjects with stable ankles with the difference in sway scores of fatigued and nonfatigued subjects with unstable ankles. While this approach is unusual in athletic training research, it is the approach that is most targeted to the exact meaning of an interaction effect.

As you can see from this short discussion, choosing a multiple comparison strategy requires a number of decisions. The most important is what your research question is. In addition, you can decide which comparisons you will make in advance of conducting the research or you can decide that you will only make specific comparisons after the occurrence of a statistically significant F. Finally, you can decide which comparisons you will consider to be a set or family of comparisons. Each of these decisions affects the power of your tests and the production of possible type I errors.

Violation of ANOVA Assumptions

Use of ANOVA involves three assumptions about the populations from which samples are drawn: (1) that the populations are normally distributed;

In the Field

Craig has just completed his statistical analysis and has a significant F. He knows that he has a difference, but he doesn't know where the difference is. As a result, he must select a post hoc test. Because of ease of use, he considers conducting a Bonferroni correction on multiple t tests. However, he has determined that he has 10 comparisons of interest. This means that the p value would have to be .005 or smaller to be significant. However, a p value that small would greatly reduce his chances of finding significance and is probably too conservative. Alternatively, Craig decides to use the Tukey honest significant difference (HSD) to control his error rate because it is accepted in the literature and is not as conservative as the Bonferroni correction.

(2) that there is homogeneity of variance among the groups; and (3) that the observations are independent. Fortunately, it has been found that the *F* test is not extremely sensitive to violations of the first two assumptions. Only when "populations are very skewed, the *n'* s are very small, or one-tailed tests" (Glass & Hopkins, 1984, p. 403) are used is there a major concern about normality of populations. Violations of homogeneity of variance also have negligible effects except under special conditions (Glass & Hopkins, 1984). The assumption of independence of observations is of greater concern. This is especially a concern when studies are done with intact groups that may involve interactions among the subjects. Subjects' scores may then become interdependent. In most research in athletic training, subjects are run individually, so this is not a concern.

Design Considerations

When building more complex research designs, several things should be considered, including research protocols, homogeneity of variance, and manipulation of variables.

Importance of Protocols

Establishing clear research protocols is an important control for experimental research. As you recall, the *F* test is composed of two variances (mean squares, in ANOVA terms) in a ratio form. Specifically, the numerator of the *F* is the factor variance (e.g., fatigue in the examples above) and the denominator is error (or the unexplained variance). From a practical framework, your goal is to maximize the numerator and minimize the denominator. This is done by controlling extraneous factors. For the denominator, this is done by minimizing differences among subjects. In a true experimental design this is best done by randomly assigning subjects to the different groups. Randomization homogenizes the different groups, i.e., makes them similar and reduces the error variance in the ANOVA. The process of homogenization can be further improved by having specific entrance criteria for the subjects. For example, you may limit subjects with ankle instability to only those individuals with third-degree sprains. Using this criterion to limit who is admitted to the study and then randomly assigning subjects to control and experimental groups would be an effective method of reducing differences among subjects (and the *F* denominator) considerably. Thus, in designing your study you should give special consideration to factors such as age, body size, sex, fitness/activity levels, and so on. Failing to control these types of factors can add unwanted variability in your data and increase the ANOVA error term to unacceptably high levels.

Another source of error in your design can be variability in the implementation of your treatments. You can create unnecessary differences among subjects by applying your treatment inconsistently. In the DOMS experiment previously described, your goal should be to apply the ice treatment consistently. For example, your protocol should include a specific interval of time for the treatment, location, and method of application of the ice. If the method of application varies from subject to subject, this will increase the variability among subjects and increase the size of the error term in your ANOVA.

Alternatively, your goal is to maximize the size of the F test numerator. Remember, the numerator represents either a main effect or an interaction in which you are interested. Put another way, the numerator represents your treatment effects. To get a significant F test, your intention should be to maximize your treatment's effect. Similar to reducing error, one way to maximize your treatment is to apply it consistently. If factors such as time of application are not consistently applied, you are in essence applying different treatments that will weaken your treatment effect. To maximize your treatment effect, it is also important to select potent treatments and/or potent treatment levels. For example, a 2-minute ice treatment will probably have the same effect (i.e., not reduce pain) as no treatment at all, because it has no potency. Similarly, ice applications of 10 minutes are not likely to reduce pain any more than ice treatments of 12 minutes because they are too similar. However, an ice treatment of 10 minutes will probably have a different effect than an ice treatment of 20 minutes. How you should make this determination is not completely straightforward. Your literature review or clinical practice standards will often suggest what the appropriate treatments are.

In the Field

Tim is studying the effects of a shoulder brace on shoulder joint reposition sense in the internal and external rotation directions. One of his concerns is natural differences among subjects. Tim suspects that healthy overhead-throwing athletes will be better than nonathletes and is concerned that if he mixes the two, he may increase the variability among subjects and reduce his chances of finding a significant difference. To solve this problem, he decides to limit his study to overhead-throwing athletes. Tim is also concerned that the quality of the brace might change over time and have a different treatment effect from one subject to another. This could also increase variability and decrease his chances of finding a difference. To better ensure consistency in the treatment, he decides to use a new brace for each subject. Finally, Tim wants to maximize the treatment effect. Because his theory suggests that compression of the brace on the skin and joint are responsible for hypothesized improvements in joint reposition sense, he decides to use a neoprene style brace to maximize the compressive effects.

Homogeneity of Variance

One of the assumptions of ANOVA is that the populations from which the samples are drawn have equal variances. Although violations of this assumption tend to have minimal effects on the F tests in ANOVA, it is of practical concern for the researcher to implement strategies that minimize heterogeneity of variance across different treatment implementations. The best way to do this is to ensure that treatments for the treatment groups are applied consistently. For example, if you are testing ultrasound treatments across different groups, you would want to standardize the treatment for each group, such as wattage, frequency, area to be treated, and so on. These can differ across groups/treatments (that may be the point of your experiment) but should not differ within the same group/treatment. If within the same group you apply the treatment inconsistently, the variance of the dependent measure will increase. Other examples would include standardizing testing positions on isokinetic dynamometers, stretching protocols, and EMG electrode placement

Manipulated and Nonmanipulated Independent Variables

As you read and conduct research in athletic training, you will encounter some independent variables that are controlled or manipulated (e.g., fatigue) by the researcher and others over which the researcher has no control (e.g., ankle instability). Manipulated variables are controlled by the researcher in four ways. First, the researcher controls who gets it by random assignment. Second, the researcher controls the exact nature of the independent variables. This is one of the reasons specific protocols are so important. Third, the researcher controls exactly when the variable is to occur. It doesn't begin before the researcher wants it to and it doesn't continue any longer than the researcher wants it to. Fourth, the researcher controls the exact duration of the independent variable. With nonmanipulated variables, the researcher has no control of these things. Manipulated variables are under the control of the researcher and include such things as tissue temperature (as with modalities research), hamstring stretching, and strength training. If fatigue is the independent variable, the researcher will control who is fatigued and who is not fatigued by random assignment of the subjects to these conditions. He or she will also specify when the protocol is to start, how long it should go on, and the level at which it is done. A variable that is manipulated in one study may not be manipulated in another study. Differences in balance after fatigue could be studied in a natural setting. After a player has played for 10 minutes, he could be brought to the sideline to measure balance. Note that in this case, players would not have been randomly assigned to fatigue and that the nature and amount of fatiguing would probably be related to position played by the player and a host of other factors. Often, we are interested in the effects of variables that either cannot be manipulated or that we are unable to manipulate. These variables may include gender, age groups, and injured versus noninjured groups. In each of these cases, the researcher selects the levels for these variables (injured versus uninjured) but doesn't actually manipulate the variable. The researcher may find that injured athletes produce less force than uninjured athletes.

While nonmanipulated independent variables provide insights to important questions, they also present a problem in attribution of causality. Is it the injury that results in lower force production? Or are weaker subjects (who produce less force) more likely to sustain injuries? As indicated in Chapter 7, for cause and effect to be determined, the researcher must have control of the variable of interest. Only then can you be sure that changes in the independent variable caused the change in the dependent variable. This is not the case with nonmanipulated variables. For example, differences between males and females in their ability to vertically jump are not necessarily related to their sex. Men don't jump higher because they are men; they jump higher because they have greater muscle mass than women. Thus, it may be more accurate to attribute the result to muscle mass. Another way to think about this is gender is acting as a proxy variable for muscle mass. In this example, this can be easily controlled by normalizing jump height by muscle mass, but it is often not that easy.

Summary

Analysis of variance (ANOVA) is the workhorse of athletic training research. In this chapter we presented the ANOVA in its basic forms: one-way and factorial. We also demonstrated that the *t* test and ANOVA are not different when only two groups are studied. Typically considered a method for experimental designs, ANOVA can be used with unmanipulated variables such as sex or injury status. The utility of ANOVA is that multiple independent variables can be tested simultaneously, and the interaction among variables can be studied. However, this versatility also adds complexity to the analysis. Since ANOVA detects differences among multiple groups but does not tell you which groups are different, post hoc tests and other methods of comparison among means are necessary. While, there is no clear choice among these methods, we have presented several common ones used in the athletic training literature.

Activities

1. Using one of the articles collected for your literature review, formulate an ANOVA table that includes the factors with levels, degrees of freedom, *F* values, and *p* values.
2. Using you own research study, develop the statistical plan outlining

independent variables, your dependent variables, design factors and levels of each factor, and post hoc (or a priori) tests you would perform.

3. Using pilot or complete data collected for your research project, conduct the statistical analysis you outlined above.

References

Glass, G. V., & Hopkins, K. D. (1984). *Statistical methods in education and psychology* (3rd ed.). Boston: Allyn & Bacon.

Bibliography

Brown, D. R., Michels, K. M., & Weiner, B. J. (1991). *Statistical principles in experimental design* (3rd ed.). New York: McGraw-Hill, Inc.

Myers, J., & Well, A. (1991). *Research design and statistical analysis.* New York: HarperCollins Publishers.

Chapter 14

Repeated Measures Designs

Objectives

After reading this chapter, you will:

- Recognize between-group and repeated measures designs.
- Explain the advantages and disadvantages of a repeated measures design.
- Distinguish between within-subjects and between-subjects factors.
- Correctly select among repeated measures, between-subjects, and mixed designs.
- Find the correct F and p values from the computer output.

Questions

While reading this chapter, think about answers to the following questions:

1. How does the repeated measures ANOVA differ from the correlated t test?
2. Can I have more than one repeated measure in a repeated measures design?
3. Can I have more than one group in a repeated measures design?
4. When should I use repeated measures?
5. Are repeated measures better than between-group designs?

Introduction

In Chapter 13, we discussed the use of analysis of variance (ANOVA) for completely randomized fixed effect designs. Each subject received only one treatment level (or combination of treatment levels). In those designs, differences between subjects were used to assess differences in the treatments to which subjects had been randomly assigned. Recall the case in which subjects were randomly assigned to two groups. A single independent variable was manipulated to make one of the groups the experimental group and the other group the control group. One measure or score was then taken on each subject. A score was hypothesized to be a function of differences attributable to being in either the control group or the experimental group and differences between individuals within the groups. An F ratio was formed composed of a between-group variance divided by a within-group variance. The within-group variance (individual differences) was the error term.

In this chapter, we consider repeated measures designs, that is, designs in which the same measures are taken on the same subjects more than once. These designs are focused on changes in subjects as well as differences between treatment groups.

We will discuss four variations of these designs, divided into two types:

Within-Group Designs

1. One-factor repeated measures designs
2. Factorial repeated measures designs

Mixed Designs

3. Mixed design with one between-group factor and one within-group factor
4. Mixed design involving combinations of between-group and within-group factors

The first two are referred to as within-group designs, since only one group of subjects is studied and there is no "between-group" factor. In one-factor repeated measures designs, there are repeated measures on one group of subjects across a single independent variable. In factorial repeated measures designs, there are repeated measures on one group of subjects across combinations of two or more independent variables.

The second two variations are referred to as mixed designs, since more than one group is studied and repeated measures are taken on the subjects in each group. So there is a mix of between-group and within-group factors. In the first of these two, there is only one between-group factor and one within-group factor. The second variation of mixed repeated measures designs could involve factorial combinations of either the between-group or within-group factors.

Within-Group Designs

One-Factor Repeated Measures Design

In one-factor within-group designs, only one group is studied across one or more independent variables. The independent variable might be two time periods with no intervening factor (as would be the case in a study of reliability); two time periods with some intervening factor (e.g., the introduction of a fatiguing protocol); or even two different angles (e.g., at which joint reposition measures are taken).

For example, 30 subjects were recruited for a study of the effect of fatigue on sway. A balance system was used to measure postural sway. The subjects stood on both feet with their eyes open on a normal stable platform. The subjects were then put through a fatiguing protocol. After fatiguing, a postfatigue measure of sway was taken while the subjects also stood on both feet with their eyes open on a normal stable platform. Our interest is in seeing the effect of fatigue on sway. The mean of prefatigue sway scores is .613 cm and the mean of postfatigue sway scores is 1.16 cm.

The results of this example are shown in Figures 14–1 and 14–2. In Figure 14–1A we have included the pre- and post-test sway scores for each subject; Figure 14–1B is a printout of the correlated t test comparing the means and the means and standard deviations for pre- and postfatigue scores. Figure 14–2 shows the same data analyzed using ANOVA to compare the pre- and post-test means. We have included the correlated t test so that you can see that repeated measures designs are an extension of the correlated t test.

First, let's look at the t test. The null hypothesis is that the population means from which the pre- and post-test means were drawn are equal. Note the subtraction in the denominator of the t test (see Formula 14–1 below).

$$t = \frac{\overline{X}_E - \overline{X}_C}{\sqrt{S_C^2 \big/ n_C + S_E^2 \big/ n_E - \left(2r \cdot S_C^2 \big/ n_C \cdot S_E^2 \big/ n_E\right)}} \qquad (14\text{--}1)$$

The correlated t test is the same test as the independent t test except that it is adjusted for the relationship between the pretest and post-test data. It has the same formula as the independent t except that the denominator has an extra term. You can see that the formula is composed of the correlation between the pre- and post-test scores and the standard error of the mean at prefatigue and postfatigue. You can also see that the subtraction term will be minimized if the correlation is zero and maximized if the correlation is 1.0. The entire subtraction term represents an adjustment for systematic individual differences from prefatigue to postfatigue. Essentially, it removes individual differences from the statistical test.

Now look at the ANOVA (Fig. 14–2B). The "sources of variance" in the summary table provide a model for variations in sway scores. Sway scores are hypothesized to be a function of differences between subjects ($MS_{Subjects}$), differences between the two time periods ($MS_{Fatigue}$), and differences between subjects across the two time periods ($MS_{Subjects \times Fatigue}$, the interactive effect). The relevant statistical test is the F test to look at differences between the pre- and postfatigue means ($MS_{Fatigue}/MS_{Subjects \times Fatigue}$). The most important thing for you to notice is that subject differences are *not* included in the assessment of differences across time. You should also see that the F test is equal to t^2 (see Chapter 13).

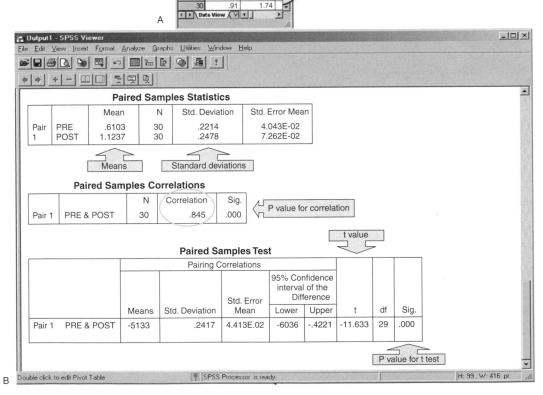

Figure 14–1 (A) Data for the correlated *t* test. (B) Output for the correlated *t* test.

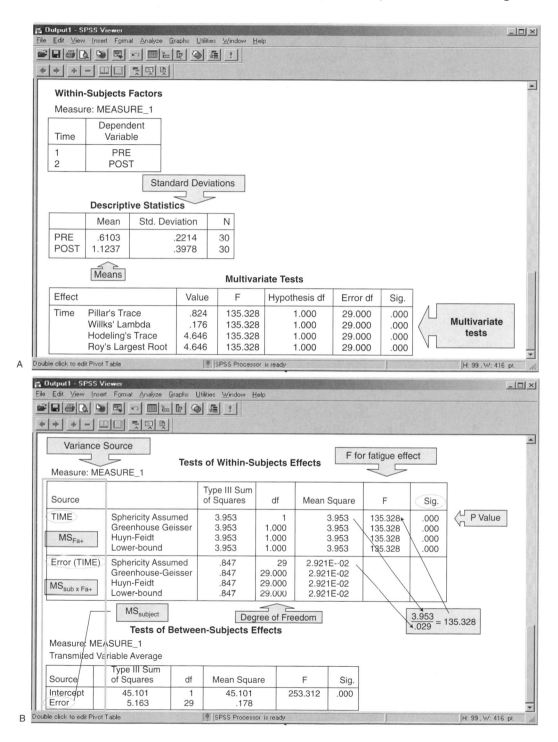

Figure 14–2 (A) Repeated measures ANOVA output.

This design is the analysis of variance analog of the correlated t test. In both the correlated t test and the F test for repeated measures, we remove individual differences from the denominator of the test. Thus, if you understand the correlated t test, you understand the basic principle of repeated measures designs. Other repeated measures designs are more complicated conceptually and mathematically, but in every case, they achieve the objective of removing individual differences, of using each individual subject as his or her own control.

The one-group, one-factor design could be extended by adding more time points or more levels (angles) to the independent variable. This could be useful for looking at increases in ROM over multiple days or weeks of rehabilitation.

Factorial Repeated Measures Designs

The second variation of the within-group design is the one-group factorial repeated measures design. The one-factor design is expanded by adding independent variables (factors). An example of this is presented in Figure 14–3. You can add as many factors as are reasonable in a given study, but remember it is usually better to "keep it simple." In the previous example, we measured sway before and after fatiguing. We took these measures with subjects standing on two feet with their eyes open on a normal stable platform. We might expect that the effect of fatigue on sway would be minimal under those conditions. What if the conditions were more difficult? We might vary whether the eyes are open or closed. We now have two independent variables: time of measure (pre and post) and eye condition (open or closed). We could then look at the effect of fatigue on sway under different eye conditions.

In this study, postural sway measures are taken with a balance system pre- and postfatigue for each of 10 subjects (Fig. 14–3). Two measures are taken each time, one with the eyes open and one with the eyes closed. In each case, the subjects stand on both feet on a normal stable platform. The interest is in seeing the effect of fatigue on sway under different eye conditions. You might expect that the effect of fatigue on sway would be greatest when the eyes are closed. By looking at the sources of variance in the ANOVA summary table, you can see that the hypothesis about factors influencing sway scores has become much more complicated. Instead of three sources of variance, there are now seven sources of variance. There are now three research questions:

1. What is the effect of fatigue (time) on postural sway scores?
2. What is the effect of eye condition on postural sway scores?
3. What is the interactive effect of fatigue and eye condition on postural sway scores?

Each of these is answered with a different F test, and each F test has a different denominator (error term). But once again, the subject factor

	Prefatigue		Postfatigue	
	Eyes Open	Eyes Closed	Eyes Open	Eyes Closed
S1	X_1	X_2	X_3	X_4
S2	.	.	.	.
S3	.	.	.	.
S4	.	.	.	.
S5	.	.	.	.
S6	.	.	.	.
S7	.	.	.	.
S8	.	.	.	.
S9	.	.	.	.
S10	X_1	X_2	X_3	X_4

Sources and Variance		F
Between		
	Subjects	–
Within		
	Pretest/Post-test Subjects x Pre/post	$MS_{Pre/post}/MS_{Subjects \times Pre/post}$
	Eyes Open/closed Subjects x Open/closed	$MS_{Open/closed}/MS_{Subjects \times Open/closed}$
	Pre/post x Open/closed Subjects x Pre/post x Open/closed	$MS_{Pre/post \times Open/closed}/MS_{Subjects \times Pre/post \times Open/closed}$

Figure 14–3 A repeated measures design with two factors.

(between subjects), which represents individual differences, has been removed from each *F* test. Although they are hidden inside the calculations, the correlations between the measures are the major influence on this term, just as they were in the one group one-factor repeated measures design. If the correlations are zero, the subject factor will be minimized. The design will reduce to a between-groups design. Instead of a single correlation between pretest and post-test, there are now correlations among all four measures. Just the addition of one independent variable has made this a much more complex design. Our advice is that you should not add factors lightly. You should have a sound theoretical or empirical basis for each factor.

Mixed Designs

One Between-Group Factor and One Within-Group Factor

Mixed designs combine the features of between-group designs and within-group designs. In a simple case, as shown in Figure 14–4, there are two groups of 15 subjects (as marked by the grouping variable shown in Figure

14–4A). One group might be subjects who have been identified to have functional ankle instability (FAI), and the other groups would not have unstable ankles. Note the data are exactly the same as in Figure 14–2, with the addition of a grouping variable. We will refer to this independent variable as stability condition.

You would measure sway of the subjects in each group before and after fatiguing (see page 233). The major interest would be to determine whether the change in sway from before to after fatiguing is the same for FAIs and non-FAIs. The means for each group at each time, the means for all subjects at time 1 and time 2, and the means (summed across time periods) for all FAI and non-FAI are given in Figure 14–4B. Visual inspection of the means suggests that the FAI group has more sway initially than the non-FAI group, that sway goes up in both groups after fatigue, and that sway goes up more after fatigue for the FAI group than the non-FAI group.

Now look at the sources of variance listed in Figures 14–4B and 14–4C. Our hypothesis is that a score is a function of stability condition (whether or not a subject has FAI), individual differences among the subjects in each of the two groups, the time of the measurement, the interaction between stability and time of measurement, and subject fluctuations across the time of measurement. The summary analysis of variance table has now been broken into within-group sources of variance and between-group sources of variance.

It should be apparent to you that we have little interest in the between-group factor in this study. We would be surprised if we did not find sway differences between the FAIs and non-FAIs. We are left with two primary research questions. First, is there an effect of fatigue on sway? Second, is the effect of fatigue on sway different for the FAI group than for the non-FAI group?

This design allows us to remove both individual differences (subject x stability) and overall group differences (stability) from our statistical analysis for the two primary questions. In general, sway goes up after fatigue (F = 173.424, df = 1,28; $p < .001$).

You will note that the p value listed in Figure 14–4B actually reads .000. Just as we explained in Chapter 13, this does not mean that the value is zero. Rather, the program truncates the value by rounding to the third decimal. To be .000 means that the fourth decimal had to be smaller than 5 or $p < .0005$. Otherwise, if the value had been $p = .0005$, the third decimal would have been round to 1, or $p = .001$. This is true of all p values listed as .000.

While sway goes up for each group, it goes up differently for the two groups (F = 9.164; df = 1,28; $p = .005$). Visual inspection once again suggests that sway following fatigue goes up more for the FAI than the non-FAI group. We have little interest in the overall means of the FAI and non-FAI groups because they are simply the average across prefatigue and postfatigue.

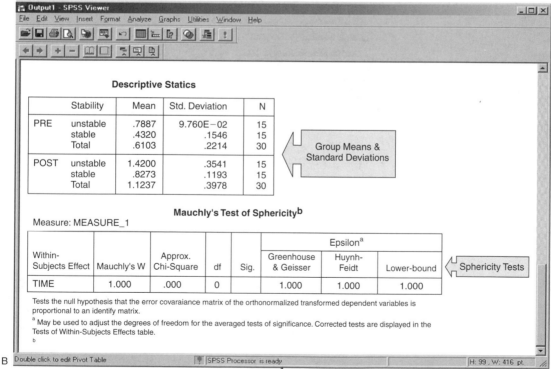

Figure 14–4 (A) Data for the mixed design ANOVA. (B) Descriptive statistics and tests of sphericity.

(*Continued on following page*)

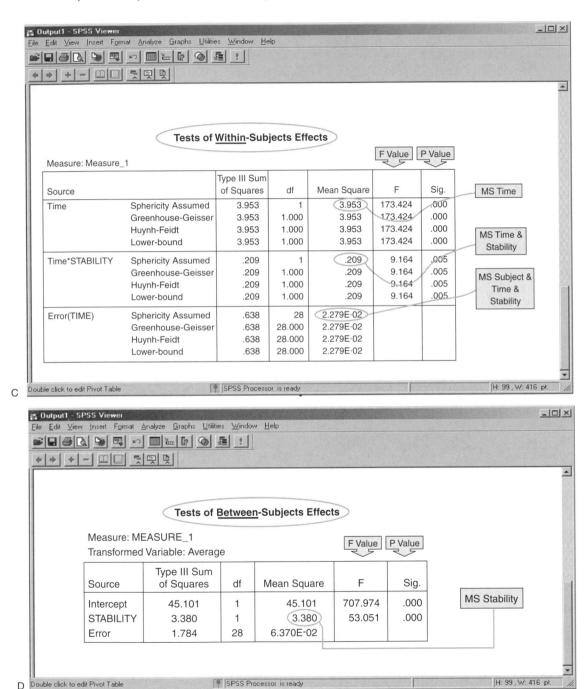

Figure 14–4 *(Continued)* (C) Within-subjects output for mixed design ANOVA. (D) Between-subjects output for mixed design ANOVA.

Mixed Designs Involving Factorial Combinations of Between-Group and Within-Group Factors

You should note that we have presented the simplest repeated measures and mixed designs here. More complex designs are possible. For example, the mixed design above could be extended. The non-FAI and FAI groups could be divided to include a balance-trained and not-trained group, adding to the between-subjects factors. Also, the Fatigue/no Fatigue condition (represented as time in Fig. 14–4C) could be divided into prebalance training and postbalance training. The final design would be a mixed design with two between-group (ankle stability and balance training) and two within-group (pre/post training and pre/postfatigue) factors.

The resulting ANOVA would be able to answer more complex questions. However, it would also be more complex to interpret. Thus, our suggestion is to build more complicated designs only because you have to, not because you can. While these complex designs appear to be more efficient and create more information, our experience is that contradictory or overly complex information can also result.

Advantages of Repeated Measures Designs

A major advantage of repeated measures designs is that they allow you to directly look at changes over time. In nonrepeated measures designs, treatment effects are measured as the difference between groups, not in terms of changes in the subjects. With repeated measures designs we can see how much change occurred. How much stronger did subjects get? How much did their balance improve? How much cognitive loss results from a mild head injury? You could take daily or weekly measures and analyze the changes. You could carefully select specific angles at which to take measures of joint proprioception sense and then determine the shape of the function, relating angle to joint proprioception sense.

A second major advantage of repeated measures designs is the ability to remove individual differences from the error term. As you saw in each of the designs presented previously, variance between subjects has been removed from the error term. The degree to which this is reduced is a result of two factors: individual differences and the correlation of scores from one measure to the next. Just as with the use of the correlated t test, the value of using repeated measures designs is affected by the magnitude of the correlation across measurements. In general, the higher the correlation, the greater the reduction in the error term. Similarly, studies with larger differences among individuals will generally result in a greater reduction in the error term if they are correlated from one measure to the next.

The reduction in the size of the error term increases the power of the F tests. This makes it possible to use fewer subjects in your study. In the simplest repeated measures design, it may be possible to use as few as half as

In the Field

> Raquel is interested in studying the effects of hamstring stretching on knee range of motion. She has decided that she needs two groups, one that uses static stretching and one that does no stretching. She will measure knee range of motion. However, she isn't sure whether she should measure subjects before stretching and create a repeated measures design. Her advisor points out that testing subjects after stretching will answer her basic question of whether the treatments produce different effects, but it won't describe how each group changed across time. Based on this, Raquel decides to include pre- and post-stretching measures, creating a mixed-design analysis.

many subjects as one would have to use in a two-group nonrepeated measures design (i.e., a design with two different groups).

Disadvantages of Repeated Measures Designs

The disadvantages of using repeated measures designs are a result of the fact that subjects are measured more than once and measured over some time period. The order in which measures are presented can affect subject learning, fatigue, and awareness. When you take multiple measures, you may not take them reliably. And as the time period of these studies lengthens, there is a greater possibility that changes are the result of natural changes in the subjects, changes in the execution of the treatment or in the compliance by subjects, subject dropout, or nonexperimental factors that are occurring coincidentally with the study. In other words, these designs are often vulnerable to threats of carryover effects, learning/practice effects, subject apprehension, instrument changes, fatigue/growth, adherence mortality, and the impact of external factors.

Carryover Effects

Treatment conditions given earlier may carry over to later treatment conditions. For example, if you were interested in the effects of heat and ice on swelling, you might compare these treatments on the same group of subjects with ankle sprains. However, if ice is applied first, decreases in tissue temperature may decrease the effect of heat and make it appear to be ineffective (assuming that you apply heat soon after each ice treatment).

Learning/Practice Effects

When you measure a person more than once, there is a likelihood that the person may learn how to take the measure or how to perform the task. Consider a study to increase the balance of subjects with functionally unstable ankles. You develop an exercise plan to improve balance. Assume that you are counting the number of touches the wobble board makes during a 30-second trial. Also, assume you are interested in knowing the effect of your exercise plan over a 6-week period. You test each subject on the wobble board 3 times per week. You know from clinical and common experience that people generally get better balancing on a wobble board the more they do it. Thus, the question becomes, is improvement in wobble board performance the result of your exercise plan or the result of repeating testing?

Subject Apprehension

Repeated measures may increase the apprehensiveness of the subjects. They may become worried that the task is too difficult, too time consuming, or even potentially harmful. In a study in which the knee is perturbed, subjects may become apprehensive about a second or third perturbation. As a result, they may tighten up the knee and respond differently.

Instrumentation

Instrumentation has to do with potential changes in the instrument. The measuring device may change from one time to the next. A machine measure may lose its calibration. Machines also fail. The machine may not be connected to the patient correctly. In studies where the experimenter is also an active recorder of the measure (e.g., using a hand-held goniometer), he or she may not take the measure the same way each time. If more than one experimenter is used, the experimenters may not take the measure the same way. Any of these factors can produce differences that are due to changes in the instrument and not the treatment.

Fatigue

While practice will tend to improve performance, fatigue will tend to decrease performance. Obviously, fatigue will result after strenuous activities such as isokinetic strength testing. If you have a design in which you would be doing repeated muscle contractions, earlier contractions may decrease performance on later contractions. For example, if isokinetic testing is done across a variety of speeds, strength may be decreased at speeds that come later in the sequence.

Natural Growth

When the taking of measures is over an extended time period, subjects may change for more natural reasons. Healing would be a common example in athletic training. Under normal circumstances, injuries tend to get better across time because of healing. Thus, some caution is needed in interpreting changes across time as being caused by your experimental treatment, because they may actually be due to natural healing. More generally, exercise (e.g., weight training) studies with adolescents may be influenced by natural growth and maturity.

Adherence/Mortality

Long-term studies (e.g., rehabilitation studies) also increase the likelihood of subject attrition and subject maintenance of protocols. Subjects may just get tired of making a special trip to your laboratory. They may get bored with the research, or they may have unrelated factors, such as illness, that force them to quit the study.

Some Solutions

First, train the subjects to use the equipment (e.g., the wobble board or balance system) or perform the task. Do not begin the study until the subject can use the equipment or perform the task. Practice data are then not part of your study and further learning from practice should be minimized. Second, check and calibrate your equipment to ensure that data are correct and being recorded correctly. Third, train all experimenters so they know how to use the equipment and take measurements. You should also check experimenters over time to ensure that they maintain the quality of the experiment and of the data. This will reduce instrument change. Fourth, minimize the number of repeated measures taken. There will be less opportunity for learning, apprehension, instrument change, fatigue, natural growth, and the interference of external factors. Add rest times in between tasks to reduce the likelihood of fatigue. Fifth, add a control group to your study and compare the amount of change of the treatment group to that of the control group on the premise that changes in the control group may be also affected by each of these problems. Sixth, in designs that occur over a long period of time (i.e., weeks instead of minutes, hours, or days), you need to work very hard to try to keep subjects in the study and to get them to continue the treatment protocols. While rare, in some studies you may be able to rule out natural growth by comparison of subjects' changes with those in other studies or in your treatment facility. Seventh, in designs where multiple measures are taken sequentially, alternate the presentation of measures across subjects. This is referred to as counterbalancing. This is the single best solution to these problems.

Counterbalancing

Obviously in the simple pre-post design you cannot reverse the order of the pretest and the post-test. But in designs where subjects receive alternate treatments (e.g., bracing studies) or in which subjects are measured at different angles, force levels, or sides, you can counterbalance the order in which these measures are taken. You need to remember that counterbalancing does not remove the effect. It just spreads it across the different measures.

Consider an example in which knee joint reposition sense is measured on nine subjects at three different angles: 20°, 50°, and 80°. A simple 3-by-3 counterbalance matrix (also known as a Latin square) is shown in Figure 14–5. Three 3-by-3 squares are presented. The first three subjects are randomly assigned to the orders of the first square, the second three subjects to the next square, and the third three subjects to the third square. The result, shown below the counterbalance, is that each angle is presented first to three subjects, second to three subjects, and third to three subjects. This does not remove the effect of multiple measures, but it does remove the order effect from the comparisons of joint reposition sense across angles. This means that the order effect (e.g., learning from practice) is not larger in one condition than another. Most of the time this is satisfactory. It is possible for an effect to be large enough in all conditions to mask the factor of interest in the study. If all of the subjects in a study on range of motion became fatigued, ROM might be reduced in all conditions and thereby minimize differences between conditions.

Assumptions of Repeated Measures Designs

It is assumed that the subjects' scores are independent from one another. When data are collected from pairs or groups of subjects, there is the pos-

	Time 1	Time 2	Time 3
Subject 1	Angle 2	Angle 3	Angle1
Subject 2	Angle 1	Angle 2	Angle 3
Subject 3	Angle 3	Angle 1	Angle 2
Subject 4	Angle 3	Angle 1	Angle 2
Subject 5	Angle 2	Angle 2	Angle 1
Subject 6	Angle 1	Angle 3	Angle 3
Subject 7	Angle 2	Angle 3	Angle 1
Subject 8	Angle 3	Angle 1	Angle 2
Subject 9	Angle 1	Angle 2	Angle 3

A

	Time 1	Time 2	Time 3
Angle 1	3	3	3
Angle 2	3	3	3
Angle 3	3	3	3

B

Figure 14–5 (A) Counterbalancing nine subjects across three treatments. (B) Resulting treatment frequency at each time point

In the Field

Henry is interested in studying the effects of ankle strength training on postural sway. His plan is to assign individuals with chronic ankle sprains to a strength training group and a no training group. He is also interested in measuring subjects' balance at five points in time. However, he is concerned that performing the balance testing multiple times is equivalent to adding a balance treatment. He expects subjects will learn to balance better from the balance test. In this case it is not possible to counterbalance the postural sway measures, since they must be done sequentially. To solve this Henry creates a third group that receives no training and is measured on balance only once, at the end of the study. By comparing this group to the no training group at the end of the study, he can determine whether the multiple balance tests acted as a treatment.

sibility that one subject's scores may affect those of another. Since in most studies in athletic training, individual subjects are tested alone, this is not usually a problem. This could be a problem when testing in a laboratory or clinic where the performance of one subject may interfere with or motivate the performance of another subject.

A second assumption is sphericity. In the example in Figure 14–4, there are two groups and each group was given a pre- and post-test. The SPSS program for repeated measures provides tests of sphericity. As you can see in Figure 14–4B, sphericity has not been violated in this case. Violations of sphericity tend to increase type 1 errors. We will reject the null hypothesis too often. SPSS provides an estimate of violation of sphericity called epsilon. SPSS also provides two corrections for violations, one by Greenhouse-Geisser and the other by Huynh-Feldt. Stevens (1992) suggests that the former underestimates epsilon and the latter overestimates it. He suggests that you use the average of the two or, if you desire to be more conservative, use the Greenhouse-Geisser. Post hoc testing may also be affected by violations of sphericity. Stevens suggests that using Tukey post hoc tests is appropriate when sphericity is not violated. When sphericity is violated, he suggests using correlated t tests corrected with a Bonferroni correction (see Chapter 13).

Summary

Repeated measures designs have many advantages. They allow you to document changes across time and they have more statistical power than between group designs. However, these advantages are offset by some disadvantages. Specifically, when subjects are pretested, the pretesting can influence any treatments and measures that follow. In athletic training research this can potentially produce a learning effect or a fatigue effect. Strategies for countering these adverse effects on the research design have been presented in this chapter.

Activities

1. Using data of your own, run a repeated measures statistical analysis with and without a between-subjects factor.
2. Compare the structure of the resulting statistical printouts and note any differences that you find.
3. For the repeated measures portion of the printout, compare the resulting F and p values for differences.

Bibliography

Brown, D. R., Michels, K. M., & Weiner, B. J. (1991). *Statistical principles in experimental design* (3rd ed.). New York: McGraw-Hill, Inc.

Myers, J., & Well, A. (1991). *Research design and statistical analysis.* New York: HarperCollins Publishers.

Glass, G. V., & Hopkins, K. D. (1984). *Statistical methods in education and psychology* (3rd ed.). Boston: Allyn & Bacon.

Stevens, J. (1992). *Applied multivariate statistics for the social sciences* (2nd ed.). Hillsdale, NJ: Lawrence Erlbaum Associates.

Chapter *15*

Correlation Analysis

Objectives

After reading this chapter, you will:
- Know the difference between correlation and regression.
- Understand how regression can be used to characterize linear and nonlinear relationships.
- Understand the connection between regression and ANOVA.
- Understand how regression can be used with multiple dependent variables.
- Understand how regression can be used in experimental designs.

Questions

While reading this chapter, think about answers to the following questions:
1. What is the difference between correlation and regression?
2. Can correlation be used to determine cause and effect?
3. Is there a connection between ANOVA and regression?
4. What types of relationships can be studied with regression?
5. Do negative relationships represent smaller relationships?
6. How big does the correlation coefficient have to be for a strong relationship?

Introduction

The word correlation means to relate together (co-relate) or to vary together (co-vary). The premise is that as the scores in one variable go up or down, scores in another variable also tend to go up or down. For example, height and weight are correlated. Taller people tend to weigh more than shorter people. Francis Galton, who was the half-cousin of Charles Darwin, first suggested the method of statistical correlation, and he used scattergrams to plot the relationship between the heights of fathers and their sons. He found two things: (1) that the taller fathers tended to have taller sons than did the shorter fathers, and (2) that the sons were not as far above or below the mean as their fathers had been. They were closer to the mean of all of the sons. He called this "regression toward mediocrity." Now we call this characteristic regression to the mean. With the help of J.D.H. Dickson, Galton plotted regression lines and developed the "index of co-relation," which came to be known as the coefficient of correlation. Later, Karl Pearson added the mathematical development for the correlation coefficient. It was represented by the symbol r, signifying regression. It estimates the degree to which two sets of scores are linearly related.

While the initial use of correlation was to assess the linear relationship between two continuous variables, the mathematical machinery was easily extended to nonlinear relationships, to relationships where one or both of the variables were noncontinuous, to relationships between three or more variables, and to relationships between categorical variables and continuous variables. We begin this chapter with a presentation of basic concepts and issues in correlation analysis. This is followed by a short discussion of the assessment of nonlinear relationships, relationships when at least one variable is categorical, and relationships among two or more variables. Finally we discuss correlational techniques that are appropriate in conjunction with the use of ANOVA.

Basic Concepts

The correlation coefficient (r) summarizes both the magnitude and the direction of the linear relationship between two variables. The r ranges from zero (no linear relationship) to 1.00 (a perfect linear relationship). The r can have a positive or a negative sign. If the sign is positive, it means that high scores of one variable are associated with high scores of the other and conversely that low scores of one are associated with low scores of the other. If the sign is negative, it means that the high scores of one variable are associated with low scores of the other and vice versa. The words "negative" or "positive" do not mean "bad" or "good." They simply refer to the pattern of co-variation of the quantitative scores of the two variables. For example, a low percent body fat might be considered a good thing. A negative relationship between amount of exercise and percent body fat would mean that subjects who exercise more tend to have a lower percent body fat than those who exercise less (which would be seen as a good thing).

We have presented four different kinds of relationships between two variables in Figure 15–1. The dots in the figures represent the paired values of two variables. Figure 15–1A represents a perfectly linear positive relationship. Note that plotting the values of the two variables results in a straight line from left to right with the paired values increasing together (co-varying). Figure 15–1B represents a perfectly linear negative relationship. Note that plotting the values of the two variables results in a straight line from left to right but that high values of one variable are paired with low values of the other variable. Figure 15–1C represents a curvilinear relationship. Initially, the values of the paired variables increase together but then increases in the values of the one variable are associated with decreasing values of the second variable. This has been referred to as an inverted U. Figure 15–1D represents no relationship at all. Note that plotting the values of the two variables results in scattered pairs that represent no apparent pattern.

The Pearson r for Figure 15–1A is 1.00 and for Figure 15–1B it is -1.00. But since the Pearson r was designed to summarize the linear relationship between two variables, it would be 0.00 or close to 0.00 for both Figures 15–1C and 15–1D. As you look at Figure 15–1C, you probably are saying to yourself that this is a very strong relationship. You are right. So is something wrong with the Pearson r? No! It is correct. There is no linear relationship between X and Y. The relationship is other than linear.

An Example of a Positive Relationship

Data for a study on the relationship between performance on the Balance Error Scoring System (Errors) and mental status assessed by the

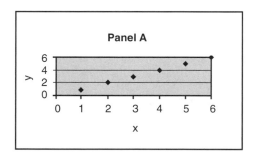
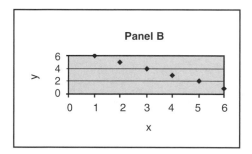
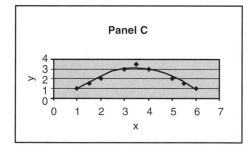
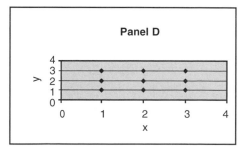

Figure 15–1 Four standard relationships between variables.

Standardized Assessment of Concussion (SAC) are given in the first two columns of Table 15–1. A scattergram of this relationship is given in Figure 15–2. For this fictitious study, Error and SAC data were obtained on 11 subjects. As you can see in the table, Error scores ranged from 12 to 19. SAC scores ranged from 22 to 29. One of the two subjects with the lowest Error score (i.e., 12) had the lowest SAC score. The other subject who had an Error score of 12 had a SAC score that was 23. You can also see that the subject with the highest Error score also happened to have the highest SAC score (see also Table 15–1). This is called a bivariate plot. A point in the figure simultaneously represents the score on both variables by one or more subjects. Note the point at the lower left corner. It indicates the scores of the subject who had a 12 on SAC and a 12 on Errors. Note also that lower postural way scores tend to be associated with lower Error scores and higher SAC scores tend to be associated with higher Error scores. The relationship appears to be "positive."

The deviation formula for calculation of the Pearson r is:

$$r = \frac{\dfrac{\sum (X - \overline{X})(Y - \overline{Y})}{n - 1}}{\left(\dfrac{\sum (X - \overline{X})^2}{n - 1}\right)\left(\dfrac{\sum (Y - \overline{Y})^2}{n - 1}\right)} \quad (15\text{–}1)$$

Throughout this text, we have avoided algebraic transformations of deviation formulae because we think they do not provide you with an intuitive understanding of the workings of the formula. You would rarely do hand calculations with deviation formulae because they are cumbersome and exhausting. But you would rarely do hand calculations at all. You would

Table 15–1 • **Data for the BESS Errors and SAC Scores Correlation**

Subject	Errors	SAC	Diff. Errors	Diff. SAC	Diff. SAC Squared	Diff. Errors Squared	Cross products
1	18.00	23.00	2.55	-2.54	6.45	6.50	-6.48
2	14.00	23.00	-1.45	-2.54	6.45	2.10	3.68
3	13.00	23.00	-2.45	-2.54	6.45	6.00	6.22
4	12.00	23.00	-3.45	-2.54	6.45	11.90	8.76
5	12.00	22.00	-3.45	-3.54	12.53	11.90	12.21
6	19.00	28.00	3.55	2.46	6.05	12.60	8.73
7	19.00	29.00	3.55	3.46	11.97	12.60	12.28
8	17.00	27.00	1.55	1.46	2.13	2.40	2.26
9	17.00	29.00	1.55	3.46	11.97	2.40	5.36
10	14.00	29.00	-1.45	3.46	11.97	2.10	-5.02
11	15.00	25.00	-.45	-.54	.29	.20	.24
Mean	15.45	25.55					Sum = 48.27

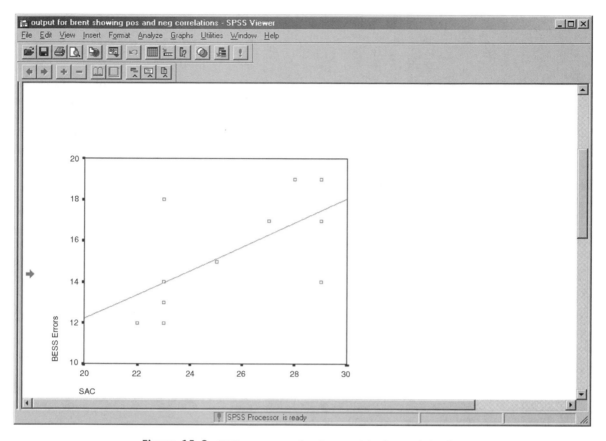

Figure 15–2 SPSS scattergram showing a positive linear relationship

use a statistical package to do the calculations. Look at the top of the formula. This is called the covariance. It is calculated from pairs of scores and focuses on the simultaneous deviation of the score of each variable from the mean of the variable.

Look again at Table 15–1. The mean of the error scores is 15.45 and the mean of the SAC scores is 25.55. The first subject is higher than average on errors (18) but lower than average on SAC (23). The first subject has an error score that is 2.55 points higher (see column 3) than the mean error score and a SAC score that is 2.54 points lower (see column 4) than the SAC mean of 25.55. Look at the other pairs of values in columns 3 and 4. In most cases subjects who are lower than the mean on errors are also lower than the mean on SAC (minus values are associated with minus values). Similarly, in most cases subjects who are higher than the mean on errors are higher than the mean on SAC (plus values are associated with plus values.). Subjects who have more errors tend to have higher SAC and subjects who have fewer errors tend to have a lower SAC. Only subjects 1 and 10 are exceptions to this.

In column 7 we have provided the "cross products" of each pair of deviations. The SAC deviation score is multiplied times the error deviation score. When both deviation scores are positive (above their respective means) or when both deviation scores are negative (below their respective means), the cross product is positive. When one deviation score is positive and other is negative, the cross product is negative. The next step is to add the values in column 7. Note that since the values for subjects 1 and 10 are negative, they will reduce the size of this sum. The sum is 48.27. We divide this by the degrees of freedom, which is 10 (the number of pairs minus one to get the covariance). The covariance is 4.827.

Now look at the bottom part of the formula. You should recognize these components from Chapter 12. The left side of the formula provides the calculation for the variance of the error scores (S_x^2). The right side of the formula provides the calculation for the variance of the SAC scores (S_y^2). The variance of x (errors) is 7.073, and the variance for y (SAC) is 8.273. If we multiply these and take the square root of the resultant value we have the square root of 58.515, or 7.65. The last step is to divide the covariance of 4.827 by 7.65. This value, .631, is the Pearson r.

It would of course have been much easier to use a program from SPSS to do this work for us. That output is given in Figure 15–3. As you can see, SPSS arrives at the same value for r as we just did, .631. The null hypothesis is that the population correlation is zero. The SPSS output also includes the two-tailed statistical probability. It is $p = .037$. It is the probability of getting an r this big or bigger (either positive or negative) by chance when the population correlation (Rho) is zero (i.e., when the null hypothesis is true). Since .037 is less than our alpha level of .05, we would reject the null hypothesis. We would conclude that there was a positive relationship between errors and SAC.

Because this study was not an experiment, we cannot conclude that this relationship is causal nor can we make conclusions about the direction of the relationship. We cannot say that errors on the Balance Error Scoring System (BESS) increase SAC or that SAC increases errors on the BESS. We simply know that for some reason balance errors and concussion scores are related. There may be some third variable that makes subjects have poorer balance and diminished mental capacity (e.g., age).

Most statistical texts will warn you about interpreting correlation coefficients as indicating a causal relationship. We would like to reinforce this admonition, but we also want to remind you that no statistic (including F tests and t tests) should be interpreted as indicating a cause-effect relationship. Confidence about drawing causal conclusions is a function of being able to rule out other causes. That is a function of research design, not the type of statistic you choose to use. The identification of relationships is very important. It is at the heart of doing research and at the heart of eventually arriving at causal conclusions. If two variables are related, one might be the

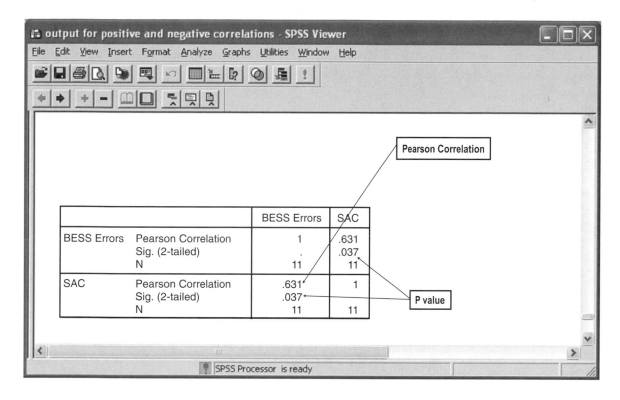

Figure 15–3 SPSS output for the Pearson correlation between BESS Errors and SAC

cause of the other. Once you have identified that a relationship exists, you may be able to design experimental studies to determine whether the relationship is causal.

Other Factors that May Affect the Size of r

Since the Pearson correlation coefficient is a measure of the linear relationship between two variables, when the relationship is other than linear, the Pearson r will underestimate the relationship between the two variables. In Figure 15–1C, the r for the curvilinear relationship would be zero or close to it in spite of the fact that the relationship is quite strong. Nonlinear alternatives can be calculated by hand or by using a statistical package such as SPSS to identify the true nature of the relationship. Other techniques are available in conjunction with the use of the analysis of variance (ANOVA).

The Pearson r can only reach its maximum (i.e., 1.00) when the distributions of the two variables are the same. If one measure is dichotomous (e.g., gender coded as male or female) and the other is continuous (e.g., height in inches), the r cannot reach 1.00. Sometimes the range of one variable or the other is restricted because of the nature of the subjects in the study. A study involving uninjured elite athletes is not likely to include subjects who are very weak or are extremely limited in flexibility. Even if strength and flexibility are indeed related, a study in which all of the subjects have very high flexibility scores will result in a lower correlation between strength and flexibility than a study that includes subjects with a wide range of flexibility.

The measurement reliability of each variable will also influence the size of the Pearson r. The maximum size of the r can only be reached if each variable has perfect reliability. If the measurement of one or both of the variables includes a lot of error (i.e., is less reliable), the maximum correlation will be reduced. We would expect, for example, that the correlation between height and weight would be lower if our measure of weight was based on guesses of subjects' weight on visual observation rather than using a reliable weight scale. This is, of course, another reason why you should be sure that you have reliable measures.

Another factor that influences the size of the r is sample size. Coefficients in small samples will tend to be larger, by chance, than coefficients from large samples. The existence of any of these factors in your study ought to give you at least pause to think. Maybe if this factor wasn't present the r would have been larger. You will minimize these factors when you plan your study. You should try to ensure that you sample appropriate subjects, that you don't accidentally or unnecessarily restrict the range of one variable or the other, that you have reliable measures, and that you have a large enough sample.

Interpreting the Size of a Pearson r

The size of the r indicates the strength of the linear relationship. Coefficients that are closer to zero indicate little or no linear relationship, while correlations approaching 1.00 indicate very strong linear relationships. Is the relationship that you have obtained strong or weak? In our example above, we found a correlation of .631. Is that a strong correlation? The first thing that we found was that it was statistically significant at $p < .05$. That allows us to reject the null hypothesis and provides evidence that there is indeed a linear relationship between flexibility and strength. A second criterion that can be used to assess the strength of the relationship is to determine the percentage of overlapping variance of the two variables. Sometimes this is referred to as the "percentage of variance accounted for." (Be careful about the use of this "causal" phrase.) The percentage of overlapping variance can be determined by squaring the r and it is called the coefficient of determination. The overlap can be represented by Venn diagrams as presented in Figure 15–4A-C. In Figure 15–4A there is no overlap. The $r = 0$ and $r^2 = 0$. None of the variance is mutual. The pattern in Figure 15–4B is like our Error/SAC example, in which the r was .631 and the r squared is .398. Forty percent of the variance is mutual. In Figure 15–4C, there is total overlap. The $r = 1.00$ and the r squared is 1.00. One hundred

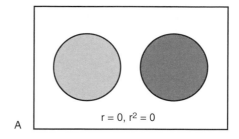

A

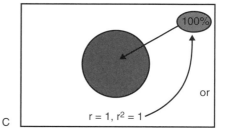

B

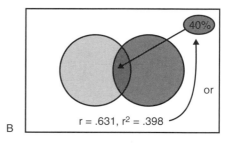

C

Figure 15–4 Venn diagram showing (A) no relationship, (B) moderate relationship, and (C) a perfect relationship.

percent of the variance is mutual. The opposite of the coefficient of determination is the Coefficient of nondetermination ($1 - r^2$). It indicates the percentage of variance that is not overlapping or "not accounted for." In our example, 60 percent of the variance is not overlapping. A substantial percent of the total variance in flexibility scores is not accounted for by strength scores. To what else is flexibility related – amount of exercise? Temperature of the muscles? Note, on the other hand, that 9 of the 11 subjects exhibited the pattern of a positive relationship between flexibility and strength.

A third way to judge the size of correlation coefficients would be to have some outside standard. If that is the average correlation that researchers find when they are really trying to identify relationships, maybe it is a good standard for researchers to use in deciding whether to pay attention to an observed r. Cohen (1988), when writing about effect sizes, has suggested the following conventions: an r of .10 is small, an r of .30 is medium, and an r of .50 or greater is large. He makes these estimates from his experience with social science data. But he points out that relationships in the physical sciences are much more predictable than those in the social sciences and that conventions used to judge the size of correlations for the physical sciences would be raised considerably. Physiological variables studied in athletic training, such as force, balance, strength, and flexibility, tend to be fairly highly intercorrelated, while educational and social variables that might be studied in athletic training research probably are more like those cited by Cohen. You may recall from Chapter 9, our suggestion that judgments about the size of reliability coefficients ought to reflect the standards within the research area. Similarly, it would be useful for you to compare a correlation from a specific research study with other studies that have been done on the same phenomena or same types of phenomena in making judgments about the size of the correlation. In athletic training research, we suggest that you use Cohen's guidelines for research on complex human behaviors (i.e., educational, psychological, and sociological variables) in nonexperimental studies, but have higher standards for physiological variables in experimental studies.

Other Measures of Relationships

You may encounter other measures of relationships in the literature. The measures can be divided into two broad categories: variations of the Pearson r and correlations calculated from ANOVA.

Variations of the Pearson r

There are three other correlation coefficients that are alternative ways to calculate a Pearson r: the point biserial r, the Phi coefficient, and the Spearman Rank correlation coefficient. The point biserial r is a Pearson correlation used when one variable is dichotomous and the other is continuous. It is calculated exactly the same as a Pearson, but the maximum value is less than 1.0 because the shape of the two distributions is not the same. Thus, referring to it as the point biserial alerts you to the limitation on its range of values.

The Phi coefficient is used when both variables are categorical. If the two distributions are the same (e.g., 2X2 table, male/female X injured/uninjured), the Phi coefficient will be equivalent to the Pearson r. If the two distributions are not the same (e.g., 2X3, male/female X first-/second-/third-degree sprain), the maximum value of the Phi coefficient is less than 1.0.

The Spearman Rank correlation coefficient is used with ranked data. It is equivalent to the Pearson r when there are no tied ranks. When there are tied ranks, the differences that result between the Pearson r and the Spearman are usually small.

Correlations Calculated from ANOVA

The intraclass correlation coefficient (ICC; see Chapter 9), used to estimate reliability, is used when one variable is categorical (test times, different testers or observers) and the other is continuous. It is typically calculated using ANOVA. It is a ratio of two variances: one to estimate the "true" score variance and the other to estimate the total variance in the scores. Unlike the Pearson r, which is sensitive only to the order of the pairs of scores, ICC 2,1 and ICC 2, k are sensitive both to the order of the pairs and to differences between the scores that were produced at different test times or by different testers.

The correlation ratio (Eta or η) is also used when one variable is categorical and the other is continuous. It is also typically calculated using ANOVA. It is a ratio of two variances: one to estimate the variance in scores that is attributable to an independent variable (e.g., experimental group/control group) and the other to estimate the total variance in the scores. When the categorical variable has only two categories, the Eta will be equivalent to the point biserial r (and therefore the Pearson r). When the categorical variable has three or more categories, the Eta will be equal to or greater than the Pearson r. We will explore the Eta later in this chapter, because of its utility in aiding in the interpretation of results from ANOVA.

Regression versus Correlation

As we have seen, correlation refers to relationship between two or more variables. If you know the correlation between two variables, you can use this information to predict the scores of one variable from the scores of the other variable. This is done through a regression equation. Formula 15–2 is the equation used to predict Y from X, assuming that the relationship is linear.

$$\hat{Y} = bX + c \qquad (15\text{–}2)$$

$$Where,\ b = r\frac{S_y}{S_x} \qquad (15\text{–}3)$$

The X in this equation is the predictor (e.g., SAC in Fig. 15–2) and the Y is the criterion (e.g., BESS Errors in Fig. 15–2). The b in this equation is the rate of change in Y for each unit change in X. It is also called the slope of the regression line. We could predict athletes' weight from their height. We could predict the likelihood that athletes would suffer an injury from their preseason fitness scores. We could predict how long it would take an athlete to return to function from scores on severity of the injury sustained. To do this we would have to know the mean and standard deviation of each variable and the correlation between the two variables.

An Example: Predicting Quadriceps Strength from Thigh Girth

Assume you have quadriceps strength and thigh girth data for 150 male college football players. The mean strength score is 185 Nm with a standard deviation of 30 Nm. The thigh girth is 56 cm with a standard deviation of 4 cm. Assume the correlation between their strength and girth is .70. There is a positive relationship. Athletes with greater girth scores tend to have higher strength scores. If we had a new athlete arriving next week and knew only the athlete's girth score, we could use this information to predict the athlete's strength score. The major factor limiting our prediction is the size of the correlation.

The higher the correlation between the two variables, the more accurate the prediction will be. If two variables have a zero correlation, there is no predictive value and the prediction would have no accuracy. On the other hand, if the correlation is .90, we could make a very accurate prediction of the player's strength score. This prediction is not dependent on whether the relationship is causal. The issue is prediction, not explanation. In many cases we might not have any idea why some relationship exists, but if it exists and if it is strong we can use it to make strong predictions. The accuracy of the prediction is dependent on whether the relationship is linear. The prediction is also dependent on whether our new athlete is a member of the same population as our original sample of 150 male athletes. If the new athlete were a female high school basketball player, we would expect that our prediction would be less accurate.

We can now use Formulas 15–2 and 15–3 to solve for the unknowns (Display 15–1). When we do this we find that $b = 5.25$ and $c = -109$. If our new athlete had a girth score of 63 cm, we would predict that he would have a strength score of 221.75 Nm.

Display 15-1

Step	Formula Number	Formula	Result
Step 1	15–3	$b = r\dfrac{S_y}{S_x}$	$b = .7\dfrac{30}{4} = 5.25$
Step 2	15–2 (rearranged and using means)	$c = \overline{Y} - b(\overline{X})$	$c = 185 - 5.25(56) = -109$
Step 3	15–2	$\hat{Y} = bX + c$	$\hat{Y} = 5.25(63) + (-109) = 221.75$

$\hat{Y}$ = Predicted Y
$\overline{X}$ = Mean of X
$\overline{Y}$ = Mean of Y

Nonlinear Relationships

Under some conditions, the relationship may not be linear. When relationships are other than linear, the use of the Pearson r can be misleading. Consider knee laxity testing with a knee arthrometer. As the ACL begins to be stretched (or other soft tissue structures if the ACL is torn), the force will continue to go up but the anterior displacement slows and then stops. A plot of the relationship between force and displacement is presented in Figure 15–5. This plot was produced using the curve-fitting function in the linear regression program in SPSS. If a researcher calculated the Pearson r

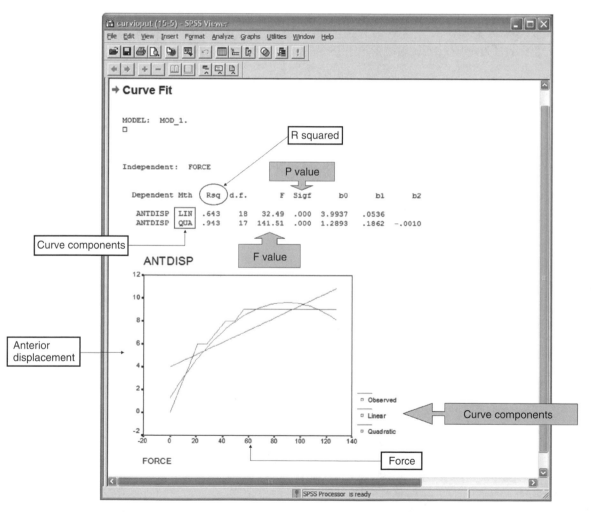

Figure 15–5 Nonlinear regression of anterior knee displacement and force.

for this relationship ($r = .801$, $r^2 = .643$), the researcher would conclude that the relationship was smaller than it actually is. While there is a statistically significant *linear* relationship, which the r indicates, the true relationship is curvilinear. The recalculated correlation is given by the SPSS curve-fitting program as .971 (r squared = .943). The correlation is almost 1.0, which is the highest an *r* can be. The equation for predicting a curvilinear relationship is:

$$Y = c + b_1x + b_2x^2 \qquad (15\text{--}4)$$

To account for curvilinear nature of the relationship, we have added x^2 into the formula.

Multiple Correlation/Multiple Regression: The Use of More than One Predictor

The correlation/regression model with one predictor and one criterion is very simple. We may be able to better predict the quadriceps strength of an athlete if we also know how active the athlete's muscle was during an isometric contraction. To get a measure of muscle activity, we could measure the EMG of the quadriceps while it is contracting. Now we could use both EMG and muscle girth together to predict muscle strength. The technique used to look at the correlation between multiple predictors and a single criterion is called multiple correlation. The equation for predicting scores on a variable using two predictors is:

$$Y = c + b_1x_1 + b_2x_2 \qquad (15\text{--}5)$$

Notice that using this equation will call for solving for two beta weights (b_1 and b_2) as well as the constant (c). Instead of using the symbol of *r*, we use *R*. If we use the multiple predictors to actually predict flexibility it is referred to as multiple regression.

Researchers often use multiple regression to try to find the "best" predictors of some variable (e.g., weight, injury, and so on). The most common way this is done is though stepwise multiple regression. In stepwise multi-

In the Field

Jerry has been interested in the relationship between EMG and strength of the peroneal muscles. In considering the relationship, some of the literature suggests that the relationship could be curvilinear. Jerry is interested in capturing the relationship as accurately as possible. To do this he decides to plot the data to assess their shape. Indeed the data are curvilinear, but he is unsure how to characterize the shape. To accomplish this he decides to conduct multiple regression using a curve-fitting function.

ple regression, the first step is to identify the predictor variable that has the highest correlation with the criterion. Subsequent steps are then used to see whether other variables can increase the predictability over and above what the first variable has done. Steps are continued as long as an additional variable increases the predictability. If not, the analysis is discontinued. This approach to entering variables is strictly mathematical. It is neither theoretically nor practically based. In contrast you might order the entry of variables for practical reasons. Clinicians may not have access to EMG equipment. However, if EMG adds little to the prediction, then EMG data may not be necessary. The determination of the "best" predictor from a set of predictors is dependent on the order of entry.

Correlational Techniques for Use in Conjunction with Analysis of Variance

Typically, researchers who do experiments and/or use the analysis of variance as their primary statistical technique tend not to do correlational analyses. This is in spite of the fact that within many experimental studies, some of the independent variables (e.g., gender, severity of injury, and functional ankle instability) may not be experimental. If they do use correlational analyses, they only tend to do so under two conditions. The first condition is to do reliability analysis using intraclass correlations (ICCs). The second is when they are analyzing data that were collected during a nonexperimental study. Examples would include a study of the relationship between injury incidence and flexibility and study of the relationship between SAT scores and grades in an anatomy course. Researchers might use the Pearson r to calculate the correlations in either of these two studies.

We believe the absence of correlational analysis of experimental data limits the understanding of experimental effects. And so, we want to alert you to this possibility. The use of the correlation ratio in conjunction with the use of analysis of variance is a special case of studying variables with restricted range. It is a special case because the restricted variable is an experimental variable and because its range has been deliberately restricted by the experimenter (e.g., treatment versus nontreatment). The "levels" of the variable are usually consciously selected and controlled by the experimenter. Remember from Chapter 13 that these are called fixed effects. In the simplest case, an experimenter might fatigue the subjects in one group (the experimental group) and not fatigue the subjects in another group (the control group) and measure the balance of each subject. A comparison would then be made between the balance scores of the two groups using ANOVA. The independent variable (fatigue) has only two levels (fatigued and not fatigued). The experimenter calculates a one-way ANOVA, which results in an $F = 38.143$ ($p < .001$). Looking back to Figure 13–2, note the R^2 given at the bottom of the table ($R^2 = .397$). One way to calculate this R is to use the correlation ratio as follows:

$$\text{Step 1} \qquad \eta^2 = \frac{\text{Sums of squares between groups}}{\text{Sums of squares total}} \qquad (15–6)$$

$$\text{Step 2} \qquad \sqrt{\eta^2} \ = R \qquad\qquad\qquad\qquad (15–7)$$

The squared Eta is usually reported in conjunction with ANOVA designs. A squared Eta, like a squared r, gives the percent of variance "accounted for" by the independent variable. In experimental designs, since the experimenter has controlled irrelevant variables, it is appropriate to use this phrase just as it is appropriate to conclude that the fatigue "had an effect on" the person's balance. The r squared is reported instead of the r because the experimenter has restricted the range of the variable. The "relationship" holds for only those particular levels of the variable and not across the range of the variable.

The correlation ratio (Eta), like the ICC calculated to estimate reliability, is a ratio of two variances. The Eta does not require the relationship to be linear. As a result, the Eta will be equal to or greater than a Pearson r calculated on the same data. The Eta can be determined in conjunction with any analysis of variance. Just as an r squared indicates the percentage of variance of one variable that is "accounted for" by the other variable, so does an Eta squared. We can calculate Eta squared using Formula 15–6.

The use of multiple regression in conjunction with ANOVA is not limited to studies with two groups. In Chapter 13, we presented an example of a study of the effect of visual reference on balance. There were three conditions: eyes open, eyes closed, and conflict dome. We conducted a one-way ANOVA (see Figure 13–5). The F of 38.446 was statistically significant at $p < .001$. Using post hoc tests, we determined that sway was greater with the eyes closed than with the eyes open or while wearing a conflict dome, and that sway was greater while wearing the conflict dome than with eyes open. But what percentage of the variance in sway is accounted for by these three visual conditions? We can calculate the Eta squared using Formula 15–6. Eta squared equals 5.722/9.963 or .574. That is, 57.4 percent of the variance in sway is accounted for by these three visual conditions. Notice the R squared at the bottom of Figure 13–5. It is .574, the same as the Eta squared that we just calculated. This is true even though the relationship is not linear and even though the independent variable is a categorical variable.

You can arrive at the same results using other methods. One way to do this is to create dummy variables to capture the levels of the independent variable (e.g., visual condition). The data presented in Figure 15–6 are the same as the data presented in Figure 13–4, except that two new variables have been added. They are given as Vector 1 and Vector 2. These are dummy variables. Subjects in the eyes-open condition are recorded as 1s on Vector 1 and 0s on Vector 2. Subjects in the eyes-closed condition are recorded as 0s on Vector 1 and 1s on Vector 2. Finally, subjects in the conflict dome condition are recorded as 0s on Vector 1 and 0s on Vector 2. Vectors 1 and 2

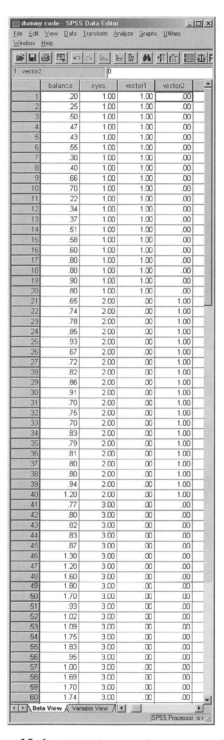

Figure 15–6 ANOVA data setup for regression analysis.

are then used as predictors in a multiple regression equation to predict balance scores. Part of the output from an SPSS Multiple Regression program is given in Figure 15–7. The model summary provides the Multiple R and Multiple R squared. Note that the R squared is the same as the Eta squared that we calculated from the ANOVA sums of squares.

These examples should point out to you that analysis of variance and correlational analyses are similar techniques. We encourage researchers in athletic training to begin to use these as companion techniques. Use analysis of variance to identify statistically significant differences and use correlational techniques to determine the percentage of variance in the dependent variable accounted for by the independent variable. This should be included as part of your efforts to judge the importance of your results.

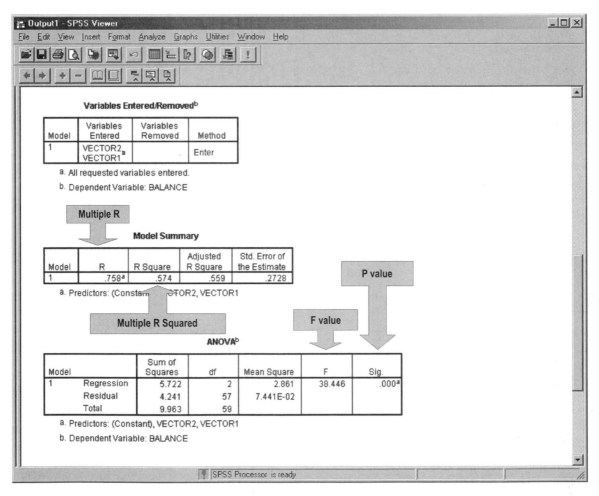

Figure 15–7 Regression analysis of ANOVA data.

In the Field

Jan is studying ankle instability. She is interested in whether there are strength differences between stable and unstable individuals with a history of injury. Her initial thoughts were to divide individuals into high-instability and low- to no-instability categories and use ANOVA. However, it occurred to her that she might be able to use regression instead. To do this, she asked individuals to rate their stability along a visual analog scale (i.e., "never gives way" to "gives way with every step"). Using this rating as the predictor variable, Jan predicts strength scores. She notices that there is a low to moderate (r = −.30) negative linear relationship. As expected, individuals reporting greater instability had weaker evertor muscles. However, in examining the data, Jan realizes there may be a curvilinear relationship. Using the same data set up, Jan reanalyzes the data using the curve-fitting function. The result is a significant curvilinear relationship with R = .82. In retrospect, Jan realizes that by using regression, her result produced a more complete description of the relationship between strength and ankle instability than she would have gotten from an ANOVA.

Other Issues

While it is beyond the scope of this text, it is possible to compare different correlation coefficients (Cohen, 1983; Pedhazur, 1982). You might calculate *r* using a linear equation and then recalculate *r* using a nonlinear equation. You would then make a statistical comparison between the two correlations to decide whether the relationship was other than linear. Similarly, comparisons could be made between two *r*'s from independent samples to see if the relationships observed in the two samples were statistically different. In complex correlation analyses where multiple predictors are included (multiple correlation or multiple regression), comparisons of different *R*'s are done both simultaneously and sequentially in successive steps of the analysis to decide which variables to add into a prediction equation. The statistical basis of these comparisons will be left for other texts. The logic of complex models and even of the statistical tests associated with them is within the grasp of the beginning researcher in athletic training. This is because that logic is as essential to the practice of the athletic training as it is to the athletic training researcher.

In recent years, researchers in many areas have attempted to go beyond the simple testing of statistical significance to assessing the importance of experimental variables. The calculation of effect sizes estimates how "big" an effect is in standard deviation units. Correlational analyses can be used to estimate the percentage of variance that an experimental variable accounts for in a dependent measure.

Researchers in athletic training tend to use correlational analyses only with nonexperimental studies or with variables that they consider to be educational or psychological. We want to encourage you to use correlational analysis with experimental studies to enhance your understanding of experimental effects. This brief presentation of the use of correlational analyses with two- and three-group ANOVA designs should alert you to the fact that this usage can be extended to very complex experimental designs. It can be used with factorial designs including repeated measures designs.

Summary

Correlation is a method by which the relationship between two or more variables can be determined. Although the reason for a relationship may be unknown, this relationship can be useful in predicting unknown values of one variable from known values of the second variable. This latter technique is known as linear regression. Linear regression is the simplest form of regression but not the only form. Curvilinear regression can be used to characterize nonlinear relationships, and multiple variables can be used to predict a single dependent variable with the multiple regression technique. Although typically used in nonexperimental research to describe relationships among variables, regression can also be used in experimental research in conjunction with ANOVA. With the proper setup, regression techniques will produce exactly the same results as ANOVA and thus are interchangeable. This emphasizes the point that the research design, not the statistical technique, defines the type of research you are conducting.

Activities

1. Discuss how a difference between groups (e.g., injured versus uninjured) could be interpreted in terms of a relationship between variables.
2. Discuss what types of relationships in athletic training research might be linear and which might be curvilinear.
3. Use a statistical package to run a one-way (three-group) ANOVA. Use the statistical output (sums of squares) to calculate the Eta.
4. Using the same data, create dummy variables and run a multiple regression. Compare the R squared with the Eta squared from Activity 3.

References

Cohen, J., & Cohen, P. (1983). *Applied multiple regression/correlation analysis for the behavior sciences* (2nd ed.). Hillsdale, NJ: Lawrence Erlbaum Associates.
Pedhazur, E. (1982). *Multiple regression in behavior research: Explanation and prediction*. Fort Worth, TX: Harcourt Brace Jovanovich.

Bibliography

Kachigan, S. K. (1986). *Statistical analysis: An interdisciplinary introduction to univariate and multivariate methods*. New York: Radius Press.
Pedhazur, E., & Schmelkin, L. P. (1991). *Measurement, design, and analysis: An integrated approach*. Hillsdale, NJ: Lawrence Erlbaum Associates.

Part 5
Writing and Publishing

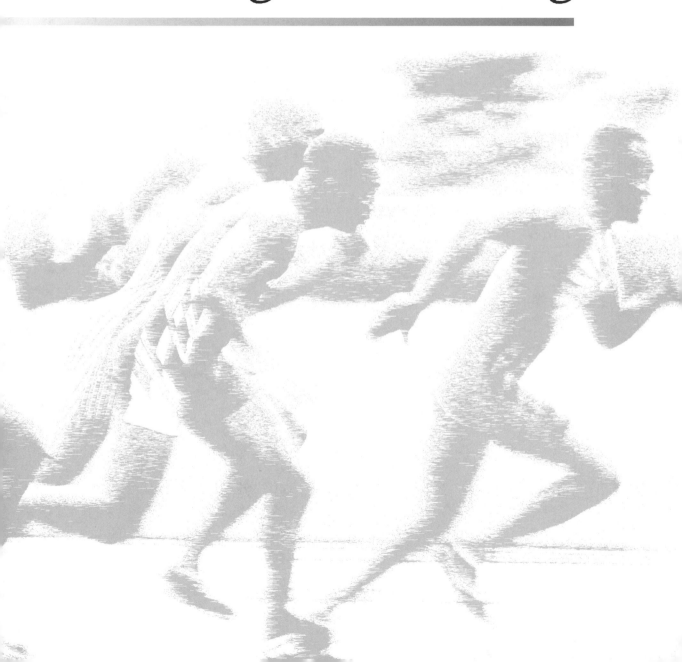

Chapter 16

Writing the Results

Objectives

After reading this chapter, you will:

- Understand how the results should be organized and presented in a manuscript to be submitted for publication.
- Know which significant and nonsignificant findings should be included in the results.
- Understand the difference between a table and a figure.
- Know how to prepare a table, a figure, and figure legends.
- Appreciate the importance of avoiding redundant presentation of results in the text, tables, and figures.

Questions

While reading this chapter, think about answers to the following questions:

1. In what format and in how much detail should the raw data be presented in the results?
2. Should only statistically significant findings be reported in the results?
3. What aspects of a particular statistical analysis are important to include in the results?
4. What are the advantages and disadvantages of presenting data in a table versus a figure?
5. Should the results be compared with other studies in this section of the manuscript?

Organizing and Writing the Results

This chapter will discuss the organization of the results section and the differences that exist between the results chapter of your thesis or dissertation and the results section of a manuscript to be submitted for publication in a scholarly journal. The preparation of tables, figures, and appendices will be discussed, and the advantages and disadvantages of each will be reviewed. Examples of presenting various forms of statistical analyses in the results will be addressed. Finally, we will emphasize the importance of presenting only the findings of your statistical analyses in the results and reserving any interpretation of the findings for the discussion chapter or section of your project.

The Results Chapter versus the Results Section of a Manuscript

The results section of your thesis or manuscript should be presented in a clear and concise manner, and only the findings that pertain to the problem statement and hypotheses of your project should be included. The results chapter of a thesis or dissertation should present the findings of your statistical analyses and should directly connect to the problem statement of the project and the hypotheses presented in Chapter 1. The means and standard deviations of the data should be presented in a table embedded within the text of the results. If an excessive number of tables are required for this purpose, the data may be presented in an appendix or appendices at the end of the thesis or dissertation. Some advisors will require that the raw data also be included in appendices at the end of the document. The findings of the statistical analyses should be completely presented, either in tables embedded within the chapter or as appendices at the end of the thesis or dissertation. For the thesis or dissertation, the statistical analyses that address each hypothesis should be presented. In contrast, the manuscript that you write from your thesis or dissertation will likely be far more focused on one or more of your hypotheses. As such, only the analyses relevant to the purpose of the manuscript should be included in the results section.

For the results section of a manuscript, the findings should also connect to your problem statement, but economy of space is essential. Only the most relevant results should be included, and examples of how to present this information in the text of the results will be presented later in this chapter. It is essential that you avoid the redundant presentation of results in the text, tables, and figures, since journal editors are very concerned about the space occupied by each manuscript (and associated cost per page!). The remainder of this chapter will address preparation of the results section for a journal manuscript.

Organization of the Results

The results section of a manuscript should begin by referring the reader to a table containing the means and standard deviations of the data having the greatest relevance to the research question. It is typically not necessary or for that matter feasible to present the raw data in the manuscript. The findings of the statistical analyses that connect to the problem statement at the end of your introduction should be presented in decreasing order of importance. Only the findings that are clearly relevant to your research question should be reported. For example, if you have used a mixed-model design analysis of variance to analyze your data, it is possible that the ANOVA includes main effects and interactions that are not necessarily all relevant to your problem statement. For example, the output in Figure 14–4C includes a main effect for time. Remember that this factor represents performance for both groups before and after fatigue. Since we are really interested in knowing about differences between the stable and unstable ankles and how these groups change after fatigue, the time factor probably does not add a great deal of additional information. In this case, it is only necessary to present the main effects and/or interactions that directly relate to your research question.

The findings directly related to your research question should be reported whether or not they are statistically significant. Tables and graphs should not be presented for nonsignificant findings. The potential reasons for nonsignificant findings may be explored in the discussion section of your thesis or manuscript (e.g., two interventions might be equally effective or perhaps there was insufficient statistical power).

In Chapters 13, 14, and 15, we discussed how to interpret the printout generated when analyses of variance and correlational analyses are computed. Most journals will not permit the entire ANOVA table or correlation matrix to be included in the manuscript, but rather require presentation of the findings in the text of the results. Journal editors may ask you to provide complete statistical tables to allow the reviewers to interpret the results. Display 16–1 shows two complete analysis of variance summary tables, and Display 16–2 illustrates the presentation of the relevant main effects and interactions in the text of the results. Display 16–3A is the complete correlation matrix from Chapter 15, and Display 16–3B is a summary table from the matrix.

Use of Text, Tables, and Figures

Text, tables, and figures (i.e., illustrations) can be used to present data or findings of the statistical analyses. If the data are not extensive and can be presented concisely, they should be included in the text of the results. A table should be used to present values that are too numerous to present in the text. A figure should be used to emphasize or convey the magnitude of differences or relationships between variables. Display 16–4 presents guidelines for using text, tables, and figures.

Tables

A table's title should clearly and succinctly identify the information to be presented in the table. The information in a table should be organized in a clear and logical manner (Display 16–5), and usually includes column and row headings, data cells, and footnotes. The column headings (left) should include the main categories of information to be presented. The row headings (right) are used to identify all items in that row. The independent vari-

Analysis of Variance Summary Table for External and Internal Rotation Perturbation: Hypothesis 1—Gender Differences in Muscle Reaction Time

Repeated Measures ANOVA with 1 Between (Gender) and 2 Within (Muscle Group and Muscle Side) for External Rotation Perturbations.

Source of Variance	Sum of Squares	df	Mean Square	F	Sig (.05)	Observed Power (.05)
Within Subjects						
Muscle Group	98590.72	2	49295.36	143.83	.000	1.000
Gender by Muscle Group	1411.92	2	705.96	2.06	.132	.417
Error (Muscle Group)	42498.02	124	342.73			
Muscle Side	2247.50	1	2247.50	41.73	.000	1.000
Gender by Muscle Side	8.46	1	8.46	.157	.693	.068
Error (Muscle Side)	3338.87	62	53.85			
Muscle Group by Muscle Side	1466.54	2	733.27	13.45	.000	.998
Gender by M Group by M Side	143.55	2	71.77	1.316	.272	.280
Error (M Group by M Side)	6762.58	124	54.54			
Between Subjects						
Gender	2475.59	1	2475.59	5.209	.026	.613
Error (Gender)	29463.87	62	475.22			

Repeated Measures ANOVA with 1 Between (Gender) and 2 Within (Muscle Group and Muscle Side) for Internal Rotation Perturbation.

Source of Variance	Sum of Squares	df	Mean Square	F	Sig (.05)	Observed Power (.05)
Within Subjects						
Muscle Group	95352.08	2	47676.04	137.85	.000	1.000
Gender by Muscle Group	886.75	2	443.38	1.28	.281	.274
Error (Muscle Group)	42887.17	124	345.86			
Muscle Side	6443.57	1	6443.57	56.62	.000	1.000
Gender by Muscle Side	9.69	1	9.69	.085	.771	.060
Error (Muscle Side)	7055.91	62	113.81			
Muscle Group by Muscle Side	5055.90	2	2527.95	26.69	.000	1.000
Gender by M Group by M Side	24.65	2	12.32	.130	.878	.070
Error (M Group by M Side)	11742.79	124	94.70			
Between Subjects						
Gender	2789.65	1	2789.65	6.642	.012	.718
Error (Gender)	26041.97	62	420.03			

ables are typically the row headings; the dependent variables, the column headings. The data cells are the body of the table, and should include means and standard deviations. The footnotes clarify any abbreviations used in the table and explain any symbols used in the body of the table to identify statistically significant findings.

Display 16-2   **Presentation of Analysis of Variance Main Effects and Interactions in the Text of Results**

We found that women responded significantly faster than men for both ER ($F_{1,62}$ = 5.209, p = .026) and IR ($F_{1,62}$ = 6.642, p = .012). Although this difference appeared to be due primarily to a shorter latency in quadriceps activation in women, no significant sex-by-muscle group (ER, p = .132; IR, p = .281) or muscle-side (ER, p = .693; IR, p = .771) interactions were found.

Source: Shultz, S.J., Perrin D.H., Adams M.J., Arnold, B.L., Gansneder B.M., & Granata K.P. (2001). Neuromuscular response characteristics in men and women after knee pertubation in a single-leg, weight-bearing stance. Journal of Athletic Training, 36, 37–43.

Display 16-3   **SPSS Correlation Output (A) and the Accompanying Summary Table (B)**

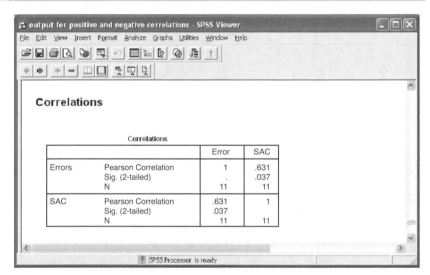

A.

Correlation between strength and flexion

	r	df	*p*
Error: SAC	.631	10	.037

B.

Display 16-4

Guidelines for Using Text, Tables, and Figures to Display Numerical Data

Uses of Text

Present quantitative data that can be given concisely and clearly

Describe simple relationships among qualitative data

Uses of Tables

Present more than a few precise numerical values

Present large amounts of detailed quantitative information in a smaller space than would be required in the text

Demonstrate detailed item-to-item comparisons

Display many quantitative values simultaneously

Display individual data values precisely

Demonstrate complex relationships in qualitative data

Uses of Figures

Highlight patterns or trends in data

Demonstrate changes or differences over time

Display complex relationships among quantitative variables

Clarify or explain methods

Provide information to enhance understanding of complex concepts

Provide visual data to illustrate findings (e.g., graphics, photographs, x-ray films, maps)

From: Iverson, C., Flanagin, A., & Fontanarosa, P.B., (Eds.). (1998). American Medical Association manual of style (9th ed.). Baltimore: Williams & Wilkins, p. 52.

Display 16-5

The Anatomy of a Journal Table

Table 3 • **Scores for three forms of the Standardized Assessment of Concussion** ← Title and table number

Form	Day 3 (n=25)	Day 5 (n=25)	Day 7 (n=25)	Day 60 (n=49) } Column headings
Row Headings { A	26.11 ± 1.91	25.72 ± 2.57	25.83 ± 1.33	26.50 ± 1.96	27.80 ± 1.32
B	26.29 ± 1.98	25.50 ± 1.69	25.11 ± 2.15	26.71 ± 2.69	26.56 ± 2.09
C	28.20 ± 1.62*	27.17 ± 1.17	27.10 ± 1.60	27.75 ± 1.75	27.19 ± 2.10

*Significantly greater than forms A and B at baseline. ← Footnote

Source: McLeod, T. C. V., Perrin, D. H., Guskiewicz, K. M., Shultz, S. J., Diamond, R., & Gansneder, B. M. (2004). Serial administration of clinical concussion assessments and learning effects in healthy young athletes. Clinical Journal of Sports Medicine, 14, 287–295.

Figures

A figure is used to present data, commonly in the form of a line or bar graph. A legend of figures is used to convey the information presented in the title and footnotes of a table. Displays 16–6A and B present a figure and legend of figures in the form they should be submitted to a journal, and Display 16–6C shows how the figure would ultimately appear in the journal. Note that the draft text in Display 16–6A differs from that in Display 16–6C. This was the result of the editorial process.

The advantage of a figure is the ability to emphasize or convey the magnitude of differences or relationships between variables. Interestingly, these differences or relationships can be misleading if the lengths of the vertical and horizontal axes are changed or if the range of possible values is reduced. These points emphasize the importance of the reader focusing on the presence or absence of statistically significant findings between the variables presented in the figure. Display 16–7 is an illustration of the same data presented in a bar graph with the y-axis scaled differently. Note that both panels show differences between the control and stretch groups, but the differences are more pronounced in Display 16–7A. The data are exactly the same, but the y-axis in Display 16–7B has been rescaled to enclose a larger range of values. In some cases you will find the effect reversed, and very small changes look significant because the y-axis is scaled to enclose too small of a range.

Figures are also used to present photographs of instruments or data collection procedures. Photographs of human subjects require the authorization of the subject. A sample consent form is presented in Display 16–8.

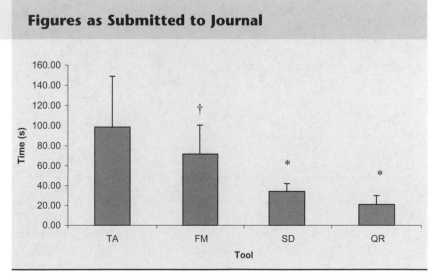

Display 16-6 A   **Figures as Submitted to Journal**

Figure 2.

Display 16-6 B **Figure Legends**

Figure–1. The helmet mounted on the force plate.
Figure–2. Mean time, in seconds, for removal of the face mask with the four tools. Error bars represent standard deviations. *SD and QR took significantly less time than the TA and FM. †FM took significantly less time than TA ($p <$ .05).
Figure–3. Mean force, in Newtons, applied to the helmet during removal with the four tools. Error bars represent standard deviations. *SD produced significantly less force than TA and FM. †SD and QR produced significantly less force than TA and FM ($p <$ .05).
Figure–4. Mean torque, in Newton-meters, applied to the helmet during removal with the four tools. Error bars represent standard deviations. *SD and QR produced less torque than TA and FM. †SD and QR produced significantly less torque than TA and FM. ‡FM produced significantly less torque than TA ($p <$ .05).

Display 16-6 C **Figure as Published by Journal**

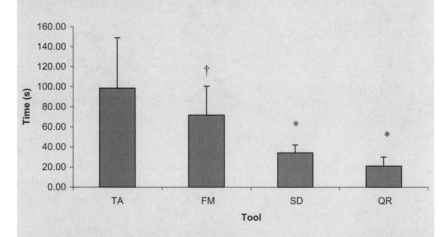

Figure 2. Mean time, in seconds, for removal of the face mask with the 4 tools. TA indicates Trainer's Angel; FM, FM Extractor; SD, Screwdriver; and QR, Quick Release System. Error bars represent standard deviations. *SD and QR took significantly less time than TA and FM. †FM took significantly less time than TA ($P < .05$)

Source: Jenkins, H.L., Valvoich, T.C., & Arnold, B.L. (2002). Removal tools are faster and produce less force and torque on the helmet than cutting tools during face-mask removal. Journal of Athletic Training, 37, 246–251.

Identical Data Reported Using Different Y-axis Scales

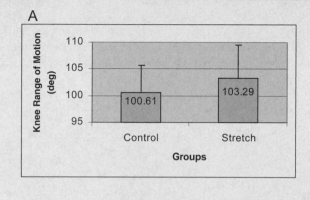

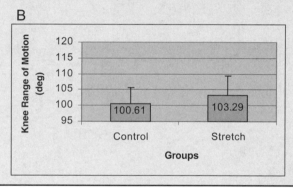

Redundant Presentation of Data

Display 16–9 illustrates the redundant presentation of data in a table and a figure. In this case it is likely a journal editor would require the author to use either the table or the figure to present the data. Since the magnitude of the differences is unremarkable, a table is the more desirable way to present these data. In reality, this is a good example of data that could be presented in the text of the results because of their simplicity and clarity.

Speculation Surrounding the Results

The results section should be just that, a presentation of the results without speculation about the findings of the study. The discussion section is used to interpret your findings and draw comparisons with other studies in the published literature.

Display 16-8

Journal of Athletic Training

RELEASE OF PHOTOGRAPHS

Date _____

I, _____, hereby give my permission for
(name of subject)
photographs and X-rays of me to be reprinted in a manuscript entitled

"_____" by author

_____

in the *Journal of Athletic Training*. I realize that my name will
remain strictly confidential.

_____

Signature of subject

_____

Signature of primary author

Source: Journal of Athletic Training Photo Release Form. Retrieved 3/25/04 from Journal of Athletic Training Website: http://www.journalofathletictraining.org.

In the Field

Jason prepared a manuscript from his thesis and submitted it for publication in the Journal of Athletic Training. *He had analyzed his data using an analysis of variance, and he included the ANOVA summary table to report the findings of this analysis. He wanted to report the actual values for the means and standard deviations of his variables, but also thought a visual comparison of the values would be helpful to the reader. To accomplish this, he reported the values in a table and used a figure to visually illustrate the differences between the variables. When he received the reviews of his manuscript, the editor requested that the relevant F values, degrees of freedom, and p values from the ANOVA table be incorporated into the text of the results, and that the summary table be deleted. The editor also suggested the table and figure presented the means and standard deviations in a redundant manner and that Jason needed to choose either the table or figure to report these values.*

An Example of Redundant Presentation of Data.

Results:

Statistical analysis produced a significant interaction for treatment across time ($F_{7,239} = 14.97$, $p < .05$) and a main effect for treatment ($F_{1,239} = 5.25$, $p = .05$). The means for the control and stretch groups are presented in Table 1. Changes in knee range of motion across time are illustrated in Figure 1. Post hoc testing revealed significant increases in hamstring flexibility for the stretch group lasting for 6 minutes. For the control group, hamstring flexibility declined across the time intervals.

Table 1 • Knee Range of Motion Means (and Standard Deviations) for the Control and Stretch Groups

Group	Pre-Str	0 mins	2 mins	4 mins	6 mins	8 mins	16 mins	32 mins
Control	40.53	42.8	43.3*	44.7*	45.4*	46.6*	48.1*	49.5*
	(11.0)	(11.3)	(11.4)	(11.5)	(11.7)	(11.8)	(12.4)	(13.1)
Stretch	38.8	31.0*	32.2*	34.5*	36.3*	37.2	39.1	40.6
	(11.2)	(9.2)	(8.5)	(8.7)	(9.5)	(9.3)	(10.2)	(11.4)

* Significantly different from the pre-stretch ($p < .05$)

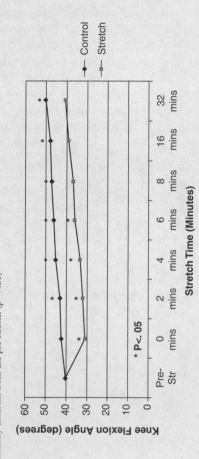

Figure 16–1. Knee range of motion means plotted across time. Adapted from Spernoga, S. G., Uhl, T. L., Arnold, B. L., & Gansneder, B. M. (2001). Duration of maintained hamstring flexibility following a one-time modified proprioceptive neuromuscular faciliation protocol. *Journal of Athletic Training, 36*, 44–48.

Summary

The results section of a thesis or dissertation should comprehensively report the statistical analyses related to each stated hypothesis. The results section of a manuscript should report only the findings most relevant to the stated purpose of the paper. Tables and figures should be used to report and illustrate the findings in a manner that is not redundant to what is reported in the text of the manuscript. Both significant and nonsignificant findings should be reported, and the reasons for nonsignificant findings should be explored in the discussion chapter of the thesis or dissertation, or in the discussion section of the manuscript. Comparisons of the results with other published studies should also be addressed in the discussion chapter or section.

Activities

1. Draft an outline or first draft of your results section.
2. Present the results in text, table, and figure formats. Discuss which method of reporting the results is most appropriate for a thesis or dissertation, manuscript, or oral presentation.
3. Compare and contrast the AMA and APA styles for preparing the results.

Bibliography

Day, R. A. (1998). *How to write and publish a scientific paper*. Phoenix, AZ: Oryx Press.

Day, R. A. (1992). *Scientific English: A guide for scientists and other professionals*. Phoenix, AZ Oryx Press.

Iverson, C., Flanagin, A., & Fontanarosa, P. B., (Eds). (1998). *American Medical Association manual of style* (9th ed.). Baltimore: Williams & Wilkins.

Chapter 17

Writing the Discussion

Objectives

After reading this chapter, you will:
- Understand how to organize the discussion.
- Appreciate the importance of focusing on the primary findings of the study.
- Know how to avoid excess speculation and overgeneralization of the findings.
- Understand how to compare and contrast the study's findings with others in the published literature.
- Know how to help clinicians apply the findings to athletic training clinical practice.
- Understand the importance of identifying and acknowledging the study's limitations.

Questions

While reading this chapter, think about answers to the following questions:
1. To what extent is speculation and generalization of the findings appropriate in the discussion?
2. Is it helpful to restate the results in the discussion?
3. Should I acknowledge the limitations of the study in the discussion?
4. Is there clinical relevance with every study, and should this be stated in the discussion?

Introduction

This chapter will provide you with guidelines about the content and organization of the discussion. The discussion chapter of your thesis or dissertation will be quite similar to the discussion section of the manuscript you write from your thesis or dissertation. You will especially enjoy writing the discussion because some speculation about your project is appropriate.

Nevertheless, it is important that your discussion relate closely to the purpose and findings of your study. You will also need to avoid generalizing the findings of your study beyond what can be justified from the design of your research and the population you studied. Finally, all studies have limitations, and it is important that you identify and address these limitations in the discussion. Display 17–1 presents a checklist for reviewing the discussion.

Organizing the Discussion

The discussion should open with a clear statement of the study's primary findings and should then address whether the results support or refute the hypotheses of the study. Comparisons with other studies in the published literature should be made, including those that support your findings and those that are in contrast with your study. If there are clinical implications of your findings, these should be pointed out, so that clinicians can apply your findings to their clinical practice. All studies have limitations, and the wise author identifies these in the discussion (rather than letting journal reviewers identify them!). The implications of your findings for future research should be identified, and the discussion should close with a concise concluding statement. It is not necessary to provide an overall summary of the study, as the opening abstract serves this purpose.

Open with the Study's Primary Findings

To help the reader focus on the primary findings of the study and to set the stage for where the discussion will go, it is helpful to open with a statement of the study's primary findings. For example, in the manuscript entitled "Relationship Between Sex Hormones and Anterior Knee Laxity Across the Menstrual Cycle," by Shultz et al., the discussion opens with this statement: "The primary findings were that estradiol, progesterone and testosterone each contribute to changes in knee laxity across the cycle, and that this relationship is stronger when changes in hormone concentrations are compared

Display 17-1 | **Checklist for the Discussion**

___ Opens with a clear statement of the study's primary findings.
___ Avoids a recapitulation of the findings presented in the results.
___ Identifies agreement or disagreement with the study's hypotheses.
___ Cites and discusses relevant research that both agrees and disagrees with the findings.
___ Generalizes the findings only to the population studied.
___ Addresses the notion of clinical versus statistical significance, if appropriate.
___ Presents the clinical applications of the findings, if appropriate.

In the Field

> *Brent is quite excited about finishing his research project and the associated manuscript that will be submitted for publication. As with many students, in his excitement he failed to recognize and acknowledge the limitations of the study in the discussion of the manuscript. In addition, he has cited and discussed only studies from the published literature that support and agree with his findings. He decides to submit his paper for review to the* Journal of Athletic Training. *When he receives his manuscript back from the journal, the editor informs him that the paper requires significant revisions before it can be considered for publication. As he reviews the comments of the reviewers, Brent notes the following reasons are given for the journal not accepting the manuscript: (1) incomplete review and discussion of the relevant literature; and (2) failure to identify and discuss the limitations of the study.*

with changes in knee laxity occurring approximately 3–4d later." This reminds the reader, in nontechnical language, that the hormones did in fact relate to observed changes in knee laxity. It is not necessary or appropriate to recapitulate the results in the discussion, and this tendency should be avoided.

Do the Findings Confirm or Refute Your Hypotheses?

In the Shultz et al. paper, the hypotheses were presented in the introduction in the following manner: "We hypothesized that (1) changes in knee laxity would occur at an identifiable time delay after a rise in hormone levels, (2) estradiol and progesterone combined would explain more of the variance in knee laxity than either hormone alone and that testosterone levels would have a negligible or negative effect on knee laxity changes, and (3) consistent with the variability in individual cycle characteristic between females, the relationship between hormone concentrations, and knee laxity would also be variable between women." The hypotheses are then explored in the discussion. For example, the authors state in the discussion: "Our findings support our hypothesis that estradiol and progesterone combined would explain more of the variance in knee laxity changes than either hormone alone, but appear to reject our hypothesis that testosterone would have a negligible or negative effect on knee laxity changes." The following paragraphs in the discussion then explore the reasons for the findings that both confirm and refute the hypotheses.

Compare and Contrast with the Findings of Others

The meat of the discussion is a comparison of your findings with others in the published literature. It is important that you avoid the tendency to discuss only the publications that support your findings. Rather, you should discuss both research that agrees with your results and research that does not support your findings. The discussion should explore the potential reasons for the differences between your findings and other reports in the published literature. In this regard, some speculation may be appropriate in the discussion, but you should avoid excessive speculation for why discrepancies between publications might exist.

Use of Tables and Figures in the Discussion

Occasionally a table or figure in the discussion may be helpful in emphasizing a point or to provide clarification to a complex concept. Display 17–2 provides an example of how the findings of several studies can be summarized in a table to facilitate a comparison and contrasting with the findings of other reports in the literature. It may be appropriate to simply refer the reader back to a table or figure in the results section of the paper or to create an additional illustration in the discussion. If an additional illustration is used, it is important that the table or figure presents new information and does not replicate material presented in the results section of the paper.

Be Cautious of Overgeneralization of Your Findings

Random selection of subjects and the use of inferential statistics in your study may permit you to generalize your findings to a larger population. That said, authors often have the tendency to overgeneralize their findings to an extent not justified by the design and findings of their study. For example, the Shultz et al. paper was part of a larger research agenda that is exploring the reasons that physically active females have a higher rate of

Display 17-2

Table 1. • **Brace and Tape Restrictions During Passive Range of Motion Testing**

	Normal Range of Motion (deg.)	Pre Exercise		Post Exercise	
		Restricted inversion (deg.)	% Restricted ROM*	Restricted inversion (deg.)	% Restricted ROM*
Eils et al.	39	14-22†	37-57†	-	-
Lohrer et al.	22	11	50	14.5	6
Vaes et al.	13.1	4.8	37	6.3	48
Vaes et al.	12.5–14.4‡	4.8–10.6†	37–78†	3.3–4.5†	52–88†
Yaggie & Kinzie	18	10-12†	55-67†	-	-
Mean	23	7.9	43.5		

* Percentage of available range of motion. Lower values represent greater restriction.
† Ranges represent differences across multiple ankle support conditions.
‡ Range represents multiple baselines across the same group of subjects.
Adapted from Arnold, B. L., & Docherty, C. L. (2004). Bracing and rehabilitation - what's new. *Clinics in Sports Medicine, 23*, 83–95.

Display 17-2   **Continued**

Table 2. • **Brace and Tape Restrictions During Trap Door Testing**

	Normal Range of Motion (deg.)	Pre Exercise		Post Exercise	
		Restricted inversion (deg.)	% Restricted ROM*	Restricted inversion (deg.)	% Restricted ROM*
Alt et al.	28–30‡	17–21†	27–42†	17–18†	62–84†
Eils et al.	39	19.89	51	-	-
Lohrer et al.	32	18	56	21–23†	66–72†
Ricard et al.	37.8	26.2–27.4	69–72	28.3-29.1	73-75
Vaes et al.	9.75	6.4	66	-	-
Mean	29.6	14.8	57.7		

* Percentage of available range of motion. Lower values represent greater restriction.
† Ranges represent differences across multiple ankle support conditions.
‡ Range represents multiple baselines of the same subjects.
  Arnold, B. L., & Docherty, C. L. (2004). Bracing and rehabilitation - what's new. *Clinics in Sports Medicine, 23,* 83–95.

injury to the anterior cruciate ligament than their male counterparts. Subjects for the study included 25 nonathletic female subjects, between the ages of 18 and 30 years; with a body mass index (BMI = weight/height^2) less than or equal to 30 years, who reported normal menstrual cycles (28–32 days) over the past six months. Consequently, it would be inappropriate to generalize the finding that changes in sex hormones mediate changes in knee laxity across the menstrual cycle beyond a population of people possessing similar characteristics. In addition, while the overall research agenda is concerned with the disparate rate of ACL injury in females, it would be inappropriate to speculate about any connection between these findings and actual incidence of injury to the anterior cruciate ligament. The study had nothing to do with injury to the ACL, but rather explored an issue that might ultimately contribute to what is known about predisposing ACL injury risk factors.

A common mistake seen in the discussion of manuscripts is the tendency to discuss nonstatistically significant findings as if they were in fact significantly different. If the statistical procedures you have used to analyze the data do not find statistically significant findings, they are not different, even if they might appear to be when comparing values in a table or figure. It is occasionally appropriate to discuss trends toward significant differences in the data, but you may be heading down a slippery slope when adopting this practice. It would probably be more appropriate to discuss the reasons why statistical significance was not achieved, such as inadequate statistical power because an insufficient number of subjects may have been included in the study. In some cases there might be "clinical significance" to the findings in the absence of "statistical significance." (In contrast, occasionally statistically significant findings are probably not very clinically meaning-ful.) Calculation of effect sizes (Cohen, 1988) can help the researcher and reader interpret the potential impact of the findings on clinical practice. As with discussing "trends" from nonstatistically significant findings, you should be cautious about suggesting that nonsignificant findings are clini-cally relevant. This concept was discussed in Chapter 12, where we pro-vided an explanation and interpretation of effect size.

Identify the Limitations and Suggest Future Research

All studies have limitations, and the wise author is forthcoming about the limitations of his or her study. In the Shultz et al. study, it was necessary to collect data every single day for a month across complete menstrual cycles. This required the collection of laxity data by more than one tester, which created a limitation addressed in the paper in this way: "An unavoidable limitation in a study of this magnitude was the need for two testers to obtain laxity measures, which may introduce more measurement error than a single tester. Although we made every effort to extensively train both testers and confirm acceptable intra- and inter-tester reliability, some variance between testers was noted. Ideally, we would have had one tester collect all measurements on a single subject, but the daily data col-lection needs of this project essentially made this impossible. Although this may have introduced greater error variance in the data, the fact that consistent trends were noted in our findings suggests this concern may be minimal."

The limitations of a study may very well establish the basis for future research. Moreover, only in very rare instances does any single study answer a question in a comprehensive and conclusive manner. In fact, many studies along the same theme are necessary to advance the scientific body of knowledge on any particular topic. In all probability, your study created more questions than it provided answers. In this regard, it is often helpful to identify for other researchers what you perceive to be logical next steps in helping to answer the questions addressed in your study, or hints to avoid repeating the limitations of your study. In the Shultz et al. paper, the authors encountered challenges with the end-to-end data procedure used in the analyses to accommodate the phase shifts across the menstrual cycle. To identify this as a limitation and to provide guidance to others conducting similar research, the authors stated this: "A second acknowl-edged limitation to this study is the end-to-end data procedure used in our analyses to accommodate the phase shifts" and "Although cycle variability is substantially less within women than between women, cycle to cycle vari-ations do exist". They also stated, "Future studies wishing to replicate these findings should collect data for a sufficient number of days preceding and following the cycle of interest to accommodate the desired range of time shifts."

Identify the Clinical Relevance of the Study

One distinguishing feature of the studies conducted by athletic training researchers is that the findings often have immediate clinical relevance to practitioners in the field. This is not always the case, but when clinical relevance does exist, it should be identified for practitioners who might read your manuscript. One good example of a study having immediate clinical relevance is seen in the paper by Valovich et al. (2003) "Repeat administration elicits a practice effect with the Balance Error Scoring System but not with the Standardized Assessment of Concussion in high school athletes." The purpose of this study was to investigate the effects of repeated administration of the Standardized Assessment of Concussion (SAC) and Balance Error Scoring System (BESS) in high school athletes. The results revealed no practice effect with the SAC and a slight practice effect with repeated administrations of the BESS. The authors present the clinical relevance of the findings in this way: "Although at this time we are unable to distinguish between improved performance on the BESS due to recovery or practice in an injured population, athletic trainers should expect their athletes to improve on subsequent test administrations. If the athlete's performance does not improve, then one might suspect a lingering abnormality, which should be followed up with an in-depth clinical examination."

It may also be appropriate to discuss and interpret for the reader the clinical versus statistical relevance of the study's findings. It is not uncommon to find statistically significant differences in the data that have little clinical meaning. Conversely, there may be instances where statistically significant differences are not found, while at the same time the findings may very well have important clinical meaning. The concept of effect size, discussed in Chapter 12, may be helpful in interpreting the clinical versus statistical significance of the findings.

Include a Concise Conclusion

The requirement of a conclusion within the discussion or as a separate subheading in the manuscript is somewhat variable among the authors' guides of journals in sports medicine. If the authors' guide does require or permit a concluding statement, it should be brief and to the point. The Authors' Guide for the *Journal of Athletic Training* states the following as related to a conclusion: "The manuscript should not have a separate summary section - the abstract serves as a summary. It is appropriate, however, to tie the article together with a summary paragraph or list of conclusions at the end of the discussion section." It might also be appropriate to include the clinical implications of your study and to offer suggestions for future research based on the questions generated from your findings in the concluding section of the discussion.

Summary

The discussion section of your thesis or the manuscript emanating from your thesis provides an opportunity to compare and contrast your findings with other research in the literature. You should write the discussion in a manner that addresses other manuscripts that both agree and disagree with your findings. Some speculation of the potential reasons for your findings is appropriate in the discussion, but it is essential that you only generalize your findings to the population you studied. Normally, findings that are nonstatistically significant are just that—not different. Occasionally it is acceptable to discuss trends in the data or the clinical implications of non-significant findings based on calculation of effect sizes. This should, however, be considered the exception rather than the rule.

Activities

1. Prepare an outline of the discussion, first identifying the general themes to be addressed.
2. Prepare a more detailed outline including a list of the published articles that will be used to compare and contrast your findings with others in the literature.

References

Cohen, J. (1988). *Statistical power analysis for the behavioral sciences* (2nd ed.). Hillsdale, NJ: Lawrence Erlbaum Associates.

Schultz, S. J., Kirk, S.E., Johnson, M. L., Sander, T. C., & Perrin, D. H. (2004). Relationship between sex hormones and anterior knee laxity across the menstrual cycle. *Medicine & Science in Sports & Exercise, 36*, 1165–1174.

Valovich, T. C., Perrin, D. H., & Gransneder, B. M. (2003). Repeat administration elicits a practice effect with the balance error scoring system but not with the standardized assessment of concussion in high school athletes. *Journal of Athletic Training, 38*, 51–56.

Bibliography

Day, R. A. (1988). *How to write and publish a scientific paper* (3rd ed.). Phoenix, AZ: Oryx Press.

International Committee of Medical Journal Editors. *Uniform requirements for manuscripts submitted to biomedical journal*. Retrieved from http://www.icmje.org

Huth, E. J. (1990). *How to write and publish papers in the medical sciences* (2nd ed.). Baltimore: Williams & Wilkins.

Chapter 18

The Publication Process

Objectives

After reading this chapter, you will:

- Understand the importance of disseminating the research findings.
- Know the various ways your findings can be published.
- Be able to prepare an abstract.
- Know how to present an abstract in slide, poster, and thematic poster settings.
- Understand how to prepare a manuscript according to the *Journal of Athletic Training* Authors' Guide.
- Appreciate how to establish who should be included as a coauthor and in what order authorship should occur.
- Know the process for submitting a manuscript for publication in a journal.

Questions

While reading this chapter, think about answers to the following questions:

1. Why is it important to disseminate the findings of a research project?
2. Is one manner of presenting an abstract more prestigious than another?
3. Is an abstract publication the same as a manuscript publication in a journal?
4. What is the difference between a refereed and a nonrefereed journal publication?
5. How do I select a journal for my manuscript?
6. Are all journal authors' guides essentially the same?
7. How do I determine who should be a coauthor and in what order should coauthors be listed?
8. How long does it take to publish a manuscript in a refereed journal?

Dissemination of the Research Findings

By the time you get to this chapter of the book, you are probably approaching the end of the research process – or at least that is what you think! In reality, the most important part of the process lies ahead, and that is to disseminate the findings of your study. Why is it important to disseminate your findings? At this point only you, your advisor or coauthors, and perhaps your classmates are aware of your study. For the study to truly have meaning, it should be disseminated to the scientific community so that it may be scrutinized for its importance (or lack thereof), and considered by others as we all attempt to expand the body of knowledge in athletic training.

There are several ways to disseminate the findings of a research project. You might have the opportunity to present your study at a state or district meeting of the National Athletic Trainers Association (NATA). The Research and Education Foundation of the NATA holds a Free Communications session at the annual meeting and clinical symposia for presentation of research by athletic trainers and other medical and allied health researchers. You have no doubt become aware of many of the journals that publish abstracts and manuscripts of clinical, basic science, and educational research related to athletic training and sports medicine. In general, there are two primary ways to disseminate the findings of your research. They include publication and presentation of an abstract and publication of a manuscript in a refereed or nonrefereed journal.

Abstracts

The term "abstract" has many meanings in the research process. It could apply to the abstract you will write for your manuscript. However, for this discussion, we are referring to the abstract that is written and submitted for publication and presentation at a scientific meeting. Perhaps you have noticed that each spring, the *Journal of Athletic Training* (*JAT*) publishes a supplement to the regular issue of *JAT*. This supplement publishes the abstracts that are presented at the Free Communications session of the annual meeting. In this section, we will review the process you would follow to write, submit, publish, and present an abstract at the annual meeting of the NATA.

Abstract Preparation

Each year the Research and Education Foundation publishes a "Call for Abstracts" in the *Journal of Athletic Training* (Display 18–1). This notice lists several categories of research and explains the guidelines under which the abstract must be written and submitted for review by the Foundation. The categories of abstracts include nonsurvey research (e.g., experimental, epidemiological), survey research, and clinical case reports. Specific instructions for preparing the structured abstract are provided, and you must closely adhere to these guidelines. For example, details related to typeface, margins, listing of authors and institution where the research was conducted, and length of the abstract are provided. The guidelines require that the abstract be submitted online. There is also a strict deadline for submission of abstracts for review and potential acceptance for presentation at the annual meeting.

Display 18-1

National Athletic Trainers' Association Research and Education Foundation Annual Call for Abstracts

NATA Research & Education Foundation CALL FOR ABSTRACTS

National Athletic Trainers' Association - Annual Meeting & Clinical Symposia
    Indianapolis, Indiana * June 12 -16, 2005
    DEADLINE FOR ABSTRACT SUBMISSION: DECEMBER 1, 2004
    All abstracts submitted for presentation at the 2005 NATA Annual Meeting and Clinical Symposia must be submitted ONLINE. See Instructions for Submission below.
          <u>***NOTICE: STRUCTURED SUBMISSION REQUIRED FOR 2005***</u>

<u>*PROCESS*</u>

    Instructions for Online Submission of Abstracts and Process for Review of All Submissions
    Please read all instructions before preparing and submitting the abstract. Individuals may submit only one Original Research abstract or Clinical Case Report abstract as primary (presenting) author, but may submit unlimited abstracts as a secondary author. All abstracts will undergo blind review. All presentations must be of original work (not previously presented). This restriction includes any electronic/internet postings. Exceptions to this restriction are limited to state and district meetings of athletic training organizations, and the NATA Athletic Training Educators' Conference.

<u>*PREPARATION OF ORIGINAL RESEARCH ABSTRACTS FOR FREE COMMUNICATIONS: EITHER ORAL OR POSTER PRESENTATION*</u>

    The Original Research abstract must be written to the generally accepted scientific standards of a research area. Abstracts not meeting these standards will not be considered. Original Research abstracts should present findings pertaining to healthcare issues of the physically active.

Instructions for Preparing Original Research Abstracts for Free Communications:

1. Provide all information requested on the online Abstract Author Information Form.
2. Top, bottom, right, and left margins of the body of the abstract (in a WORD file) should be set at 1.5" using the standard 8.5" × 11" format. Use a regular font no smaller than 12 pt. Provide the title of the paper or project starting at the left margin.

(Continued on following page)

Display 18-1

**National Athletic Trainers' Association
Research and Education Foundation
Annual Call for Abstracts** *(Contd.)*

3. On the next line, indent 3 spaces and provide the names of all authors, *with the author who will make the presentation listed first*. Enter the last name, then initials (without periods), followed by a comma, and continue the same format for all secondary authors (if any), ending with a colon.
4. On the same line following the colon, indicate the name of the institution (including the city and state) where the research was conducted.
5. Double space and begin entering the body of the abstract flush left in a single paragraph with no indentions. *The text of the body must be structured* (i.e., with the headings as indicated below). Do not justify the right margin. Do not include tables or figures. *The body must not exceed 400 words.*
6. Original Research abstracts must include the following headings as running headings within a single paragraph:

   For non-survey research (e.g. experimental, epidemiological)
   a. *Objective:* Provide a clear purpose statement establishing a need for the study.
   b. *Design and Settings:* Explain the experimental methods and materials utilized. Provide validity and reliability information on any novel instrumentation. Describe the underlying target population.
   c. *Subjects:* Describe the final subject pool and criteria for selection.
   d. *Measurements:* Describe the types of measurement and instrumentation utilized, data analysis procedures, statistical tests and significance level.
   e. *Results:* Provide the data that supports the stated aims and objectives.
   f. *Conclusions:* The statement of your findings must be consistent with the results as reported.

   For survey research
   a. *Objective:* Provide a clear purpose statement establishing a need for the study.
   b. *Design and Settings:* Explain the process of survey development (formative research and pre-testing). Provide validity and reliability information on any instrument utilized. Provide a description of the sampling methods and underlying target population.
   c. *Subjects:* Describe the final subject pool and response rates.
   d. *Measurements:* Describe any categorization or manipulation of data, statistical tests and significance level.
   e. *Results:* Provide the data that supports the stated aims and objectives.
   f. *Conclusions:* The statement of your findings must be consistent with the results as reported.

MOST COMMON REASONS CONTRIBUTING TO REJECTION OF ORIGINAL RESEARCH ABSTRACTS

*Information requested within structured heading is not provided
*The abstract is of a pilot study or preliminary data
*Poor overall clarity of writing
*Unclear specific aim or objective

(Continued on following page)

*Data does not match/support specific aim and/or conclusion

*Lack of operational definitions of primary independent and dependent variables

*Necessary definitions are excluded: of groups (e.g., training vs. non), conditions (e.g., fatigue, DOMS), variables (e.g., TTS, EMG onset, etc.)

*No demographic data describing the subjects, including number of subjects

*Methods used do not address specific aim or objectives

*No data in the results section

*No information on survey development process and available psychometric data

*Validity and/or reliability of instrument not established

*Poor or no description of sampling methods

*No description of statistical tests used

*Inappropriate use of statistics

*No presentation of measures of dispersion (variance, standard deviation, confidence intervals, etc.) associated with results

*No specific identification of the dependent variable(s) measured: e.g., what EMG, kinematics, kinetic variables exactly (values/labels would be very beneficial)

*No description of how dependent variable(s) were measured: e.g., scapula ROM, how they trained, how they loaded the extremity, etc.

*Results: are they significant, p values, direction of differences

*Inaccurate conclusion or clinical relevance of data

*Inaccurate depiction of the degree of generalizability of the data

*Research not unique

PREPARATION OF CLINICAL CASE REPORT ABSTRACTS FOR FREE COMMUNICATIONS: EITHER ORAL OR POSTER PRESENTATION

The Clinical Case Report abstract must be written to the generally accepted scientific standards of a research area. Abstracts not meeting these standards will not be considered. Clinical Case Report abstracts should present a unique individual athletic injury case of general interest to the NATA membership.

Instructions for Preparing Clinical Case Report Abstracts for Free Communications:

1. Provide all information requested on the online Abstract Author Information Form.

2. Top, bottom, right, and left margins of the body of the abstract (in a WORD file) should be set at 1.5″ using the standard 8.5″ × 11″ format. Use a regular font no smaller than 12 pt. Provide the title of the clinical case report starting at the left margin. The title should not contain information that may reveal the identity of the individual. An example of a proper title for a clinical case report is "Chronic Shoulder Pain in a Collegiate Wrestler."

3. On the next line, indent 3 spaces and provide the names of all authors, *with the author who will make the presentation listed first.* Enter the last name, then initials (without periods), followed by a comma, and continue the same format for all secondary authors (if any), ending with a colon.

4. On the same line following the colon, indicate the name of the institution (including the city and state) where the research was conducted.

5. Double space and begin entering the body of the abstract flush left in a single paragraph with no indentions. *The text of the body must be structured* (i.e., with the headings as indicated below). Do not justify the right margin. Do not include tables or figures. *The body must not exceed 600 words.*

6. Clinical Case Report abstracts must include the following headings as running headings within a single paragraph:

(Continued on following page)

National Athletic Trainers' Association Research and Education Foundation Annual Call for Abstracts *(Contd.)*

a. *Background:* Include the individual's age, sex, sport, pertinent aspects of their medical history, a brief history of their complaint and physical findings from the examination.

b. *Differential Diagnosis:* List all possible injuries or conditions based on history and physical findings. Include all possible diagnoses present prior to physician evaluation, diagnostic imaging and laboratory results.

c. *Treatment:* State the results of diagnostic imaging and laboratory results, final diagnosis of the injury or condition and the treatment and clinical course followed. Pertinent and unique details should be included, as well as the final outcome.

d. *Uniqueness:* Briefly describe the uniqueness of this case.

e. *Conclusions:* The statement of your findings must be consistent with the results as reported, and should concisely describe the most pertinent points of your clinical case.

MOST COMMON REASONS CONTRIBUTING TO REJECTION OF CLINICAL CASE REPORT ABSTRACTS

*Information requested within structured heading is not provided
*Poor overall clarity of writing
*Case reprot not unique
*Case report mismanaged

ABSTRACTS WILL NOT BE ACCEPTED AFTER DECEMBER 1, 2004

Retriered from NATA Research and Education Foundation: https://secure.e-builders.net/forms/efa.htm

---

The manner in which the abstract is written is somewhat similar to the abstract that accompanies the manuscript you will prepare for submission to a journal. In general, the abstract should include the purpose of the study, the basic procedures, main findings, and principal conclusions. Authors are required to use a structured abstract format that includes subheadings throughout the abstract. For an original research abstract, these subheadings might include objective, design and settings, subjects, measurements, results, and conclusions.

You will note from the Foundation's Call for Abstracts that the abstract is limited to no more than 400 words. This will require you to write succinctly and to avoid including unnecessary verbiage. For example, a problem statement could be shortened from "The purpose of the present study was to examine the effects of..." to "This study examined...." It will be important for you to "economize" your writing and to present only the most pertinent details of your study. The preparation of your abstract is a key to the successful review and acceptance of your study for presentation at a scientific meeting. The following list presents some keys to consider in writing your abstract:

Keys Points for Writing an Abstract

- Avoid writing and submitting an abstract until the data collection, analysis, and interpretation are completed.
- Clearly indicate the purpose of the study and significance of the findings.
- Be certain to address each component of the research project in the abstract, i.e., the purpose, methods, results, discussion, and conclusion.
- Include some data in the results to help convince the reviewers the study is actually finished.
- Generalize your findings only to the extent justified by the study population and methods.

Appendix 18–1 provides an example of an abstract that was published in the *Journal of Athletic Training* supplement and presented at the Free Communications session of the annual meeting.

Abstract Submission

As previously noted, most professional societies place a strict deadline for the submission of abstracts. You must plan well in advance to allocate sufficient time to write the abstract and to provide your coauthors with ample opportunity to read and provide feedback on your writing. Always provide all coauthors with the opportunity to review any abstract or manuscript submitted on which their name appears. You must pay extremely careful attention to detail, since errors in the abstract can lead to rejection by the reviewers or, if the abstract is accepted, these errors will appear when the abstract is published in the journal supplement or meeting proceedings.

In most cases, the abstract submission should precede the submission of the full manuscript that is written from your study. The abstract publication and presentation are considered to be the original presentation of the findings of the research project. Most professional societies consider it inappropriate, and in some cases even unethical, to present an abstract after the study has appeared as a full manuscript publication in a journal. Does this mean you cannot write and submit your manuscript for review by a journal until after you have presented your abstract? You will learn later in this chapter that the process of submission and review for publication of a manuscript in a refereed journal is a lengthy one. So, if you wait until the abstract is published and presented, you will lose precious time in the preparation, review, revision, and publication of your manuscript. It is important, however, that you carefully consider the timing of your abstract and manuscript submissions to avoid any chance that publication of the full manuscript might precede the abstract publication and/or presentation.

Presenting an Abstract

The presentation of your abstract can be an unnerving one, especially knowing that the audience likely includes some of the foremost authorities on your topic. The options for presenting your abstract usually include oral or poster formats, or a combination of the two (thematic poster). Some professional societies let you indicate your preference for oral or poster formats, while others provide no opportunity for input into this aspect of the abstract presentation. In either case, the preparation of a poster or oral presentation is somewhat of an art, and these formats for presentation of your research carry the same level of prestige in the scientific community.

Oral Presentations

The first step in preparing the oral presentation of your abstract is to determine how long you will be permitted to speak. The meeting moderator will strictly adhere to the time limitations, and so it is very important that you rehearse your presentation until you are absolutely certain you will adhere to the time allotted. In general, the presentation should adhere to the traditional order of presenting a study, which should be the same as the components of your abstract. These components include a short introduction and statement of purpose, methods and procedures, main findings, and principal conclusions. A very common mistake is to spend too much time reviewing the literature as part of the introduction. The audience is primarily interested in hearing and learning about your study and not what has been previously published in the literature. Table 18–1 provides an approximation of the amount of time that should be devoted to each component of the presentation.

Your slide or PowerPoint presentation should be prepared in a manner that facilitates good visualization throughout the room. Use a large font and limit each slide to no more than six or seven lines of text. For oral presen-

Table 18–1 • **Suggested Allocation of Time for a 15-Minute Abstract Presentation**	
Component	**Time (min.)**
Introduction with use of only a few key studies to set up the problem	3
Statement of the problem (purpose statement)	1
Methods	3
Results	3
Discussion	2
Questions from the audience	3
Total	15

tations, figures are much more effective at presenting data and conveying relationships among groups or variables than tables with numbers.

Advances in technology permit the creation of flashy and colorful slides with any number of backgrounds and points of entry of the text on each slide. Our recommendation is to minimize the use of these distracters–especially for a scientific presentation—and to use clear and crisp slides with a minimum of extraneous material. The following list summarizes some of the key points to making a successful oral presentation of your research:

Keys to a Successful Oral Abstract Presentation

- Organize the presentation by the traditional components of an abstract, i.e., purpose, basic procedures, main findings, and principal conclusions.
- Rehearse the presentation so you can present all of the material in the allocated time without rushing. If you have to rush, reduce the amount of material.
- Assume your audience is reasonably well informed about the topic, but be sure to include key points and details.
- Avoid a lengthy review of the literature and focus instead on your study.
- Select and focus on the main points and avoid unnecessary details.
- Use figures (graphs) rather than tables to present and illustrate data

In the Field

Carl realized the goal of conducting research was to share his findings with his peers. The thought of sharing his findings for the first time was intimidating and downright scary. The first opportunity he had to orally present research findings to his peers was following the completion of his masters' degree. He had practiced his oral presentation with his advisor, who assured him he was ready. However, he wondered if he was ready, and if there would be any opportunity for him to fall flat on his face?

Prior to taking the stage at the NATA Research and Education Free Communications oral research presentations, Carl knew the other presenters were students like himself. At the last moment, a prominent scholar of athletic training entered to present in the absence of one of his students. The scholar's presentation was on the topic of cryotherapy, and he was a renowned expert on this topic. Carl's initial impression was that he was doomed for failure. He thought he certainly couldn't compete, and that the scholar surely would highlight any personal weakness and the limitations in Carl's research study. Neither occurred. While he was frightened, the presentation went fine and the atmosphere of the session was professional and nonthreatening. Carl entertained a few questions from the audience, and the scholar was his always professional and compasionate self. Carl has now witnessed hundreds of oral presentations, and realizes the forum to present one's research findings should not be fraught with personal anxiety but should be looked upon as an unintimidating opportunity to share with one's colleagues.

Posters

Posters convey essentially the same information as the oral presentation, except that the poster replaces the slide or PowerPoint presentation. The poster includes the abstract that was submitted and accepted for presentation at the meeting. The poster then presents the introduction, methods, results, figures and tables, discussion, and conclusion. The information in the poster is the same as would be used for an oral presentation, except that a larger, bold (32 point) typeface is used. The poster is usually available for review by the audience for several hours, and authors of each poster are asked to be present for questions and discussion for 1 hour (Fig. 18–1).

Thematic Posters

Thematic posters are a combination of an oral and poster presentation. Preparation of the poster follows the same guidelines as presented above. The session is normally 3 hours in length, with the first hour unstructured for viewing of posters by the audience. In the remaining time, each author makes a 7-minute presentation, followed by 3 minutes of questions and answers. The session concludes with a 30-minute panel discussion with a moderator and each of the poster presenters. Audiovisual aids are not used for the thematic poster session.

Manuscript Preparation

The final phase of the research process is preparation and submission of a manuscript from your study. This process involves selection of a journal by you and your coauthors, preparation of the manuscript according to that journal's author guide, and submission of the manuscript. The journal's author guide will dictate the specific style manual you need to follow. For example the *Journal of Athletic Training* uses the American Medical Association's *Manual of Style*. Other journals may use the Publication Manual of the American Psychological Association.

Refereed versus Nonrefereed Journals

Journals are generally categorized as refereed or nonrefereed periodicals. The primary distinction is that refereed journals use a process of peer review. Peer review means the articles submitted to the journal are reviewed by a collection of experts on the topic. These experts then make a recommendation to the editor regarding the manuscript's suitability for publication in the journal. Figure 18–2 is a flow chart of the peer-review process. Refereed, or peer-reviewed, publications carry greater weight in the scientific community, since they provide some level of assurance that experts have scrutinized the manuscripts before the materials are published. We should

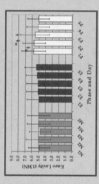

Figure 18–1 Example of a poster presentation.

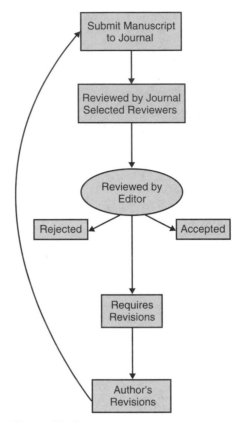

Figure 18–2   Flow chart of the peer-review process.

also note that abstracts don't undergo the same rigor of peer review and author revision as a full manuscript. Abstracts are therefore considered a preliminary presentation of a study, and a peer-reviewed journal publication is considered the normal standard for disseminating the findings of a study.

Selecting a Journal

Before beginning the actual preparation of your manuscript, it is important to determine the journal to which you intend to submit your paper. Many factors go into this decision, including the journal's selectivity and backlog of articles, compatibility of the journals' mission with the topic of your paper, readership of the journal and your target audience, and the exposure you will gain from publication of your work in a particular journal.

One measure of a journal's selectivity is the ratio of articles accepted to those rejected. It is not uncommon for the top scholarly journals to have an accept/reject ratio as low as 10 percent. This simply means that you have one chance in 10 that your paper will be accepted for publication in the journal. Naturally, it will be important for you to realistically assess the magnitude of your research before deciding to submit your manuscript to a highly selective journal.

Some researchers assess a journal's scientific prestige by its impact factor rating. The impact factor is calculated from the number of citations of a journal's articles in the preceding 2-year period divided by the number of citable materials published by that same journal within the same period (Kurmis, 2003). The journal impact factor ratings are issued by the Institute for Scientific Information (ISI) in Philadelphia for approximately 8000 journals in ISI's *Journal Citation Report*. Unfortunately, the impact factor is fraught with limitations and biases, and is often inappropriately interpreted and applied.

Some journals also have a substantial number of articles that have been accepted for publication, but not yet published. This backlog of articles may or may not be related to the quality of the journal. The balance between quality of the journal, backlog of articles, and your interest in publishing the findings in a timely manner should be considered in selecting the journal. You can obtain information related to accept/reject ratios and backlog of manuscripts by contacting the journal's managing office.

You should also review the subject matter of the journal to ensure compatibility of the journal's mission with your topic. For example, if you have studied the incidence of eating disorders in female athletes, the *International Journal of Sport Nutrition* might be a more appropriate outlet for your research than the *American Journal of Sports Medicine*, the periodical of the American Orthopaedic Society for Sports Medicine. On the other hand, if you have studied the relationship of eating disorders to the female athlete triad, the *American Journal of Sports Medicine* might be very appropriate for your work. The following list summarizes some of the factors to be considered in selecting a journal for submission of your manuscript:

Factors to Consider in the Selection of a Journal

- What is the journal's accept/reject ratio?
- Where is the journal indexed?
- Is the readership of the journal representative of your intended target audience?
- Is the topic of your manuscript consistent with the mission of the journal?
- What is the size of the journal's circulation?
- What is the average time from submission of a manuscript to publication of an article?
- What is the magnitude of the journal's backlog of articles?

Journal Author Guides

After you have selected a journal, you will need to carefully review that journal's authors' guide. Unfortunately, all journals do not use the same authors' guide, which can add confusion to the process of manuscript

Display 18-2

The Journal Impact Factor

- The impact factor, a simple mathematical formula reflecting the number of citations of a journal's material divided by the number of citable materials published by that same journal, has evolved to become one of the most influential tools in modern research and academia.
- The impact factor can be influenced and biased (intentionally or otherwise) by many factors.
- Extension of the impact factor to the assessment of journal quality or individual authors is inappropriate.
- Extension of the impact factor to cross-discipline journal comparison is also inappropriate.
- Those who choose to use the impact factor as a comparative tool should be aware of the nature and premise of its derivation and also of its inherent flaws and practical limitations.

From: Kurmis, A. P. (2003). Understanding the limitations of the journal impact factor. Journal of Bone and Joint Surgery, 85A, 2449–2454.

preparation. However, several common elements can be found in most author guides, including items related to copyright, use of human subjects, and writing and reference format:

Elements Common to Most Journal Authors' Guides

- An author statement that the manuscript is original and not under simultaneous review by another journal
- A transfer of copyright from the author to the journal
- Disclosure of potential conflict of interest
- Institutional approval for use of human subjects
- Writing style and reference format
- Procedures for submission of the manuscript to the journal office

In the Field

Doug is putting the final touches on the manuscript from his dissertation. As part of this he has begun to consider to which journal he should submit his paper. He is aware that journals indexed in MEDLINE are considered to be upper tier. His next step is to select a journal that represents his research topic. From this he narrowed the list to three journals. In consulting with his advisor as well as others who had submitted manuscripts to these three journals he discovered that although two of them had high impact factors, the rejection rates for manuscripts were also high. The third journal had a lower impact factor and a lower rejection rate, but had a slow review process and a year's backlog of articles. Because Doug is interested in being hired in a tenure-track faculty position and he would like to get some publications under his belt as soon as possible, he decided to look at some other journals. By expanding his search to include journals indexed in Sport Discus and PubMed Central, he was able to find some sports medicine journals with shorter review and publication timelines but at the cost of lower impact factors. Nevertheless, based on his current career goals, this seemed to be the best option.

Two manuals commonly used as the basis for the authors guide for journals in sports medicine and athletic training are from the Council of Biology Editors and the American Medical Association. Appendix 18–2 presents the authors' guide used by the *Journal of Athletic Training*. Regardless of the journal you select for submission of your manuscript, you will need to use that journal's authors guide as the bible for all policies and procedures related to manuscript preparation and submission.

Authorship

In reality, the determination of who will be your coauthors should have been decided long before it is time to begin writing the paper. In general, the members of the research team who had involvement in the formulation of the topic, the design of the study, the analysis and interpretation of the data, and preparation and review of the manuscript should be included as coauthors (see Display 18–3). Some journals require the submission of an authorship form as evidence that all contributors have met the criteria for authorship. One definition of authorship has been provided by the Vancouver Group, a prominent collection of scientists involved in the publication process as editors and authors. At a meeting of the group in Copenhagen, a revised criterion for authorship was provided that includes substantial contributions to conception and design, acquisition of data, or analysis and interpretation of data. This was a modification of an earlier position that recommended participation in each of these areas of manuscript preparation.

The order of authorship is normally determined by the magnitude of each author's contribution to the study. The researcher who had the primary role in the study—from formulation of the topic to preparation and submission of the manuscript—should be the primary author and listed first. Some professional societies, such as the American College of Sports Medicine, tend to list the senior author last when he or she is not the primary author. This might be the researcher who served as the faculty mentor for the project or the laboratory director of the facility in which the research took place. In any event, each coauthor should have played a substantial role in the research process. People having a lesser role, but nonetheless deserving of recognition, should be included under acknowledgments at the end of the article. Display 18–4 provides two examples of criteria that can be used to determine authorship of a scientific paper.

Manuscript Submission

Before submission to the journal of your choice, you should give each coauthor an opportunity to review and comment on the paper. It is also a good idea to ask a colleague who is somewhat removed from the study to read

Display 18-3   **Journal of Athletic Training Authorship Form**

JAT# _____ Title of the manuscript _____

Please write or type in each author's last name, and then indicate the contributions of that person in the appropriate categories.

Contributors who do not meet the criteria for authorship should be thanked in the Acknowledgments section.

	Contribution*										
Author's Last Name	Conception & design	Acquisition of data	Analysis & interpretation of the data	Drafting of the article	Critical revision of the article for important intellectual content	Final approval of the article	Provision of study materials or patients	Statistical expertise	Obtaining of funding	Administrative, technical, or logistic support	Collection & assembly of data

Name of author completing checklist_____ Date_____

Contribution descriptions reprinted with the permission of the Annals of Internal Medicine.

and comment on the paper's clarity. Once you have completed these steps and all authors are comfortable with the quality and accuracy of the manuscript, you are ready to submit your paper.

Author Letter

Your manuscript must be accompanied by a letter, signed by all authors, stating that the material is original, not under simultaneous review by another journal, and will not be submitted to another journal until it is released back to the authors (in the case of rejection). The letter should also transfer copyright ownership of the paper, should it be published, to the journal or in some cases the journal's professional society. The issue of copyright is an important one, because it means that even though it is your

Display 18-4

Examples of Criteria for Authorship

From "Uniform requirements for manuscripts submitted to biomedical journals." *The New England Journal of Medicine* 336:309–315, 1997:

"Authorship credit should be based only on substantial contributions to (a) conception and design, or analysis and interpretation of data; and to (b) drafting the article or revising it critically for important intellectual content; and on (c) final approval of the version to be published."

From: *Journal of Athletic Training* Authors' Guide:

"Each author must have contributed to the article. This means that all coauthors should have made some useful contribution to the study, should have had a hand in writing and revising it, and should be expected to be able to defend the study publicly against criticism."

study and that you wrote the paper, the journal has ownership after the manuscript is published. This means that if you want to use any material from the article for your future work (such as illustrations or tables), you must obtain permission from the original source and reference the article accordingly in all subsequent publications.

Receipt by the Journal Office

When your manuscript arrives at the journal's office, it will be screened to ensure compliance with the authors' guide and that the author letter (with all signatures) accompanies the paper. If either of these requirements is not met, the manuscript will be returned to the authors. If all preliminary requirements have been met, the paper will be assigned to a panel of expert reviewers.

The Review Process

The editor, or in some cases an associate editor, will oversee your manuscript during the review and revision process. Normally two or three content experts will be assigned to review the paper in a blind or double-blind manner. The blind format means the author is unaware of the identity of the reviewers, and the double-blind format means both the authors and reviewers are unaware of each other's identity. The blind format is used to reduce the likelihood of reviewer bias and to enable the reviewer to be uninhibited in providing an honest assessment of the paper. Once the content experts have completed their reviews, the manuscript is returned to the editor, who will make a decision regarding the disposition of the paper at this point.

The editor will review the comments and recommendations of the reviewers, and then decide to (1) accept without revisions, (2) accept with revisions, (3) request revisions before making a decision, or (4) reject. It is very unusual for a manuscript to be accepted without revisions. More commonly, the paper will be returned to you along with the reviewers' comments and a request to revise the paper before a decision regarding its suitability for publication will be made. Often, the process of review and revision occurs over multiple occasions before the paper is ultimately accepted for publication. It is in the authors' best interest to carefully address each reviewer's comments either by making the recommended changes or by carefully articulating in a response letter the rationale for not making any recommended changes. If the manuscript is rejected for publication, the editor will usually provide the reasons that are the basis for this decision.

Common Reasons for Rejection of Papers Submitted for Publication

- The manuscript does not contain new, unpublished information that will expand the body of knowledge.
- The authors are unwilling to address the suggestions of the reviewers.
- The design of the study is inappropriate to answer the research question.
- The statistical analyses are incorrect.
- The authors have failed to establish the reliability and validity of the instrumentation and the data collection procedures.
- The conclusions of the paper cannot be supported by the findings of the study.

If the manuscript is rejected, the authors are free to submit it to another journal. If the manuscript is accepted for publication, it will be moved into the production phase.

Manuscript Acceptance and Publication

After your manuscript is accepted for publication, it will be copyedited and typeset by the journal's managing editor and often by the company that publishes the journal. When this phase is completed, you will receive galley proofs of your manuscript, which are pages of text exactly as the paper will appear in the journal. This is your last chance to carefully examine the manuscript for any errors in the text, tables, and figures. You should painstakingly review the galley proofs, since missed mistakes will appear in your journal article forever.

After the production process is complete, your manuscript will be ready for publication. Several factors influence the timing of the publication, including the backlog of articles accepted by the journal and the potential of publishing a group of articles related by topic or theme in the same issue.

Table 18–2 • **Realistic Timeframe of a Research Project from Development of a Topic to Publication in a Refereed Journal**	
Fall 2004:	Development of the topic and preparation of the proposal
Spring 2005:	Collection and analysis of data
Summer 2005:	Interpretation of findings and preparation of an abstract
Fall 2005:	Submission of abstract for June 2006 annual meeting, and preparation of a manuscript
Spring 2006:	Submission of manuscript and receipt of reviews from the journal editor
Summer/June 2006:	Presentation of abstract at Free Communications session
Summer 2006:	Continued revision and review of the manuscript
Fall 2006:	Acceptance, copyediting, and typesetting of the manuscript for publication; review of galley proofs
Spring or Summer 2007:	Journal publication of the research project

It is not unusual for a period of 3 months to 1 year to pass before your accepted manuscript actually appears as an article in a journal. Table 18–2 illustrates a realistic timeframe from conception of the study topic to when it appears as a journal publication.

It should be quite clear by this point that the process of conducting a research project, preparing it for dissemination to the scientific community, and ultimately publishing it in a refereed journal is a lengthy one. However, the process is one of the more gratifying experiences you will have in your academic life and one that will contribute significantly to expanding the body of knowledge in athletic training.

Summary

The process of disseminating and publishing research findings typically involves three primary steps. The first step is to prepare your findings in abstract form. This abstract is submitted to a professional organization (e.g., NATA or American College of Sports Medicine) for publication in their journal's research supplement. The second step is presentation of your research at the organization's annual meeting. This step is directly tied to the first. In order to be invited to present your findings, your abstract must be accepted for publication. If the abstract is published, you will then be required to present your findings in one of three forms: an oral presentation, a poster, or a thematic poster. Although some organizations allow researchers to request a preferred format, the ultimate decision is made by the organization. The final step is submission of a complete manuscript to a refereed journal for publication. In general the scientific community regards this last step as the most important, and research that is not published in a journal as a full manuscript (i.e., only published as a research abstract) has minimal scientific impact.

Activities

1. Using the research findings from your project, write an abstract following the format prescribed by the NATA Foundation.
2. Using the research findings from your project, prepare a poster following the format prescribed by the NATA Foundation.
3. Using the research findings from your project, prepare a slide presentation for presentation at a professional conference.
4. Using the research findings from your project, begin converting your Introduction, Methods, Results, and Discussion into a manuscript according to the *Journal of Athletic Training* authors guide.

References

Kurmis, A. P. (2003). Understanding the limitations of the journal impact factor. *The Journal of Bone and Joint Surgery, 85A*, 2449–2454.

Bibliography

International Committee of Medical Journal Editors. *Uniform requirements for manuscripts submitted to biomedical journals: Writing and editing for biomedical publication.* Retrieved 3/25/04 from the International Committee of Medical Journal Editors Website: http://www.icmje.org

Iverson, C., Flanagin, A., & Fontanarosa, P. B. (Eds.). (1998). *American Medical Association manual of style* (9th ed.). Baltimore: Williams & Wilkins.

Appendix 18–1

Example of an Abstract Published in the *Journal of Athletic Training* Supplement and presented at the Free Communications Session of the NATA's Annual Meeting and Clinical Symposia

Lower Extremity Muscle Activity and Kinetic Patterns Differ Between Double-leg Drop Landings and Drop Jumps

Ambegaonkar JP, Shultz SJ and Perrin DH: University of North Carolina at Greensboro, Greensboro, North Carolina

Objective: Drop landings (DL) and drop jumps (DJ) are used to study neuromuscular and biomechanical demands on the lower extremity during physical activity. Little is known about how muscle activation and kinetics may differ between these tasks. Our objective was to compare lower extremity muscle activity and kinetic patterns during the initial landing phase of a double-leg DL and DJ. *Design and Settings:* Subjects performed 10 drop landings and 10 drop jumps each from a .45m box (order counterbalanced). Surface electromyography recorded muscle activity and a forceplate recorded kinetic data of the dominant leg. *Subjects:* Fifteen physically active females (21.2±4.1 yrs, 167.4±8.6 cm, 67.4±13.5 kg). *Measurements:* Onset of muscle preactivity (ON) and integrated muscle activation amplitudes 150 ms before ($IEMG_{pre}$) and after ($IEMG_{post}$) impact were recorded for the medial and lateral quadriceps (MQ, LQ), hamstrings (MH, LH), and lateral gastrocnemius (LG) muscles. Peak Ground Reaction Forces (GRF_{pk}) and time to GRF_{pk} (GRF_{tpk}) were also recorded. Two separate repeated measures ANOVAs for ON and IEMG compared muscles (MQ, LQ, MH, LH, LG) by task (DL, DJ), and in the case of IEMG, also by impact phase (pre, post). Paired samples t-tests compared DL & DJ on GRF_{pk} and GRF_{tpk}. Alpha level was set *a priori* at .05. *Results:* ON differed by muscle and landing task ($P=.006$). While in both tasks MH, LH, & LG activated earlier than MQ & LQ, the LG activated earlier in DL (190.3±116.6ms) than DJ (125.1±35.5ms). For IEMG, muscle activation differed by muscle, landing task and impact phase (i.e. a 3-way interaction). Post-hoc analyses using separate 2-way ANOVAs for $IEMG_{pre}$ and $IEMG_{post}$ followed by main effects testing revealed greater $IEMG_{pre}$ for DL vs. DJ in MQ (38.3 vs. 32.6%MVIC) and LG (59.2 vs. 53.6%MVIC; $P=.049$), but greater $IEMG_{post}$ for DJ vs. DL in all muscles ($P=.006$). GRF_{pk} was greater in DJ vs. DL (1.10 vs. .82BW; $P=.038$), but occurred much later upon landing (GRF_{tpk}=238.6 vs. 91.4ms; $P<.0001$). *Conclusions:* When performing a DL as compared to a DJ, subjects demonstrated greater preactivity of the LG and MQ, and earlier activation of the LG before impact, and then reduced muscle activation in all muscles and a more abrupt increase in GRF upon landing. These finding suggest that lower extremity muscle activity and kinetic patterns during landing may differ considerably depending on whether a subsequent task is anticipated.

Condensed Version of the *Journal of Athletic Training* Authors' Guide (Revised January 2000)

The complete text of the Authors' Guide can be found at the *Journal of Athletic Training* web site (www.journalofathletictraining.org) It is also available from the editorial office. The American Medical Association's Manual of Style served as the basis for this Authors' Guide.

The mission of the *Journal of Athletic Training* is to enhance communication among professionals interested in the quality of health care for the physically active through education and research in prevention, evaluation, management, and rehabilitation of injuries.

Submissions

Submit 1 original and 5 copies of the entire manuscript (including figures and tables) to *Journal of Athletic Training* Submissions, Hughston Sports Medicine Foundation, Inc, 6262 Veterans Parkway, PO Box 9517, Columbus, GA 31908–9517.

All manuscripts must be accompanied by a letter signed by each author and containing the following statements: "This manuscript 1) contains original, unpublished material that has been submitted solely to the *Journal of Athletic Training*, 2) is not under simultaneous review by any other publication, and 3) will not be submitted elsewhere until a decision has been made concerning its suitability for publication by the *Journal of Athletic Training*. In consideration of the NATA's taking action in reviewing and editing my submission, I, the undersigned author, hereby transfer, assign, or otherwise convey all copyright ownership to the NATA, in the event that such work is published by the NATA. Further, I verify that I have contributed substantially to this manuscript as outlined in the current Authors' Guide." Manuscripts that are not accompanied by such a letter will not be reviewed. Accepted manuscripts become the property of the NATA. Authors agree to accept any minor corrections of the manuscript made by the editors.

Each author must have made some useful contribution to the study, should have had a hand in writing and revising it, and should be able to defend the study publicly against criticism.

Financial support and provision of supplies must be acknowledged. Include grant or contract numbers whenever possible. Give the complete name of the funding institution or agency, along with the city and state in which it is located. If individual authors were fund recipients, list their names parenthetically.

Authors must specify whether they have any commercial or proprietary interest in any device, equipment, instrument, or drug that is the subject of the article in question. Authors must also reveal if they have any financial interest (as a consultant, reviewer, or evaluator) in a drug or device described in the article.

Signed releases are required to verify permission for the *Journal of Athletic Training* (1) to reproduce materials taken from other sources, including text, figures, and tables; (2) to reproduce photographs of individuals; and (3) to publish a case report. A case report cannot be reviewed without a release signed by the individual being discussed in the report. Release forms are available on the *JAT* web site and from the editorial office, or authors may use their own forms.

The *Journal of Athletic Training* uses a double-blind review process. Authors and institutions should not be identified in any way except on the title page.

Published manuscripts and accompanying materials cannot be returned. Unused manuscripts will be returned if a stamped, self-addressed envelope is submitted.

Text Preparation

Each page must be printed on 1 side of 8-by-11-inch paper, double spaced, with 1-inch margins in a font no smaller than 10 points. Include line counts on each page and page numbers to facilitate the review process. Do not right justify pages.

Organize manuscripts as follows, with each section beginning on a separate page:

a. Title page
b. Acknowledgments
c. Abstract and Key Words
d. Text (body of manuscript)
e. References
f. Tables (each on a separate page)
g. Legends to figures
h. Figures

Titles should be brief within descriptive limits. A 16-word maximum is recommended. The title page should also include the name, title, and affiliation of each author and the name, address, phone and fax numbers, and e-mail address of the corresponding author.

A structured abstract of no more than 250 words must accompany all manuscripts. Required items differ by type of article. **Original Research**: Objective, Design and Setting, Subjects, Measurements, Results, Conclusions, and Key Words; **Literature Review**: Objective, Data Sources, Data Synthesis, Conclusions/Recommendations, and Key Words; **Case Report**: Objective, Background, Differential Diagnosis, Treatment, Uniqueness, Conclusions, and Key Words; **Clinical Technique**: Objective, Background, Description, Clinical Advantages, and Key Words. Key Words should include 3 to 5 words that do not appear in the title.

Begin the manuscript text with an introductory paragraph or two in which the purpose or hypothesis of the article is clearly stated and developed. Tell why the study needed to be done or the article written and end with a statement of the problem or controversy. Reserve a detailed review of the literature for the discussion section.

Write in the active voice (for example, instead of "Subjects were selected," use "We selected subjects") and in the first person (for example, instead of "The results of this study showed," use "Our results showed").

The body of the manuscript varies according to the type of article. The body of an **Original Research** article consists of a methods section, a presentation of the results, and a discussion of the results. The body of a **Literature Review** should be organized into subsections in which related thoughts of others are presented, summarized, and referenced. The body of a **Case Report** should include personal data (age, sex, race, marital status, and occupation when relevant – but not name), chief complaint, history of present complaint (including symptoms), results of physical examination, medical history, diagnosis, treatment and clinical course, criteria for return to competition, and deviation from expectations. The body of a **Clinical Technique** should include both the *how* and *why* of the technique: a step-by-step explanation of how to perform the technique, supplemented by photographs or illustrations, and an explanation of why the technique should be used.

A separate summary section should not be included. However, it is appropriate to tie the article together with a summary paragraph or list of conclusions at the end of the discussion section.

Units of measurement should be recorded as SI units, as specified in the *AMA Manual of Style*, except for angular displacement, which should be measured in degrees rather than radians.

Percentages should be accompanied by the numbers used to calculate them.

Communications articles, including official Position Statements and Policy Statements from the NATA Pronouncements Committee; technical notes on such topics as research design and statistics; and articles on other professional issues of interest to the readership, are solicited by the *Journal*. An author who has a suggestion for such a paper should contact the editorial office for instructions.

Number references consecutively, using superscripted Arabic numerals, in the order in which they are cited in the text. Reference citations are formatted according to the *AMA Manual of Style*. Journal title abbreviations conform to *Index Medicus* style.

Figure and Table Preparation

Figures: All black-and-white line art should be submitted in camera-ready form. Line art should be of good quality and should be clearly printed on white paper with black ink, sans serif typeface, and no box. Computer-generated art should be printed on a laser printer. Figures that require reduction for publication must remain readable at their final size (either 1 column or 2 columns wide). Photographs should be glossy black-and-white prints. Do not use paper clips, write on photographs, or attach photographs to sheets of paper. Prepare write-on labels with the figure number, author name, and an arrow indicating the top, and affix the labels to the reverse of each figure. Submit 1 original and 5 copies suitable for review.

Tables: The title is bold, and the body and column headings are roman type. Units are set above rules in parentheses, and numbers are aligned in columns by decimal. Footnotes are indicated by symbols *, †, ‡, §, ||, ¶. Capitalize the first letter of each major word in titles; for each column and row entry, capitalize only the first word.

Please keep in mind that this Authors' Guide is a condensed version of the full text, which is available on the *JAT* web site and from the editorial office. It is important to refer to the complete version when preparing an article for submission to *JAT*. Any further questions should be directed to the editorial office.

Part 6
Additional Issues

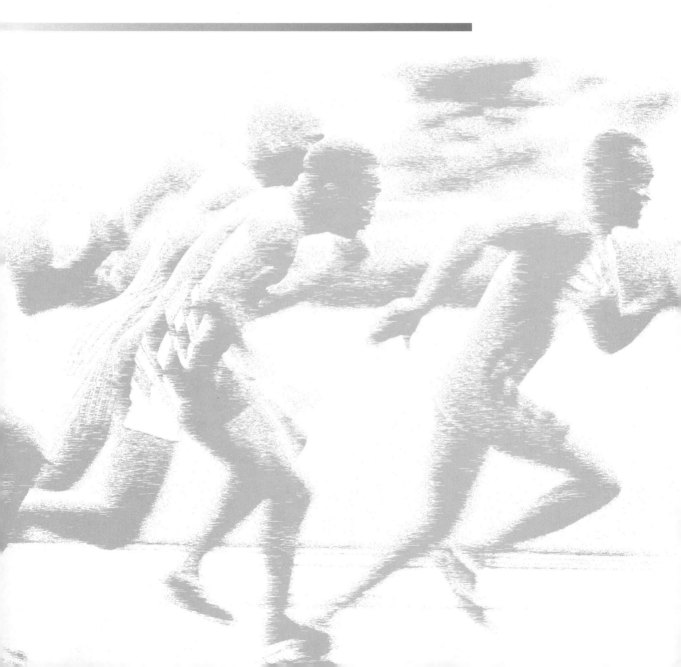

Chapter 19

Introduction to Grant Writing and Research Funding Sources

Sandra J. Shultz PhD, ATC, CSCS

Objectives

After reading this chapter, you will:

- Describe the purpose, goals, and benefits of seeking funding for research.
- Appreciate the variety of funding sources and grant mechanisms that support sports medicine research.
- Describe the process by which to identify appropriate granting agencies to seek funding for your research idea.
- Describe the essential elements and steps in the grant application process.
- Appreciate the importance and role of the institution and collaborators in the application process.

Questions

While reading this chapter, think about answers to the following questions:

1. How do I find an appropriate funding source for my research?
2. What types of grants are available to fund my research?
3. How do I know whether my project is fundable?
4. What kind of time and effort are required to write a winning proposal?
5. What can I expect once the proposal is submitted?
6. Who will benefit if my proposal is funded?

 Introduction

One stumbling block frequently encountered in the research process is a lack of funding and/or resources needed to carry out the research project. While you may feel you have a great research idea, you may not have the resources available in your program or research laboratory to cover the required personnel time, equipment, and/or supplies needed to conduct the project. In such cases, you are forced to either change your research direction or to seek out potential funding sources from which to request the necessary costs.

Writing a competitive grant proposal is a skill that requires considerable time and effort beyond the initial research proposal. If successful, however, a grant has the potential for many benefits and rewards. A grant award need not always be for a substantial monetary amount to benefit faculty members or students in their research endeavors. While some projects are dependent on significant financial support, others may only require a few hundred dollars for needed supplies that would otherwise not be available unless paid for out of pocket. Even in situations where resources are adequate, smaller grant awards can provide additional flexibility for such things as student support, lab supplies, and travel and presentation expenses. Furthermore, there are a number of nonmonetary personal and professional rewards that are realized through seeking grants, regardless of the amount awarded.

This chapter is intended to introduce you to the grant-writing process by exploring the goals and benefits of seeking grants, the variety of resources and mechanisms from which funding can be sought, and the basic elements and considerations in the grant application process. Although this chapter is not intended to provide instruction on how to successfully write a research grant proposal, a number of resources are provided from which this information can be obtained.

Goals and Benefits of Seeking Research Funding

In addition to the obvious financial support a grant award provides, there are other important goals and benefits associated with the grant-writing and award process. Moreover, these goals and benefits are not limited to the individuals seeking the award, but also extend to benefit the program, institution, and/or discipline to which the awardees are affiliated.

Individual Goals/Benefits

For individuals seeking an award, grant funds serve to promote and support their research agenda as well as their educational and career goals. Grant awards can be used to support the individuals conducting the research, to cover the equipment and supply costs of the research, or both.

Whether you are a student working on a thesis or dissertation, a clinician interested in investigating the efficacy of a treatment or rehabilitation protocol, a teacher or clinical instructor wishing to develop new curricula and opportunities for your student interns, or a tenured faculty member striving to develop and support an independent research agenda, your project will likely have expenses. In many cases, sufficient funds and resources are not available at the institution to cover the substantial costs of a particular project, requiring one to seek money from outside the program area or institution. In other cases, a grant may simply supplement current resources, providing additional funds for student, faculty, and laboratory activities that would not otherwise be covered. These additional funds may offset travel to a professional meeting to present the research findings, cover expenses for presentation development (i.e., printing or slide or poster production), provide a summer stipend or wages, or may simply free up or "pay back" laboratory supplies so that they can be available for other projects. In each of the above cases, individuals who know where and how to obtain additional funds through grant writing can achieve goals that would otherwise not be attainable at their institution.

Grants can also meet educational and career goals by supporting a particular position. Grant awards are often used to support additional student, research, and faculty positions that otherwise would not exist at the institution. These positions may fulfill a variety of purposes, including training of undergraduate and graduate students or interns, funding of research assistants or technicians for a particular project, research and clinical training experiences for postgraduates, and provision of additional faculty positions required for a particular project or program. These positions are often referred to as "soft-money" positions, since they are not directly supported by the institution and are lost once the grant funds are exhausted. Although these positions may seem tenuous, they clearly provide opportunities and experiences that would otherwise not exist were it not for grant funds. In fact, it is quite possible that your own assistantship may be supported by grant funds.

For the tenure-track faculty member, grant writing can play a vital role in both obtaining a faculty appointment and maintaining job security through promotion and tenure. At many institutions, the ability of faculty members to write grants and bring in external funding to support their research is not only desirable but also expected. Take a moment to review some of the recent job announcements for faculty positions in athletic training and sports medicine. You will often see a statement to the effect that the "ability to secure external funding and develop and maintain an independent research agenda" as an expectation for the successful applicant. Thus, for a faculty member to be successful in achieving promotion and tenure at these institutions, he or she must have a good understanding of the grant-writing process and be able to write a competitive grant proposal. Moreover, the ability to demonstrate grant-writing experience or success when applying for the position can provide a considerable "leg up" and set the applicant apart from others who may be competing for that position.

Equally important but less tangible individual benefits derived from the grant-writing process include promotion and recognition from others outside the institution and within the profession at large. When students or faculty members receive funding for their research, this essentially says that others also feel their research is important and serves to legitimize and validate their research question within the sports medicine community. In other words, it is one thing for you to think your research question is important, but when others (i.e., grant reviewers) consider your research question important enough to support it financially, this brings greater confidence that the research is credible and clinically relevant.

Program/Institutional Goals and Benefits

Grant writing also serves to meet departmental and institutional goals, bringing recognition and prestige to the university. For example, federal granting agencies pay the indirect costs associated with funded research. These indirect costs support the use of facilities and administrative costs of the research. Grants supplement institutional support to promote training and research activities. For athletic training programs, these activities may expand research and clinical opportunities for students. On a larger scale, grant funds also serve to meet program area, department and school-wide goals to attract external funding, which can improve national college rankings, enhance institutional prestige, and ultimately attract better students.

Professional Goals/Benefits

Finally, the goals and benefits of grant writing reach beyond the local institution to the profession at large. When funding is provided to support and promote a particular research agenda, new knowledge is gained from that research. For example, grant funding may allow for the development and testing of a new treatment or rehabilitation protocol, which leads to faster or safer recovery from an injury. A new educational model may be evaluated, leading to an improved method of learning and student education. A new research model may be tested, which may serve to validate a new assessment instrument or improve scientific inquiry in the future. When these findings are then communicated in a public forum through abstract presentations and lectures at professional meetings and through publication in professional journals, the knowledge within the profession is ultimately advanced. This newfound knowledge will ultimately improve the services to the physically active, the educational preparation of students, the clinical skills for practitioners, and the science by which we evaluate our research questions. Clearly, the goals and benefits of grant funding extend well beyond the individual who may be submitting the grant proposal.

Types of Funding Agencies and Grant Mechanisms

Numerous resources are available to assist your grant-writing efforts and to identify potential funding agencies and mechanisms. The Internet is a powerful and time-efficient tool to search for these resources. To gain a perspective of the wealth of information the Internet provides, simply type in the word "Grant" using one of the search engines on your web browser. Display 19–1 provides just a sampling of grant resource links that may be

Display 19-1	**Grant Resources: Links to Pertinent Web Sites**

Grant Search Engines

- Foundation Directory. A comprehensive directory providing descriptions of more than 74,000 grantmakers, including private grant-making foundations, community foundations, operating foundations, and corporate grantmakers. Retrieved 3/25/04: http://fconline.fdncenter.org
- Foundations and Grantmakers Directory. Retrieved 3/25/04: http://www.foundations.org/grantmakers.html
- Grant Select Online Grant Resource Database. Retrieved 3/25/04: http://www.grantselect.com
- Community of Science Funding Opportunities. Retrieved 3/25/04: http://fundingopps.cos.com

Grant-Writing Resources

- How to Write a Winning Proposal and Get Those Grants!: A Beginner's Guide to the Proposal Writing and Submission Process at the University of Virginia. Retrieved 3/25/04: http://trc.virginia.edu/Publications/Grants.htm.
- National Institute of Arthritis and Musculoskeletal and Skin Diseases (NIAMS) division of the National Institute of Health 2000–2004 Strategic Plan. This document assists the grant writer by providing the topical areas and research initiatives of particular interest to NIH and NIAMS. Retrieved 3/25/04: http://www.niams.nih.gov/an/stratplan/overview.htm
- Barrett, E. Hints for Writing Successful NIH Grants. University of Miami School of Medicine. Retrieved 3/25/04: http://chroma.med.miami.edu/research/Ellens_how_to.html
- Grant-Writing Resources. Provides a comprehensive list of grant writing resources. Retrieved 3/25/04 from A+ English Writing and Editing Network: http://www.writingnetwork.com/grantlinks.htm

Granting Agencies for Sports Medicine Research

- Aircast Foundation: Orthopaedic Research and Education. Retrieved 3/25/04: http://www.aircastfoundation.org/funding/index.html
- American College of Sports Medicine Research Grants. Retrieved 3/25/04: http://www.acsm.org/GRANTS/grants.htm#ACSMFoundation.
- American Orthopaedic Society for Sports Medicine. Retrieved 3/25/04: http://www.aossm.org/research/default.htm
- Center for Disease Control and Prevention (CDC) Funding. Retrieved 3/25/04: http://www.cdc.gov/funding.htm
- National Athletic Trainers' Association Research and Education Foundation. Retrieved 3/25/04: *http://www.natafoundation.org.*
- NATA District Grants:
  - Eastern Athletic Trainers' Association. Retrieved 3/25/04: http://www.goeata.org
  - Mid-Atlantic Athletic Trainers' Association. Retrieved 3/25/04: www.maata.org/
  - Great Lakes Athletic Trainers' Association. Retrieved 3/25/04: http://www.glata.org
  - Mid-America Athletic Trainers' Association. Retrieved 3/25/04: http://www.maata.net/
  - Far West Athletic Trainers' Association. Retrieved 3/25/04: http://www.fwata.org/
  - Southeast Athletic Trainers' Association. Retrieved 3/25/04: http://www.seata.org/

(Continued on following page)

Display 19-1

Grant Resources: Links to Pertinent Web Sites
(Contd.)

Application Forms and Instructions

- National Institute of Arthritis and Musculoskeletal and Skin Diseases (NIAMS) division of the National Institute of Health (NIH) Grants and Contracts. Retrieved 3/25/04: http://www.nih.gov/niams/grants/
- National Institute of Health. Lists Research Training Opportunities for Undergraduate, Pre-doctoral and Post Doctoral Awards. Retrieved 3/25/04: http://grants.nih.gov/training/extramural.htm. Applications and Instructions can be downloaded from: http://grants.nih.gov/grants/funding/416/phs416.htm
- National Strength and Conditioning Association (NSCA). Retrieved 3/25/04: http://www.nsca-lift.org
- Women's Sport Foundation. Retrieved 3/25/04: http://www.womenssportsfoundation.org
- Applications and instructions available for downloading for NIH grant applications. Retrieved 3/25/04: http://www.niams.nih.gov/rtac/grantapps/index.htm
- Grant agency electronic forms available for downloading in MAC, PC, and PDF formats. Retrieved 3/25/04: http://tram.east.asu.edu/

useful to students, faculty, and researchers in athletic training. It includes a variety of grant search engines that allow you to do a customized search for funding sources based on your research topic. You can limit your search by the type of agency (i.e., federal versus foundation), type of grant (e.g., research, training, equipment, and so on), funding range, and topical key words that will target agencies and grant mechanisms potentially compatible with your line of research. Many of these search engines allow you to set up a custom profile, providing you with weekly or daily updates of new grant mechanisms that match your inquiry.

Funding Agencies

There are a wide variety of agencies from which funding can be sought. Websites for some of the funding agencies that support sports medicine research are listed in Display 19–1. These agencies vary considerably in the scope of research they are interested in funding, the amount of money they may have available, and the mechanisms of support they are willing to fund. Granting agencies are typically categorized as institutional, federal, foundations, professional, or private.

Institutional

The first place to look for funding is within the academic institution with which you are affiliated. Some institutions offer small grants with the primary goal of supporting students and faculty. For instance, there may be a pool of money for which students can apply to attend a conference or to cover miscellaneous costs for their thesis or dissertation. New faculty may be able to apply for seed money to initiate their research agenda until external funding can be obtained. An example may be to apply for 1 or 2 months of summer salary to focus on grant-writing and research efforts. In most cases, institutional reserves for these "internal grants" are fairly limited and are intended to support only short-term or small projects. While these institutional grants are competitive, they have a high probability for funding. Unfortunately, many students and faculty are unaware that these funding opportunities exist at their institution, so they never apply. Students and faculty are encouraged to search their university's research funding web sites to discover the potential funding sources available at their institution. An excellent starting point is a visit to the institution's office of sponsored programs or office of research services that provides a wide range of services to encourage and support research, creative, and scholarly activities.

Federal

Federal granting agencies are funded by the United States government, and usually represent large money sources that support a broad array of research and educational initiatives. Examples of federal agencies include the National Institutes of Health (NIH), the Centers for Disease Control and Prevention (CDC), and the Department of Education (DOE). Within each of these federal agencies are multiple institutes or divisions that offer a variety of mechanisms for funding, including opportunities for student awards. One need only search the Websites of these federal agencies to appreciate the breadth and depth of the funding opportunities offered.

While federal granting agencies provide millions of dollars in funding annually, applying for federal grants is highly competitive and has a lower probability of funding compared to other types of granting agencies. The application process is often quite complicated and tedious, and there can be considerable delay (e.g., as much as a year or more) between the time of application and notification of a funding decision. However, for the applicant who is successful in obtaining a federal grant, it is well worth the effort and patience, and it brings considerable financial support, prestige, and recognition to both the individual and the institution.

Foundations

Foundations are nonprofit organizations that offer grants to individuals, institutions, and other nonprofit organizations. They may represent the philanthropic or research arm of a company or professional organization, or may be stand-alone entities. The primary reason for their existence is to award grants and give away money. As such, they often have a higher probability of funding, more streamlined application process, and faster timeline for review and funding notification than other types of granting agencies. Foundations vary widely in the range of funding they offer as well as the type of research or activities they wish to fund. While some have very specific funding interests, others are quite general. Examples of foundations that are particularly targeted to support sports medicine research are listed in Display 19–1.

For athletic training professionals, the National Athletic Trainers' Association (NATA) established the Research and Education Foundation in 1991 to support and advance the athletic training profession through research and education. The goals of the foundation are listed in Display 19–2.

There are also a number of other professional and private foundations that support athletic training and sports medicine research. The Aircast Foundation is one such private foundation that was established in 1996 to promote scientific research and education in the area of orthopedic medicine and science. Other potential foundation funding sources include the American College of Sports Medicine (ACSM), the American Orthopaedic Society for Sports Medicine (AOSSM), and the Women's Sport Foundation. Conducting an online search coupling key words such as "orthopedic," "sports medicine," and "athletic training," with "foundation" will yield a number of potential private foundation funding sources.

Professional (District and State Athletic Training Organizations)

Many district and state athletic training associations have limited funds available to promote student and faculty research and educational interests within the profession. These awards are typically less than $3000 and are ideal when project costs are small or when seeking funds to support initial

Display 19-2	**National Athletic Trainers' Association Research and Education Foundation**
FOUNDATION GOALS	• Advance the knowledge base of the athletic training profession. • Encourage research among athletic trainers who can contribute to the athletic training knowledge base. • Provide forums for the exchange of ideas pertaining to the athletic training knowledge base. • Facilitate the presentation of programs and the production of materials providing learning opportunities about athletic training topics. • Provide scholarships for undergraduate and graduate students of athletic training. • Plan and implement an ongoing total development program that establishes endowment funds, as well as restricted and unrestricted funds, that will support the research and educational goals of the foundation.

Retrieved 3/25/04 from National Athletic Trainers' Association Foundation: http://www.natafoundation.org

pilot work for a future proposal. Students and faculty are encouraged to visit their NATA district and state association Websites or contact their respective grants and scholarship committees often to learn of available grant and scholarship opportunities.

Private

Private industries and corporations may also set aside funds to support research projects or programs that may directly or indirectly advance the products or interests of the company. In contrast to federal and foundation grants, their purpose in awarding grants is less philanthropic and more self-serving, with the primary goal of testing, evaluating, or promoting their products. Private corporations may provide funding by donating a piece of equipment or a drug for the research project and may also provide seed money for smaller projects. They represent an excellent source of potential funding if the project you are working on uses equipment or products that may either promote recognition of the product or further validate its use.

While some corporations may have a formal application mechanism for requesting funding, other companies may award funds based on a developing partnership with the investigator. According to Gitlin and Lyons (1996), one of the most important factors in obtaining funding from a corporation is the investigator's ability to form a mutually beneficial and trusting research partnership with a company. For example, over time an individual may have developed a relationship with a particular company, offering clinical expertise to improve the quality of the company's product. The company becomes aware of the individual's research skills and asks the individual to evaluate a new product that is in development, providing the necessary funding to support the research and personnel. Another example may be a researcher who wishes to test the efficacy of a particular brace in limiting motion during sport activity. The researcher then approaches the company who manufacturers the brace, asking it to support the research project by donating the braces.

The only caution when seeking funds from private corporations who may have a vested interest in the investigator's research is to make sure that academic and research integrity are maintained. Obviously, if the research findings demonstrate the brace is effective, or more effective if tested against other braces, that company will ultimately benefit from this independent research. However, the findings may not always be in the company's favor. In order to protect research integrity, an agreement between the investigator and private company should be made prior to the project ensuring that (1) the investigator will have complete ownership of all data, (2) the investigator is free to disseminate the results through presentations, abstracts, and manuscripts, regardless of findings, and (3) at no time can the company use the name of the university or any of its students or faculty to market its product.

Types of Funding Mechanisms

Just as there are multiple purposes for seeking funding, there are also multiple mechanisms through which one can apply for funding. While some mechanisms are designed to support a particular individual's education or training, others are intended to support a particular research project or to purchase large pieces of equipment. On a larger scale, grant mechanisms are also available to fund a collaborative research center or program to advance a comprehensive research agenda.

Educational and Training Grants

Education and training grants are designed to support students, faculty, or clinicians seeking to enhance or promote their education, research, or clinical training in a particular discipline. Scholarships support the educational preparation of both undergraduate and graduate students by providing funding for tuition, fees, and living expenses. Although these scholarships are intended to support the student rather than a specific research project, the funds provided can help free the student's time from other wage-earning activities so that he or she can devote time to research and scholarly efforts. The NATA Foundation provides more than 50 scholarships annually, each in the amount of $2,000. Table 19–1 provides information on the variety of student scholarships (and grants) available through the NATA Foundation.

Table 19–1 • NATA Foundation Student Scholarships and Grants Available

Award Type	Awards Given Annually	Eligibility Requirements
Scholarships • Undergraduate • Graduate • Doctoral	60 Awards $2,000 each	• Application deadline Feb. 10th annually • NATA member • Minimum 3.2 GPA (4.0 scale) • Must be sponsored by an NATA certified athletic trainer
Osternig Masters Grant	Multiple Awards $1,000 max. each	• Must be NATA member at time of application submission • Full-time masters student during term of grant • Deadline May 1st and Nov 1st annually
Doctoral Research Grant	Multiple Awards $2,500 max. each	• Must be NATA certified member at time of application submission • Full time doctoral student during term of grant • Deadline March 1st annually

Retrieved 3/25/04 from National Athletic Trainers' Association Foundation: http://www.natafoundation.org

Fellowship or research training grants are intended to promote the development of researchers, clinicians, and scholars through funding of intensive or specialized training programs. These grants primarily cover salary support, travel, and tuition, but may also cover minimal supplies and equipment. Predoctoral training awards (undergraduate and graduate) are designed to support early research experiences (i.e., thesis or dissertation) or clinical experiences. The NATA's Osternig Masters Grant and Doctoral Research Grant programs are examples of predoctoral training awards that support athletic trainers working on a master's thesis or doctoral dissertation, respectively. Information about these awards, including eligibility criteria, submission deadlines, and application procedures, can be found at http://www.natafoundation.org (see also Table 19–1).

Postdoctoral training awards promote additional research training immediately after the completion of a terminal degree and before full-time employment. Clinician-researcher training awards assist health professionals to gain new knowledge or specialized skills through intensive research training experiences. Career development awards are intended to provide money for an investigator to concentrate a large percentage of their effort to develop or advance a particular research agenda. Career development awards assist new investigators in getting their research agenda off the ground and seasoned investigators who could benefit from an intensive period of research focus to advance their career. Career development awards are available through the National Institutes of Health and National Science Foundation and may also be offered by individual institutions.

Research Grants

Granting mechanisms designated as research grants are intended to fund a particular project through salary support; research team support; costs of materials, supplies and operating expenses; and presentation/travel expenses to present the findings at a scientific or professional meeting. Research grants are further delineated by the type of research they support. Typically, research grants are categorized as either basic science, clinical/applied, educational, epidemiological, or qualitative in nature (Table 19–2).

Project Grants

Project grants are large, comprehensive awards that support collaborative efforts focused on a broader research agenda. These are typically large-scale, multi-year, multi-million-dollar projects and are highly competitive. They create the opportunity to bring together researchers from a variety of disciplines and backgrounds (e.g., athletic trainers, orthopedists, biomechanists, and engineers) to pool their expertise in an attempt to answer a more comprehensive research question than each could adequately address alone.

Table 19–2 • **Types of Research Grants**	
Basic Science	Controlled laboratory studies that answer a specific scientific question that adds to the theoretical body of knowledge of a particular discipline (i.e., exercise physiology, biomechanics, motor learning, biomedical engineering)
Clinical/Applied	Studies that are carried out in the field where scientific theory is applied to a particular clinical practice or problem. Includes assessment of the efficacy of a particular preventative measure, intervention/treatment technique, rehabilitation program, or use of a new clinical device. The goal is to investigate a particular outcome associated with the clinical intervention.
Educational	Tests the application or effectiveness of learning strategies, educational materials, instructional technique or curricula. May support the planning and implementation of a new educational program, revising or updating of a curriculum, or recruiting and retention of students.
Epidemiology	Collection of injury rate data to describe the frequency, incidence and injury patterns associated with a particular subgroup, body region or condition.
Qualitative/Observational	More descriptive in nature, including surveys and observational studies.

Essential Elements and Steps in the Grant Application Process

Grantsmanship = Art + Science + Luck

Grantsmanship is a combination of art, science, and perhaps a bit of luck. In order to "sell" your research idea to a granting agency, the proposal must be creative and present your ideas in such a way that it clearly demonstrates the significance of the project and why it should be funded over any other application received.

Developing the Research Idea: Desirable Characteristics and Potential for Funding

Obviously, the first step in the grant application process is the development of a research idea. But what is it that determines whether a research idea is potentially fundable? To appreciate the desirable characteristics of a fundable research idea, let's consider the following scenario of Shaniqua (see "In the Field," p. 331), who wishes to propose her research idea to a granting agency for funding.

While there are similarities between writing a grant proposal and writing a research proposal, there are also clear differences. Whether you are proposing your research idea to your faculty advisor or a granting agency, both require strong scientific or technical writing skills. However, in order to obtain funding, the grant proposal requires more than just an adequate presentation of the research purpose and plan; it must also create excite-

In the Field

Shaniqua is a graduate student working toward her master of science degree in Athletic Training. She has a keen interest in trying to understand why more female athletes sustain injury to their anterior cruciate ligament compared to male athletes. After reviewing the literature, she has the theory that female sex hormones may influence knee laxity and injury risk, and wishes to compare knee laxity in collegiate athletes at selected time points across one complete menstrual cycle. To do this study correctly, she realizes that she will need to take blood samples and purchase ovulation kits to determine hormone levels accurately. Her advisor has read her proposal and is excited about the research idea. However, he indicated that the costs of this project would be about $1,500 and unfortunately, there are not sufficient funds in the lab budget to fund her project. She decides to submit her research proposal to a granting agency to obtain external funding.

ment and demonstrate a clinical or scientific need that the granting agency can identify with. While your research idea may have merit and importance to you and your faculty advisor, you will also need to sell the granting agency on its merit and importance to be successful in obtaining funding. To demonstrate these qualities, the proposal should possess the following characteristics.

Descriptive versus Hypothesis Based

Research that is hypothesis driven rather than just descriptive will typically make for a stronger proposal. With a hypothesis-driven proposal, there is a clear research question and expected finding that can be well supported by current theory or knowledge. A descriptive purpose on the other hand, doesn't necessarily define or answer a specific question or result, and simply aims to establish whether two or more variables may be related. While it is true that you may not know whether a relationship exists in some cases, particularly when previous research is lacking, this may give the appearance that you do not have a clear understanding of the literature and are not sure what you expect to find. For your research question to have purpose, you must have some idea that a specific relationship exists and has clinical meaning, otherwise you are just simply satisfying your curiosity. Let's continue with the example of Shaniqua (see "In the Field," p. 332).

Although the difference in this example may seem subtle, a clear hypothesis will better demonstrate the intent, direction, and significance of the project to the granting agency.

Developing a Theoretical Model

For a research question to be hypothesis driven and justifiable, it must be based on the current state of knowledge and what can be logically theorized based on that knowledge. To form the basis for your hypothesis, you will

In the Field

Shaniqua submits a draft of her proposal to her advisor for feedback. Her purpose is clearly stated: "To explore the influence of fluctuating female sex hormones on knee joint laxity across the menstrual cycle." However, under expected findings, she writes, "Knee laxity will differ across the phases of the menstrual cycle." This would indicate she expects there to be a relationship between the two variables, but she offers no indication what the direction of that relationship may be. Probing further, her advisor asks why she expects this to occur. Shaniqua explains that the literature indicates that estrogen appears to have an effect on collagen tissue, making it more elastic, and this leads her to believe that this would cause the ligament to be more lax when estrogen levels substantially increase around ovulation. Thus, based on her knowledge of previous literature, she expects to find that "females will demonstrate increased knee laxity at high estrogen phases of the menstrual cycle." This statement more clearly indicates a hypothesis-driven research proposal and adds considerable clarity to her research purpose.

need to develop a "theoretical model" that lays out for the granting agency how your research question fits into the existing knowledge base related to your area of research, and what might logically be concluded. Consider again the example of Shaniqua.

A research question based on theory that can be adequately supported and justified by relevant literature makes for a much stronger proposal than one merely based on supposition. Presentation of a strong theoretical model will also better illustrate your understanding of the literature and the rele-

In the Field

For Shaniqua's research question and hypothesis to have meaning, she must be able to justify why she would expect to find increased knee joint laxity at higher estrogen phases of the menstrual cycle. Moreover, she must have a reason for why she would think increased knee laxity may potentially play a role in the increased incidence of ACL injury in females. Through her literature search, she has found several studies that have demonstrated that females have increased joint laxity compared to males. She has also found that changes in collagen content, metabolism, elasticity, and tensile strength have been demonstrated in various tissues and animal models in the presence of estrogen. Based on this literature, she theorizes that estrogen may have a similar effect on the anterior cruciate ligament and may be the reason females have increased joint laxity compared to males. Furthermore, she proposes that (1) structural changes in the ACL caused by estrogen fluctuations may weaken its tensile properties and (2) greater laxity may allow the ligament to stretch farther before sufficient tension is developed to provide proprioceptive feedback and a protective muscular response to joint stress. While her current proposal will not address all of the questions in this theoretical model, it establishes how the knowledge gained from the current proposal will lead to this understanding.

vance of your research question to the general problem under study. This is an important concept when "selling" your research idea to a granting agency.

Demonstrates Clinical Significance

In addition to establishing the theory and justification for the research question, the grant proposal must also demonstrate the clinical relevance of the findings to the granting agency. In other words, the grant proposal must also answer the "so what" factor by answering "why" or "how" the findings will impact our understanding and/or change clinical practice. For example, Shaniqua will need be able to explain how understanding the influence of estrogen on knee joint laxity may help in identifying potential ACL risk factors and ultimately lead to prevention of ACL injury. Ultimately, the proposed research must be able to demonstrate a benefit, whether it is to the agency, the population under study, or the discipline's greater knowledge.

Addresses a Particular Need

For a granting agency to fund your research, it must address a particular need. This goes back to understanding the goals and interest of the granting agency, and whether your research question addresses one of its interest areas and fulfills a clinical, scientific, or educational need that it feels to be important. For instance, a granting agency may have identified that it has an interest in funding research that promotes women's health issues or that addresses gender-related factors in musculoskeletal injury. If Shaniqua applies to this agency, she would be remiss not to clearly state that the ultimate goal of her research is to identify gender-related factors in knee injury in order to prevent knee injuries and promote safer inclusion of women in sports participation. The bottom line is that if the research question doesn't fulfill or address a particular need that benefits the populations or areas of interests to the agency, the purpose of your proposal will likely be of little interest to them.

Vision – Potential for Future Funding

Another characteristic that granting agencies look for is whether the proposal asks a question that is of sufficient scope that it will lead to further knowledge and research. In most cases, a single research question or project will not make monumental strides in our knowledge of a particular injury or treatment, but rather provides a piece to a larger puzzle. Shaniqua's research project will not be sufficient in itself to answer why more females injure their ACLs than males, but it will add to the accumulating body of knowledge in sorting out potential gender-related risk factors in ACL injury. Moreover, identifying the next steps of where the research may lead will also add to its significance. Shaniqua must acknowledge that her research plan will only be able to establish whether a relationship exists between fluctuating estrogen levels and knee joint laxity. To lend greater credibility and significance to her findings, she should briefly discuss in her proposal how these findings might lead to additional research questions and our understanding of ACL injury in females.

Identifying an Appropriate Funding Source to Submit Your Proposal

After you have identified a list of potential agencies that may have an interest in your area of research, the task is then to determine to which agency it is most appropriate to submit your proposal. While it is possible to submit your proposal more than one agency, because of the tremendous amount of work that goes into writing a proposal and the fact that agencies vary considerably in their grant application format, it is unlikely that you will have sufficient time to prepare more than one proposal. Thus, you want to find the agency that provides the closest match with your abilities and research goals to maximize your probability for funding. This section addresses some of the key considerations in identifying an appropriate funding agency.

Purpose, Missions, Goals, and Areas of Interest of the Granting Agency

When evaluating a particular agency, go directly to that agency to learn of its mission and goals and to determine its areas of interest or priorities. Many times, the agency will list the areas of research or type of activities (i.e., mechanisms) it wishes to fund. If after reading the materials you are still not sure whether the agency may be a good match for your particular area of research, don't be afraid to call and speak to a person directly and ask more specific questions. Remember, the agency's goal is to award grants, and its staff are generally very helpful and willing to provide additional information. Be particularly watchful for program announcements (PAs) or request for proposals (RFPs) through which agencies invite proposals to address a particular area of research. Submitting an application in response to a PA or RFP can significantly enhance the probability of funding versus submitting a proposal through a general application process.

Mechanisms and Level of Support Available

Agencies will also indicate the type of grants they award and the level of funding that is available. For example, you may wish to conduct a clinical studies research project that will cost about $25,000 to complete. First, you must find agencies that express or identify interest in the type of clinical study you wish to conduct. Then, from those agencies, target those that have sufficient funding to cover the cost of your project. For a $25,000 project, you will likely wish to target an agency that has significantly more than $25,000 available, unless you are confident your grant is the only one that they will wish to fund (that's a lot of confidence). To further refine your search in regard to the type and level of funding of a particular agency, review each agency's list of award recipients, which will tell you exactly what they have funded in recent years.

Eligibility Requirements

Carefully read the application materials for application criteria and eligibility requirements. Usually, the grant application will clearly state who is eligible to apply, what credentials are required, and what is expected of the applicant. It may be that the agency either does not fund student research or, conversely, may state that you must be a student at the time of the award. Some awards are restricted to a particular geographical area, profession or population (e.g., women or minorities). The more specific the eligibility requirements and the more closely you match the agency's eligibility criteria, the greater your chance may be for funding.

Investigator Expertise Required

Before applying, you should determine what level of research or clinical experience is required or desired of the applicant. This may be specific to a particular grant mechanism or the agency as a whole. If you are a doctoral student trying to obtain funding for your dissertation, you will have much better success applying for an award such as the NATA Doctoral Dissertation Award than a federal NIH grant. To be competitive for an NIH grant, the applicant must have a terminal degree and demonstration of a well-developed track record of previous funding and research success at the time of the award. Young investigators within a few years of completing their doctoral studies and who have yet to develop a track record would do well to seek grant mechanisms that support postdoctoral fellowships or new investigators. Whatever your research experience or track record may be, try to identify grant mechanisms that specifically target your level of expertise. Your chance for success will be much greater if you are competing against others of similar experience levels than against those with significantly more research experience than yourself. Building a track record and funding success takes time. Although the funding success of each researcher is unique, Figure 19–1 illustrates a likely continuum of funding potential based on an individual's track record and level of expertise.

Application and Award Timelines

An often overlooked but critical consideration is the application and award timelines for a particular grant. If you are in the second semester of your first year of a 2-year Master's program and are on target to complete your

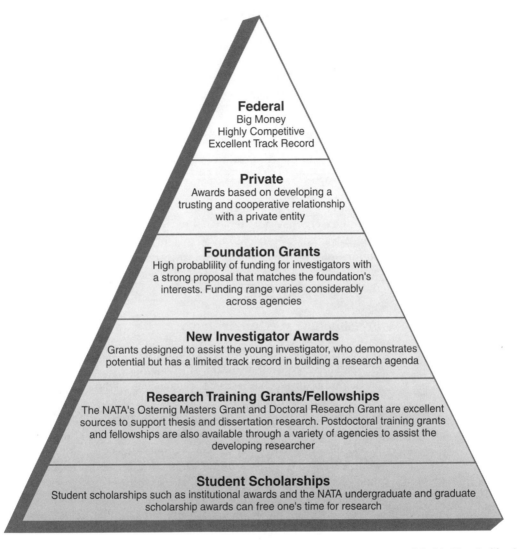

Federal
Big Money
Highly Competitive
Excellent Track Record

Private
Awards based on developing a
trusting and cooperative relationship
with a private entity

Foundation Grants
High probablility of funding for investigators with
a strong proposal that matches the foundation's
interests. Funding range varies considerably
across agencies

New Investigator Awards
Grants designed to assist the young investigator, who demonstrates
potential but has a limited track record in building a research agenda

Research Training Grants/Fellowships
The NATA's Osternig Masters Grant and Doctoral Research Grant are excellent
sources to support thesis and dissertation research. Postdoctoral training grants
and fellowships are also available through a variety of agencies to assist the
developing researcher

Student Scholarships
Student scholarships such as institutional awards and the NATA undergraduate and graduate
scholarship awards can free one's time for research

Figure 19–1 Building a track record of successful funding. This figure illustrates a continuum of the likelihood of funding through various agencies and grant mechanisms from the student researcher to the experienced investigator.

thesis the following year, you will need to identify a granting agency that will review your grant and make a decision on funding within approximately 9 months (i.e., by the fall of your second year). In this case, it doesn't make much sense to apply to an agency whose next application deadline is not for 6 months and has a review timeline of almost 9 months before a funding decision is made. Thus, you need to think ahead and find an agency or mechanism whose timing is consistent with your research progression and goals, in order to prevent significant delays in the completion of your project.

Track Record and Award Rates

A careful search history of an agency's funding track record provides additional valuable information as to your chance of funding through that particular agency. Most agencies will provide information on the number of applications received and the type and level of grants that have been awarded in recent years. Reviewing the award rate (number of applications received versus the number funded) will give you an idea of how competitive the application process is for a particular agency or grant. Reviewing the list of past award recipients will also help you get a better sense of the type of research they truly have an interest in funding and to what level they are willing to fund these projects. While an agency may indicate it has broad research interests in orthopedic research, if its track record indicates that 9 out of the last 10 awards went to physicians assessing surgical procedures, it may not be a good source of funding for your ankle rehabilitation research. Further, if the funding range seems sufficient to cover the costs of your research of $15,000, but you find that the majority of the past recipients were only funded for $10,000 or less, your proposal may be a hard sell for this particular agency. Clearly, the more that you know about the funding history of a granting agency, the better your chances of identifying the agency that best suits your research goals and that maximizes your funding potential.

Application Process: Elements of the Proposal

As you are beginning to appreciate, the writing of a grant proposal requires a significant effort. In order to develop a strong proposal, you will need to start early, preferably months in advance of the application deadline. A proposal that is hastily thrown together will not only produce incredible stress, it will also likely receive a poor review. Consider for a moment that your application is one of 10 or more being reviewed by a panel of expert reviewers for scientific merit and potential funding. The more clearly and succinctly you can convey your research intentions and identify the significance of the research, the more competitive your proposal will be. A proposal that is well thought out, creatively presented, and founded on solid theory will stand apart from the other applications and, frankly, will be a much more enjoyable read for the reviewer. While it is beyond the scope of this chapter to provide instructions on how to write a proposal, this section will briefly describe the typical elements that go into a grant proposal to help you better appreciate the effort that is involved, should you wish to apply for funding at some point in your career.

Pre-Proposal

To avoid wasting significant time and effort on the part of both the granting agency and the applicant, many agencies require that applicants submit a pre-proposal that briefly describes the proposed research. This process will allow the agency to determine if the project is consistent with the goals, mission, and interests of the agency and whether a full proposal would be invited. While approval of a full proposal submission does not in any way indicate a commitment to funding, it at least assures the applicant that the grant is of interest to the agency before spending many hours in preparing the grant application. The pre-proposal is typically limited to one to two pages, and should briefly and concisely describe the research purpose, specific aims and hypotheses, and provide an overview of the research design and methods. It should also include the credentials and contact information of the investigators and their sponsoring institution. Even if an agency does not require a pre-proposal approval process, it will typically welcome a preliminary inquiry such as this and be willing to provide feedback as to its level of interest.

Abstract

The abstract is an essential element of the proposal that succinctly describes and summarizes the scope of the proposal. It is typically limited to one page and should identify the purpose of the research, a general description of the subjects and methods to be used, the primary hypotheses and expected outcomes, and the potential benefits or clinical relevance of the study to the sports medicine community. The abstract should be well thought out and carefully developed, since it is often the first page read by the reviewer. An abstract that is well worded and sufficiently descriptive can serve to "hook" the reviewer and build excitement for the proposal that lies ahead.

Proposal Justification

The proposal justification is that section of the proposal where you essentially "sell" your idea to the granting agency by clearly stating the need for the project, the intent of the project, and the potential benefits that may emanate from the research. This may very well be the most important section of the proposal. As previously stated, it must be well thought out, clearly presented, and justifiable based on previous literature. This section is typically the first section of the proposal and can set the "tone" for the remainder of the proposal, potentially determining to what level of interest the reviewer may continue reading.

The primary sections of the proposal justification include the background and significance, purpose statement, and specific aims and research hypotheses. In the background and significance, the need and theory behind the proposed research is clearly defined, based on current knowledge and previous literature. This section should demonstrate what is currently known, what is still unanswered, and how your research will assist in filling this void. This section should also justify the significance or importance of your question and the methods by which you plan to answer the question. The purpose statement should then logically flow from the background and significance and should clearly indicate the scope and intent of the project. The research hypothesis and specific aims (what you expect to find and how you intend to address each hypothesis) should also be justifiable and intimately linked to the background and significance section. As you can see, the background and significance is foundational to your grant proposal. It must provide sufficient information to support your research question and plan, but not so much detail that it becomes unfocused and causes the reviewer to lose interest. When the background and significance is written well, the need for the research question will be well justified and the reviewer should essentially be able conclude what the purpose, specific aims, and expected findings of your research will be.

Research Design and Methods

To be successful in obtaining funding, it is not enough to just have a great research idea, you must also be able to demonstrate how you intend to carry out the research project. The research design and methods section will be fairly consistent with the research proposal already prepared for your thesis or dissertation. This section should clearly identify how you plan to answer the research question and derive your findings. The project narrative should include a description of the subjects (including power analysis to justify the number of subjects), instrumentation to be used, testing procedures, and how the data will be collected and analyzed. It must be sufficiently detailed so that the independent and dependent variables are clearly identified and one could essentially replicate the research based on the information provided. The more descriptive your research plan, the more confident the reviewer will be in your expertise and ability to carry out the project.

Preliminary/Previous Research

A grant applicant who can demonstrate previous research or pilot data relevant to the project can enhance the reviewer's confidence in the applicant's ability to carry out the project. There are three primary goals that can be achieved through presentation of preliminary research: (1) to support the research hypotheses or theoretical model, (2) to establish reliability and validity, and (3) to demonstrate the ability and competency of investigators to conduct the proposed research

Previous studies may serve to further justify the purpose and need for the research question based on previous findings in your laboratory. Preliminary studies can also be instrumental in establishing reliability and validity of any new instrumentation that will be used, as well as the investigators' proficiency in measuring the variable(s) under study. Finally, when evidence of previous work relating to the proposed area of research can be demonstrated, this will lend considerable weight to the credibility and expertise of the researchers to carry out the current project successfully. Given two equally justifiable and worthwhile research proposals, the proposal that can provide evidence of previous work in the area will further enhance its potential for funding.

Supportive Documentation

Supportive documentation that provides particular assurances to the granting agency as to the personal and institutional commitment to the project is desirable and often required. A research proposal that has already been reviewed and approved by the institution's review board (IRB) for the protection of human subjects will provide further assurance to the granting agency that the methods meet the appropriate research and subject protection standards. While many agencies do not require IRB approval until funding is received, it is advantageous to provide this assurance as part of the proposal, to prevent any questions or concerns in this regard. A description of the facilities and resources, including any support letters from the laboratory directors, will provide the assurance that the facilities are adequate to carry out the project and that the institution will make the necessary space and equipment available as needed. Personnel and biographical sketches are also included as supportive documentation that provide the reviewer/agency with adequate information regarding the researcher's educational and professional background, level of experience, previous scientific contributions and research efforts, and other professional contributions that may be pertinent. Letters of support from faculty advisors, department chairs, or deans will provide further assurances of institutional commitment to both the project as well as the researcher.

Timeline, Budget Proposal, and Budget Justification

The timeline, budget proposal, and budget justification will delineate to the agency the time and resources that will be required to carry out the research project successfully. The timeline should be realistic and should include all aspects of the project: piloting and subject recruitment, all phases of data collection and analyses, manuscript preparation and submission, and oral presentation of the results at a scientific meeting. It is important to realize that your effort on the project does not end with the collection of data and that sufficient time and resources must be allotted to prepare the results for presentation.

The budget should also be realistic and carefully considered. Trying to submit a budget that is too lean in an effort to increase the chances of funding can be potentially dangerous if you run out of funds before the completion of the project. Conversely, a budget that appears "padded" or excessive based on the scope of the research proposed will be poorly viewed. Thus, each aspect of the budget should include a justification that clearly indicates why the funds are needed. Figure 19–2 shows a sample budget form that includes the more common sections that must be considered and delineated when determining the cost of a research project. Specific budget categories and instructions on how to prepare a budget for a particular grant, including allowances for indirect costs (discussed later in this chapter), will be included in the grant application instructions provided by the agency.

| DETAILED BUDGET FOR 2 YEAR BUDGET PERIOD
DIRECT COSTS ONLY | | | | FROM
06/01/00 | | THROUGH
08/31/01 | |

| PERSONNEL(*Applicant Organization*) | | | | DOLLAR AMOUNT REQUESTED | | | |
NAME	ROLE ON PROJECT	TYPE APPT (*months*)	% Effort FUNDED ON PROJECT	INST. BASE SALARY	SALARY REQUESTED	FRINGE BENEFITS	TOTALS
Investigator A, PhD	Principal Investigator	9	15.0%	$42,000	$6,300	$1,481	$7,781
		3(summer)	33.0%	$13,860	$4,574	$320	$4,894
Investigator B, PhD	Co-Investigator	9	10.0%	$60,000	$6,000	$1,410	$7,410
PhD Student	Research Technician	10	100.0%	$9,000	$9,000	$630	$9,630
SubTotals					$25,874	$3,841	$29,715

CONSULTANT COSTS

| Consultant A, PhD | Statistician | (1 Day @ $359/day) | $359 | |
| B | | | $0 | $359 |

EQUIPMENT (*Itemize*)

None Requested

$0

SUPPLIES (*Itemize by Category*)

EMG Electrodes (80 subjects x $10.00 each)	$800	
Office, Copying, Computer and Printing Supplies	$500	
C		
D		
E		
F		$1,300

TRAVEL

| One trip for PI to present findings at NATA Annual Meeting | $900 | $900 |

OTHER EXPENSES (*Itemize by Category*)

| PhD Student Tuition @ $5100/yr | $5,100 | |

| | | $5,100 |
| **TOTAL DIRECT COSTS FOR THE BUDGET PERIOD** | | **$37,374** |

Figure 19–2 Sample budget form.

Submission Process: What to Expect After the Grant Is Submitted

After the grant is submitted, considerable time may elapse before any word is received on the reviews or decision for funding. Much effort goes into the review of grant applications and it is helpful for applicants to have an understanding of this process as they patiently await word on their proposals. There are typically three primary steps that a grant application will go through once submitted: a mechanical review, a scientific review, and a review for funding decision.

Mechanical Review

After a grant application is received, it will first go through a mechanical review. The mechanical review will check each section of the grant application to insure that all sections are included and complete, and that the proper format has been followed. At this stage, the proposal is not evaluated for specific content. Hence, the mechanical review highlights the importance of carefully following all application instructions to the letter. Think of the frustration you will feel if your grant is rejected simply because you failed to follow directions and it is never given the opportunity for review on its merit. Careful attention to application criteria will help avoid wasted effort and unnecessary rejections.

Scientific Review

After completion of the mechanical review and assurance that the application is complete, the agency will assign reviewers to critique the grant on its scientific merit. Depending on the agency, the review panel may consist of an established review committee and/or may include two to three external (invited) reviewers selected for their expertise in the area of research. For all committee members to review each of the grant applications received in a given funding cycle would be overwhelming and inefficient. Thus, each grant is typically assigned a primary and secondary reviewer to conduct an in-depth, critical review of the grant. The reviewers will critique the quality of each section of the grant proposal based on established criteria of the granting agency. Display 19–3 lists some of the general evaluation criteria that are typically considered by reviewers.

After sufficient time has been provided to review each grant individually, the review committee will then convene at a specified date to review the grants collectively. The assigned reviewers for each grant will present a summary of the review to the entire panel, briefly describing the project and highlighting any strengths and weaknesses. The committee will then have the opportunity to ask questions and further discuss what they believe to be the grant's strengths and any concerns they may have. Thus, in many cases, whether a committee decides to approve a proposal for funding is based on how well the grant proposal is received by the primary reviewers and how

| Display 19-3 | **Grant Evaluation Criteria** |

General Evaluation Criteria for Grant Proposals often include:

- The extent to which the proposal meets the purpose.
- The extent to which the background and rationale supports the proposed project.
- The extent to which the project's objectives are realistic, clearly stated and achievable.
- The extent to which the methods meet the project objectives, including feasibility.
- The evaluation plans and procedures if applying for a training grant.
- The perceived ability of the applicant to carry out the proposed project.
- The commitment of the institution, including administrative support, facilities, and resources available to the applicant.
- The extent to which the budget is reasonable, cost effective and justified.

Adapted from Gitlin, L. N., & Lyons, K. J. (1996). Successful grant writing: Strategies for health and human service professionals. New York: Springer Publishing, p. 28.

well they are able to summarize the proposal for the committee. To increase the likelihood of a positive review, Display 19–4 lists some tips for a successful review.

Based on the reviewer's comments and committee discussion, a decision is then made whether to approve or defer the proposal for a funding decision. Generally, a grant will come out of the scientific review with a particular score or one of six recommendations for funding (see Display 19–5).

| Display 19-4 | **Keys to a Favorable Review** |

- Ask a researcher who has been successfully funded to read and critique your proposal before you submit it.
- Be hypothesis driven.
- Clearly state the benefit and impact your project will have on the field
- Don't be overly ambitious...keep the proposal focused on no more than 3–5 specific aims.
- Always include preliminary data.
- Be considerate of reviewers...use readable fonts and spaces between paragraphs for easier reading.
- Convey your excitement and enthusiasm for the project.
- Discuss data interpretation and alternate hypotheses.
- Avoid trying to fill the allotted pages...use only the number of pages necessary to clearly and succinctly convey your ideas.
- Be organized...use headings and diagrams to help reviewers get organized and oriented.

Source: Hopkin, K. (1998). How to wow a study section: A grantsmanship lesson. The Scientist, 12, 11.

Display 19-5

General Recommendations for Funding

Following the review process, a grant application will typically be assigned one of the following recommendations:

- Unacceptable—resubmission not recommended
- Unacceptable—resubmission okay
- Acceptable—fund after revisions are made and as funding is available
- Acceptable—recommended for funding as funds are available
- Excellent—recommended for funding after requested revisions are addressed
- Excellent—recommended for immediate funding

Funding Decision

At the completion of the scientific review, each grant proposal will have been rated or scored based on its scientific merit, and a recommendation is made whether funding should be considered. If a proposal is approved for funding, this does not in itself guarantee that the grant will be funded. Grant proposals that score well and are recommended for funding are then prioritized and go through a final review for a funding decision.

Decisions on funding may be made by the same committee, but are often determined by a separate committee. For instance, the board of a foundation may make all funding decisions, but it establishes a research committee to conduct the scientific review of the grant applications and make recommendations to the board. It may be that the review committee has identified 10 grant proposals that score well and are recommended for funding, but the foundation only has enough money to fund 5 of the proposals. The foundation's board will then make the final decision of who will receive funding based on the scientific review and recommendations of the research committee, as well as the foundation's initiatives, interests and available funds.

Applying for a research grant is a competitive process. How well you present your proposal and clearly and succinctly lay out the significance of the project and research plan to the reviewers are paramount to receiving a favorable review. The specific criteria by which a grant application is reviewed may differ somewhat from agency to agency. Review criteria are often described, at least in general terms, as part of the application instructions, program announcements, or request for proposals. It is always advisable to read these documents carefully to determine what the reviewers will be specifically looking for and to ensure that your proposal addresses the essential elements of the review criteria.

Other Considerations When Seeking Research Funding

Very few quality research projects are successful as an individual effort and often require the expertise and assistance of others. Many agencies today recognize that more can be accomplished collectively than can be accomplished by a single individual and as such, view collaborative, cross-disciplinary efforts favorably. Selecting others to collaborate on your research project will not only strengthen the quality of your research, it will also strengthen the quality of your grant proposal. Further, the institution will play a vital role as a resource both in identifying potential granting agencies and in assisting in the grant application process.

Importance of Collaboration and Research Team Selection

There are many benefits to collaboration. Collaborating with other researchers with like or similar expertise provides the ability to bounce ideas off one another and brainstorm ideas that may open your mind to new research questions and avenues. Collaboration with complementary disciplines allows you to pursue an integrated approach to answer a specific question or may allow you to answer a bigger or broader question than what you could answer alone given your expertise. This is particularly true of a graduate student who is learning the research process. Clearly, collaborating with your faculty advisor or other faculty with an interest in your research question will provide valuable feedback and expertise in the design and development of your study and grant proposal. Moreover, their involvement as members of the research team can also assure the granting agency that you have the expertise needed to carry out the project successfully.

Roles and Responsibilities of Collaborators

When submitting a grant proposal, research team members should be named and their roles and level of effort identified:

- *Principal Investigator*: This is the individual who will serve as the lead investigator, overseeing all aspects of the grant. The PI is typically the individual who conceived the project and has invited others to assist with aspects of the proposal. The PI serves as the primary contact with the granting agency during the application process.
- *Co-Principal Investigator*: While some agencies will only recognize one person as the principal investigator, others will allow Co-PIs. For there to be more than one principal investigator means that both are equally responsible for development, planning, and implementation of the project. As a graduate student applying for a research grant, it is likely that your faculty advisor will serve in this capacity. In fact, the faculty member may be required to serve as a Co-PI on student-initiated grants for institutional purposes. Further, including them as Co-PI may lend the necessary experience and expertise to be competitive for funding.
- *Project Coordinator*: When a research project is fairly large and involves multiple collaborators, the principal investigator may enlist

the assistance of an individual to serve as the project coordinator. The role of the project coordinator is to assist in overseeing the day-to-day operation of the grant, coordinate efforts between team members, and keep the PI abreast of project progress and any difficulties encountered.

- *Co-Investigator*: Co-investigators indicate members of the research team who will make a substantial contribution to the research project. Co-investigators will typically make a contribution to one or more of the following: (1) concept and design, (2) analysis and interpretation of the data, (3) provision of study materials or participants, (4) assistance with conducting a particular measurement or procedure, and (5) statistical assistance.

- *Research Technician or Assistant*: The research technician or assistant is someone who will assist with data collection, but otherwise does not make a significant contribution to those listed under co-investigator. A research assistant who simply collects or collates the data in preparation for analysis does not necessarily have to have a knowledge of the area of research or contribute to the research design or interpretation of the data.

- *Consultant*: The consultant is an individual who lends a specific area of expertise or fulfills a specified role on a particular aspect of the project. This individual need not be an expert or even have an interest in the area of study. The addition of a consultant is usually contractual in nature, compensated on an hourly basis rather than by percent effort. For example, the study may require the use of a new piece of equipment, and the investigators need to be trained on its use by someone familiar with the equipment. The individual may have no involvement in the development of the research plan or in carrying out the project, other than to provide two or three training sessions. After the consultant has provided the training on the equipment, he or she is no longer needed or involved in the project.

Selection of Research Team Members

Selection of the research team should be done with great care. To follow are some of the more important considerations when selecting the research team:

- *Required Expertise*: Identify the type and level of expertise required to carry out the project. If your research project involves measuring hormone levels, it may be advisable to have an endocrinologist as a co-investigator to assist in interpreting the lab results. If you are measuring muscle responses with electromyography and there is a faculty member with expertise in EMG assessment, that individual may be a valuable contributor to the research design and measurement procedures. When considering the level of expertise, consider what level of expertise is needed to be competitive for funding. Perhaps you wish to pursue a district grant, but you have no previous research experience or record of funding. Teaming up with an experienced investigator can enhance your chance for funding by providing sufficient assurance that the expertise required to carry out the project is present.

- *Potential for Contribution:* Obviously, individuals you select to participate on the project should be able to contribute in a meaningful way. When considering potential collaborators, identify what role or responsibility they will fill and how their participation will enhance the project. Also determine whether the individual has the interest and time available to contribute to the project. Even if they have the needed expertise, if they don't have the time available to put forth the effort, they will be of little benefit to you.
- *Workability:* Consider each individual's personality and how well they will mesh with the other members of the research team. When working together, there is always the potential for disagreement, and how well team members are able to work cooperatively to resolve problems can mean the difference between success and enjoyment or failure and frustration. Identify individuals who will be team players and will check their ego at the door. Avoid those who demonstrate a selfish ambition and are concerned more with their own professional advancement than contributing to the team. Consider those who are sensitive to deadlines and committed to meet the expectations of the project.

Role of the Institution

The institution plays an integral role in the grant application process. Agencies rarely fund or pay individuals directly. Typically, the contract is made with the institution with which the investigator is affiliated. Once the award is made and the contract is signed, the funds are paid to the institution, and a separate account is set up from which the funds are administered. This provides assurances that there is a record and adequate reporting of how and when the funds are spent. Because the award and contract are made with the institution, a representative of the institution must sign off on all grant applications before they are submitted. This ensures that the institution is supportive of the research effort and willing to provide the release time and resources for the investigator to complete the project, that the budget is consistent with current institutional rates and allowances, and that the investigator has met all institutional requirements.

Direct versus Indirect Costs

Conducting a research project does not occur without some cost to the institution. These costs include light, power, temperature regulation, and maintenance of the space, facilities, or equipment utilized during the research project. It may also include administrative resources and costs such as telephone, secretarial, and administrative support. To offset these costs to the institution, many granting agencies agree as part of the grant contract to provide additional funds to reimburse for these "overhead" or indirect costs. Typically, indirect costs are determined based on a percentage of the direct or actual research project costs. Indirect cost allowance can vary widely, depending on the granting agency and type of grant, and is usually negotiated or stipulated in advance of application submission. Federal research grants usually have the highest rate of indirect cost recovery, ranging as high as 80 percent of the applicable direct costs, while other agencies may limit this cost recovery to 10 to 20 percent. In many cases, nonprofit organizations (i.e., foundations) will not pay any indirect costs. Additionally, research grants that rely heavily on institutional facilities and resources will have a significantly higher indirect cost allowance than a training grant that is primarily designed to support an individual. Although an institution is not likely to approve or stifle a grant proposal submission based on the indirect cost recovery rate, they must be willing to absorb the overhead costs associated with a research project when very limited or no overhead cost recovery is funded.

Institutional Support

Most institutions have an office of sponsored programs that is willing and available to assist the investigator in the application process. It is the business of this office to be aware of the proper procedures to follow and will ensure that all granting agency and institutional application requirements are met. The office can assist with obtaining and filling out the proper application forms and in preparing the budget. It is a valuable resource for obtaining information on set institutional rates for faculty and student wages, fringe benefits, tuition, consulting, and indirect cost recovery rates that are needed in preparing the budget. It can also be instrumental in the early stages of proposal development in helping investigators seek out potential agencies appropriate for submitting their proposal.

Summary

After reading this chapter you should have a better sense of the goals and benefits that arise from writing a grant proposal, as well as the work that is involved in submitting a quality grant application. Although writing a grant proposal represents a significant effort, receiving an award, not to mention the experience gained from the application process, can be very rewarding. Writing a successful grant takes skill, time, patience, and sufficient resources to seek out the most appropriate funding source and mechanism and to develop a quality proposal that clearly defines the purpose, aims, procedures, and significance of the project. Being aware of the many resources available to identify appropriate grant agencies and mechanisms is the first step in the grant-writing process and can be of great benefit when seeking funding to support your research ideas. Understanding the essential elements and steps in the grant-writing process will allow you to be realistic of the time and effort required when you are ready to seek funding for your research and will assist you in putting together a solid proposal.

Activities

1. Identify and explore a general search engine for funding sources on the Internet.
2. Identify potential funding sources for a particular area of research.
3. Obtain and review an application form from a potential funding source.
4. Obtain and review a completed grant application that has been successfully funded.
5. Invite or visit a representative from the institution's office of sponsored programs to become better acquainted with resources and assistance available for prospective grant applicants and the role they play in the application submission process.

References

Gitlin, L. N., & Lyons, K. J. (1996). *Successful grant writing: Strategies for health and human service professionals*. New York: Springer Publishing.

Hopkin, K. (1998). How to wow a study section: A grantsmanship lesson. *The Scientist*, *12*, 11.

National Athletic Trainers' Association Research and Education Foundation. Retrieved 3/25/04: http://www.natafoundation.org

Chapter 20

Ethical Considerations in the Research Process

Objectives

After reading this chapter, you will:

- Know how to avoid committing scientific misconduct in the research and publication process.
- Appreciate the importance of citing the work of others to avoid committing plagiarism.
- Know the importance of obtaining informed consent from human subjects.
- Understand the guidelines that constitute authorship on a manuscript.
- Appreciate the problems associated with multiple submissions of abstracts and manuscripts.
- Understand the concept of copyright as related to the publication process.
- Know the definition of "duplicate" or "redundant" publication.
- Know how to avoid the appearance of conflicts of interest.

Questions

While reading this chapter, think about answers to the following questions:

1. How do I gain approval to conduct my research and use human subjects for data collection?
2. What is scientific misconduct?
3. What is plagiarism and how do I cite the work of others to avoid committing this serious offense?
4. Who should be included as authors on my manuscript, and in what order should the authors be listed?
5. What are the conflicts of interest that might occur in the research process, and how can I avoid committing them?
6. Who has copyright ownership of my manuscript after it is submitted for publication with a journal?
7. Can I submit my manuscript to more than one journal at the same time?
8. Can I draw from the data of one study to prepare and submit more than one manuscript for publication?

This chapter will discuss ethical considerations in the research and publication process, and how you can avoid committing these serious offenses. Ignorance of the ethical and legal considerations guiding the research process is not an excuse for committing scientific misconduct. It is essential that you carefully read and understand the concepts presented in this chapter.

Scientific Misconduct

Scientific misconduct is defined as plagiarism, fabrication, or falsification during the process of research and publication. Plagiarism is the failure to attribute the work of others to the original source of the work. Fabrication occurs when a researcher makes up data or presents findings that are not the result of the actual research process. Falsification is changing the data or results of the research process. In each case, the researcher has misrepresented the actual findings of a study or failed to properly reference the work of others, and a serious case of scientific misconduct has occurred.

Plagiarism results when an author presents the work of others without properly citing the original source of the work. This "work" includes ideas, language (actual sentences or phrases), protocols, data, figures, or other sources or products of the work of others. You must avoid plagiarism by referencing the work of others in your writing and in the presentation of your study. If you are presenting the ideas of others, you must reference the work with a citation of the actual source. If you are using the exact language (sentence or phrase), you must place this material in quotations and reference the original source of the work. If you are making a verbal presentation of your study you should also cite the work of others, just as you would in a written communication. A good rule of thumb is to assume the authors of the other work are in your audience. Would they be satisfied that you have sufficiently acknowledged and given credit to their work?

You might wonder why a researcher would fabricate or falsify data. However, the process of research and publication creates all kinds of stresses that can result in acts of very poor judgment.

Imagine that you have completed collection and analysis of your data. You find that the data are very close to being statistically significant. To

In the Field

Sally is approaching the end of data collection for her study, and deadlines for completing requirements for graduation are fast approaching. Her last subject doesn't show for data collection, and she has exhausted all efforts for subject recruitment. It would be easy to view the data for the subjects she has tested and to plug in values for the final subject that fall within the range of these data points. Sally's data collection thus would "appear" to be completed and she would be on her way to analysis of the data and completion of the project. This would represent a serious act of fabrication of data.

increase the values for just one or two subjects would in all probability produce a statistically significant finding and in your judgment add more credibility to your research project. However, doing this would represent a serious act of falsification of data.

What are the implications of fabricating or falsifying data, or committing acts of plagiarism? If you are a student and the scientific misconduct is detected before graduation, you place in jeopardy the awarding of a degree from the institution at which you are studying. Acts of scientific misconduct are grounds for dismissal from an institution of higher learning. Institutions even have the right to revoke degrees from former students found to have committed acts of scientific misconduct. If you are a faculty member in a college or university, scientific misconduct can result in very serious ramifications, ranging from public disclosure and discipline by your supervisor to dismissal from your position. Scientific misconduct is one offense that can justify the firing of a tenured professor.

If scientific misconduct is alleged after publication of a manuscript emanating from the research project, the editor of the journal will inform the senior research administrator at the institution where the alleged perpetrator is employed. If the allegations are found to be true, the penalty will include a public disclosure in a subsequent issue of the journal. The journal's editor may also sensor the author from further submission or publication for a period of time or perhaps even permanently. The actions by the author's supervisor can range from public disclosure and discipline to dismissal. You can see that scientific misconduct is a very serious offense and one that should be avoided at all costs.

Protecting Individuals' Rights in Research

To protect the rights of individuals in the research process, investigators must have study protocols approved by an Institutional Review Board for the Protection of Human Subjects. The purpose of this process is to protect individuals' rights in research and assure that the risks of the research are compatible with the expected benefits. (Please note that research involving the use of animals also requires appropriate institutional review and approval by the institution's animal protection board.) The contemporary guidelines for protecting the safety and dignity of human subjects resulted from abuses in the 20th century. These abuses led to the doctrines known as the Nuremberg Code (Appendix 20–1) and the World Medical Association's Declaration of Helsinki (Appendix 20–2).

An additional purpose of an Institutional Review Board for the Protection of Human Subjects is to assure compliance with federal and institutional regulations, whether or not the research is federally funded, privately funded, or not funded. Details pertaining to federal regulations in the use of human subjects can be found at http://www.ohrp.osophs. dhhs.gov/humansubjects/guidance.

Faculty and students are sometimes unclear about which class projects and research protocols require review and approval by an institutional review board. In general, if the goal of the project is to disseminate information through presentation or publication, the project requires approval by the institutional review board. In some cases, the research can be exempted from the requirements for obtaining informed consent. Examples of research that might be eligible for exemption from review include the collection or study of existing data. In any event, the research must be reviewed by the institutional review board to receive exempted status. Appendix 20–3 presents an example of research that might be eligible for exemption from review by an IRB, along with the process for obtaining this exemption.

To assure that individuals' rights have been protected in scientific publication, most journals require authors to include a statement that subjects provided informed consent to participate in protocols approved by an Institutional Review Board for the Protection of Human Subjects. The *Journal of Athletic Training* Authors' Guide (see Appendix 18–2) includes the following statements:

"For experimental investigations of human or animal subjects, state in the Methods section of the manuscript that an appropriate institutional review board approved the project."

"For investigations of human subjects, state in the Methods section the manner in which informed consent was obtained from the subjects."

Use of Human Subjects and Obtaining Consent

The tenets of the process of obtaining consent are that subjects:

- Must provide informed consent
- Have the right to privacy and anonymity
- Have the right to withdraw from the research at any time without penalty

Informed consent means that the nature, purpose, risks, and benefits of the research must be explained to the subjects in a manner that is comprehensible by a layperson. Subjects should also be assured that the appropriate steps have been taken to protect their privacy and anonymity, and only in instances of potential risk to the researcher (e.g., exposure to the subjects' body fluids) would the subjects' identify be revealed to the appropriate medical personnel. Finally, the subjects should be assured that they are free to withdraw from the study at any time without penalty. Appendixes 20–4 and 20–5 provide sample templates for research of a medical nature and a scientific nature, respectively. Keep in mind that these are only examples and that researchers must follow the guidelines of their respective Institutional Review Board for the Protection of Human Subjects.

Research protocols involving the use of minors as subjects must include the consent of both the subject and the parent or legal guardian of the minor. Appendix 20–6 provides an example template of a consent form for the use of subjects less than 18 years of age.

Authorship

Perhaps the first step in the research project is to delineate the roles of the people who will be involved with the study. This delineation of roles should include a discussion of what constitutes authorship and who will be included as an author on papers emanating from the research project. The order in which authors will be listed on these manuscripts should be included as part of this discussion. Some flexibility should be permitted in determining authorship, since sometimes people intending to play a major role in the research project ultimately do not. In other cases, the expertise of someone not involved initially might need to be added during the course of the study, and this person could very well be deserving of authorship.

Most journals delineate the requirements for authorship in their authors' guide. Many journals have adopted the authorship guidelines of the International Committee of Medical Journal Editors (ICMJE). In short, the policy of ICMJE was developed to discourage the inflationary increase in the number of authors listed on manuscripts and to end the practice of "gift" authorship (Perrin, 2001). The ICMJE guidelines (International Committee of Medical Journal Editors, 2003), which serve as the basis for the Uniform Requirements for Manuscripts Submitted to Biomedical Journals (URMSBJ), are:

> **Authorship credit should be based only on 1) substantial contributions to conception and design, or acquisition of data, or analysis and interpretation of data; 2) drafting the article or revising it critically for important intellectual content; and 3) final approval of the version to be published. Conditions 1, 2, and 3 must all be met. Acquisition of funding, the collection of data, or general supervision of the research group, by themselves, do not justify authorship.**

An authorship form can be helpful in the early delineation of the roles of the research team and determining who is deserving of authorship at the conclusion of the study (see Display 18–3 in Chapter 18). The members of the research team who do not meet the requirements for authorship, but who contributed in some smaller way, can be thanked in an acknowledgment section at the conclusion of manuscripts emanating from the project.

Determining the order in which authors appear on manuscripts can also be confusing, and the philosophy on this issue varies among professional societies. For example, some societies tend to list the two individuals contributing the most to the study first and last among all authors listed. The recommendation of the Uniform Requirements for Manuscripts Submitted to Biomedical Journals is:

> **The order of authorship on the byline should be a joint decision of the coauthors. Authors should be prepared to explain the order in which authors are listed.**

The authors' guides of most journals follow a manual of style, such as the American Psychological Association guidelines, the Council of Science Editors, and the *American Medical Association Manual of Style*. The recommendation of the AMA's Manual is that all authors should be listed in order of actual contribution made to the work. Regardless of the manner in which order is determined, the recommendation of the URMSBJ that order should be a joint decision of the coauthors is a good one, and this decision should be made earlier rather than later in the research process.

Manuscript Submission and Scientific Misconduct

Most journals require that submitted manuscripts contain original material that has not been simultaneously submitted or previously accepted elsewhere. The most common acts of scientific misconduct as related to the manuscript submission process include multiple submission and duplicate or redundant publication.

Multiple Submission

Multiple submissions occur when an author submits one article to two or more journals. The rationale for doing this might be a perceived greater likelihood of acceptance of the article by one of the journals, or perhaps the author is interested in hastening the time from submission to acceptance by selecting the journal that moves the paper along the fastest. In either case, multiple submission of a manuscript is an example of scientific misconduct. Moreover, journals such as the *Journal of Athletic Training* require the following or similar statements: "This manuscript (1) contains original unpublished material that has been submitted solely to the *Journal of Athletic Training*, (2) is not under simultaneous review by any other publication, and (3) will not be submitted elsewhere until a decision has been made concerning its suitability for publication by the *Journal of Athletic Training*."

Nearly all journals require a statement from the authors that the manuscript is an original submission and not under simultaneous review by another journal. Display 20–1 presents the statement that the *Journal of Athletic Training* requires of its authors. A key element to this letter is that all authors sign it, to ensure that all authors are aware of the submission of the article.

You will also note in the letter in Display 20–1 that the author conveys copyright ownership of the article to the professional society associated with the journal. If the journal rejects the manuscript, the copyright is returned to the author. If the author wishes to recover the copyright ownership of the manuscript before a publication decision is made, he or she can request that the journal's editor release the paper back to the author. If the editor agrees to do this (be sure to get this in writing), the author is free to submit the article elsewhere. Of course, if the manuscript is rejected by a journal, the author is also free to submit the paper to another journal.

Submission of Abstracts and Manuscripts

Chapter 18 describes the process of writing and submitting an abstract from a research project for presentation at a scientific meeting. It is quite com-

Display 20-1 | **Example of a Letter That Must Accompany the Submission of an Article to a Journal**

Copyright Form

Journal of Athletic Training

Date_____

Manuscript title_____

_____

    This manuscript 1) contains original unpublished material that has been submitted solely to the *Journal of Athletic Training*, 2) is not under simultaneous review by any other publication, and 3) will not be submitted elsewhere until a decision has been made concerning its suitability for publication by the *Journal of Athletic Training*. In consideration of the NATA's taking action in reviewing and editing my submission, I the undersigned author hereby transfer, assign, or otherwise convey all copyright ownership to the NATA, in the event that such work is published by the NATA. Further, I verify that I have contributed substantially to this manuscript as outlined in item #3 of the current Authors' Guide.

    Author's Name_____ Author's Signature_____

    Author's Name_____ Author's Signature_____

    Author's Name_____ Author's Signature_____

    Author's Name_____ Author's Signature_____

    Please submit this form with your manuscript to the following address:

Journal of Athletic Training
Hughston Sports Medicine Foundation, Inc.
6262 Veterans Parkway
Columbus, GA 31909

In the Field

    Kelly's manuscript is under review with the Journal of Athletic Training. After 3 long months, he received the comments of the reviewers and disagreed with the majority of their recommendations. He decided that rather than revise the paper and respond to the reviewers, he would submit the manuscript to the Journal of Orthopaedic and Sports Physical Therapy. When he received the reviews of his manuscript from JOSPT, the comments were far more favorable than from the JAT reviewers. He revised the manuscript and returned the paper to JOSPT, and it was published 3 months later. Shortly after publication, he received a letter from the editor of JAT saying that the copyright for the paper was with JAT, since Kelly had accompanied the original submission with a letter saying that it had been submitted solely to JAT and was not simultaneously under review by another journal. The editor of JAT contacted the person who oversees scientific misconduct at Kelly's university.

mon for authors to first write and present an abstract, and then to submit a full manuscript of the research project for publication in a journal. Is the simultaneous submission of the abstract and the manuscript considered to be a multiple submission? The answer depends to some extent on the professional society associated with the submission and presentation of the abstract.

Some, and probably most, professional societies require that the publication and presentation of the abstract be the original dissemination of the research project. For example, the NATA Research and Education Foundation policy states:

> All presentations must be original (not previously presented). This restriction includes internet and worldwide web postings. Exceptions to this restriction are limited to state and district meetings of athletic training organizations.

In Chapter 18 you learned that the process of submission and publication of a manuscript is a lengthy one. This begs the question of whether it is acceptable to submit the full manuscript simultaneously with the abstract or before the abstract has been published and presented. It is probably common practice for most researchers to do this, and so long as the full manuscript is not published before the abstract is published and presented, it is probably acceptable. The risk to the author is that the manuscript review process might be more expedient than anticipated. If this happens, you are at the mercy of the journal's editor to delay publication of your manuscript until after presentation and publication of the abstract. In some professional societies, the manuscript publication may precede presentation and publication of the abstract. For some professional societies, the penalty is censorship from future abstract submissions and/or journal publications for a specified period of time.

Duplicate and Redundant Publication

Violation of a journal's policy related to the original submission of manuscripts is known as duplicate or redundant publication. According to the Council of Science Editors (www.councilscienceeditors.org):

> Violating this requirement by reporting substantially the same work more than once, without attribution of the original source(s), has been variously called duplicate, repetitive, or redundant publication. Of these terms, duplicate and, to a lesser extent, repetitive, connote identicality, and 2 papers need not be identical to be substantially the same. Thus, "redundant publication" is probably the favored term to describe this practice, and the term applies whether or not publication has actually occurred (that is, it includes submission in hopes of redundant publication).

The determination of redundant publication is not always clear cut. For example, it is not unusual for a research project to have primary purposes and secondary purposes that encompass so much data collection that publication of the entire project in one manuscript is impossible. Display 20–2 provides excerpts from the Council of Science Editors' policy that can help

| Display 20-2 | **Keys to Avoiding an Accusation of Redundant Publication** |

Ask if the reader of one paper would gain any new insights or perspectives from reading the other, at least with respect to those elements common to both papers.

Identify specifically to the editor any potential overlap with other manuscripts, published, submitted, or in preparation, and provide a copy of any relevant paper(s).

Mention, in the text of a paper, one's own work that is, at the very least, closely related.

Modified from Council of Science Editors. (1996). CBE Views, 19, 76–77, published by the Council of Science Editors, Reston, VA © 1996.

you determine how to avoid redundant publication. The entire policy is included in Appendix 20–7.

Conflicts of Interest

A potential conflict of interest exists when a researcher's objectivity is compromised by an interest in a device or instrument used in the study or when the researcher has a financial interest in some aspect of the study or serves to benefit from the study's findings. This is not to say a researcher cannot have any association with the manufacturer of a product associated with the study. Indeed, the appearance of a conflict of interest is as troublesome as an actual conflict of interest. For this reason, researchers should disclose the presence of any potential conflict of interest associated with the research project. Display 20–3 presents two elements of the *Journal of Athletic Training* Authors' Guide that address the disclosure of potential conflict of interest.

| Display 20-3 | **Disclosure Statements Related to Potential Conflicts of Interest** |

Financial support or provision of supplies used in the study must be acknowledged. Grant or contract numbers should be included whenever possible. The complete name of the funding institution or agency should be given, along with the city and state in which it is located. If individual authors were the recipients of funds, their names should be listed parenthetically.

Authors must specify whether they have any commercial or proprietary interest in any device, equipment, instrument, or drug that is the subject of the article in question. Authors must also reveal if they have any financial interest (as a consultant, reviewer, or evaluator) in a drug or device described in the article.

Source: (2001). Journal of Athletic Training Authors' Guide, 36, 450–451.

It is not uncommon for manufacturers to loan or donate equipment and instrumentation for athletic trainers to conduct research. It is imperative that both the researcher and the manufacturer come to an understanding before the donation that the research team must be free to design the research, conduct the study, and disseminate the findings independent of scrutiny or censorship by the manufacturer. The research team should also disclose the donation or gift by the manufacturer in all presentations and publications emanating from research in which the device was used.

Summary

Many of the issues and examples of scientific misconduct addressed in this chapter would seem obvious to responsible people conducting research. Yet the literature is replete with examples of violations of scientific misconduct. It is imperative that you have a thorough understanding of these principles and avoid even the appearance of violating scientific misconduct at all costs. Your research mentor, the chief research officer of your institution, and perhaps a journal editor can be helpful in clarifying any questions you might have about possible violations of scientific misconduct.

Activities

1. Discuss the ethical implications of submitting the same or similar manuscript to different journals simultaneously.
2. Discuss your decision-making process for deciding who deserves authorship on your submitted manuscript.
3. Discuss your process for determining the order of authorship on your submitted manuscript. What resources would you use justifying your decision?

References

Call for Abstracts. Retrieved 3/25/04 from the NATA Research & Education Foundation: http://www.natafoundation.org/

Council of Science Editors. (1996). *CBE Views, 19,* 76–77.

International Committee of Medical Journal Editors. Retrieved 3/25/04: http://www.icjme.org/

Perrin, D. H. (2001). Guidelines for authorship in JAT. *Journal of Athletic Training, 36,* 15.

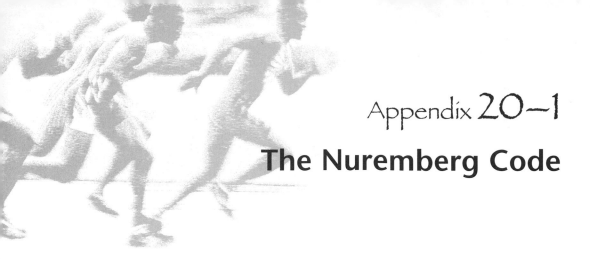

Appendix 20–1
The Nuremberg Code

1. The voluntary consent of the human subject is absolutely essential. This means that the person involved should have legal capacity to give consent; should be so situated as to be able to exercise free power of choice, without the intervention of any element of force, fraud, deceit, duress, over-reaching, or other ulterior form of constraint or coercion; and should have sufficient knowledge and comprehension of the elements of the subject matter involved, as to enable him to make an understanding and enlightened decision. This latter element requires that, before the acceptance of an affirmative decision by the experimental subject, there should be made known to him the nature, duration, and purpose of the experiment; the method and means by which it is to be conducted; all inconveniences and hazards reasonably to be expected; and the effects upon his health or person, which may possibly come from his participation in the experiment.

   The duty and responsibility for ascertaining the quality of the consent rests upon each individual who initiates, directs or engages in the experiment. It is a personal duty and responsibility which may not be delegated to another with impunity.

2. The experiment should be such as to yield fruitful results for the good of society, unprocurable by other methods or means of study, and not random and unnecessary in nature.

3. The experiment should be so designed and based on the results of animal experimentation and a knowledge of the natural history of the disease or other problem under study, that the anticipated results will justify the performance of the experiment.

4. The experiment should be so conducted as to avoid all unnecessary physical and mental suffering and injury.

5. No experiment should be conducted, where there is an a priori reason to believe that death or disabling injury will occur; except, perhaps, in those experiments where the experimental physicians also serve as subjects.

6. The degree of risk to be taken should never exceed that determined by the humanitarian importance of the problem to be solved by the experiment.

7. Proper preparations should be made and adequate facilities provided to protect the experimental subject against even remote possibilities of injury, disability, or death.

8. The experiment should be conducted only by scientifically qualified persons. The highest degree of skill and care should be required through all stages of the experiment of those who conduct or engage in the experiment.

9. During the course of the experiment, the human subject should be at liberty to bring the experiment to an end, if he has reached the physical or mental state, where continuation of the experiment seemed to him to be impossible.

10. During the course of the experiment, the scientist in charge must be prepared to terminate the experiment at any stage, if he has probable cause to believe, in the exercise of the good faith, superior skill and careful judgment required of him, that a continuation of the experiment is likely to result in injury, disability, or death to the experimental subject.

Source: *Trials of War Criminals before the Nuremberg Military Tribunals Under Control Council Law No. 10, Vol. 2, pp. 181–182.* Washington, DC: U.S. Government Printing Office, 1949. Retrieved 3/26/04 from Office of Human Subjects Research, National Institutes of Health: http://www.nihtraining.com/ohsrsite/guidelines/nuremberg.html

The Declaration of Helsinki

The Helsinki Declaration in Norwegian. Ethical Principles for Medical Research Involving Human Subjects
Adopted by the 18th WMA General Assembly
Helsinki, Finland, June 1964 and amended by the
29th WMA General Assembly, Tokyo, Japan, October 1975
35th WMA General Assembly, Venice, Italy, October 1983
41st WMA General Assembly, Hong Kong, September 1989
48th WMA General Assembly, Somerset West, Republic of South Africa, October 1996
and the 52nd WMA General Assembly, Edinburgh, Scotland, October 2000

■ A. INTRODUCTION

1. The World Medical Association has developed the Declaration of Helsinki as a statement of ethical principles to provide guidance to physicians and other participants in medical research involving human subjects. Medical research involving human subjects includes research on identifiable human material or identifiable data.

2. It is the duty of the physician to promote and safeguard the health of the people. The physician's knowledge and conscience are dedicated to the fulfillment of this duty.

3. The Declaration of Geneva of the World Medical Association binds the physician with the words, "The health of my patient will be my first consideration," and the International Code of Medical Ethics declares that, "A physician shall act only in the patient's interest when providing medical care which might have the effect of weakening the physical and mental condition of the patient."

4. Medical progress is based on research which ultimately must rest in part on experimentation involving human subjects.

5. In medical research on human subjects, considerations related to the well-being of the human subject should take precedence over the interests of science and society.

6. The primary purpose of medical research involving human subjects is to improve prophylactic, diagnostic and therapeutic procedures and the understanding of the aetiology and pathogenesis of disease. Even the best proven prophylactic, diagnostic, and therapeutic methods must continuously be challenged through research for their effectiveness, efficiency, accessibility and quality.

7. In current medical practice and in medical research, most prophylactic, diagnostic and therapeutic procedures involve risks and burdens.

8. Medical research is subject to ethical standards that promote respect for all human beings and protect their health and rights. Some research populations are vulnerable and need special

protection. The particular needs of the economically and medically disadvantaged must be recognized. Special attention is also required for those who cannot give or refuse consent for themselves, for those who may be subject to giving consent under duress, for those who will not benefit personally from the research and for those for whom the research is combined with care.

9. Research Investigators should be aware of the ethical, legal and regulatory requirements for research on human subjects in their own countries as well as applicable international requirements. No national ethical, legal or regulatory requirement should be allowed to reduce or eliminate any of the protections for human subjects set forth in this Declaration.

▪ B. BASIC PRINCIPLES FOR ALL MEDICAL RESEARCH

10. It is the duty of the physician in medical research to protect the life, health, privacy, and dignity of the human subject.
11. Medical research involving human subjects must conform to generally accepted scientific principles, be based on a thorough knowledge of the scientific literature, other relevant sources of information, and on adequate laboratory and, where appropriate, animal experimentation.
12. Appropriate caution must be exercised in the conduct of research which may affect the environment, and the welfare of animals used for research must be respected.
13. The design and performance of each experimental procedure involving human subjects should be clearly formulated in an experimental protocol. This protocol should be submitted for consideration, comment, guidance, and where appropriate, approval to a specially appointed ethical review committee, which must be independent of the investigator, the

sponsor or any other kind of undue influence. This independent committee should be in conformity with the laws and regulations of the country in which the research experiment is performed.

The committee has the right to monitor ongoing trials. The researcher has the obligation to provide monitoring information to the committee, especially any serious adverse events. The researcher should also submit to the committee, for review, information regarding funding, sponsors, institutional affiliations, other potential conflicts of interest and incentives for subjects.

14. The research protocol should always contain a statement of the ethical considerations involved and should indicate that there is compliance with the principles enunciated in this Declaration.
15. Medical research involving human subjects should be conducted only by scientifically qualified persons and under the supervision of a clinically competent medical person. The responsibility for the human subject must always rest with a medically qualified person and never rest on the subject of the research, even though the subject has given consent.
16. Every medical research project involving human subjects should be preceded by careful assessment of predictable risks and burdens in comparison with foreseeable benefits to the subject or to others. This does not preclude the participation of healthy volunteers in medical research. The design of all studies should be publicly available.
17. Physicians should abstain from engaging in research projects involving human subjects unless they are confident that the risks involved have been adequately assessed and can be satisfactorily managed. Physicians should cease any investigation if the risks are found to outweigh the potential benefits or if there is conclusive proof of positive and beneficial results.
18. Medical research involving human subjects

should only be conducted if the importance of the objective outweighs the inherent risks and burdens to the subject. This is especially important when the human subjects are healthy volunteers.

19. Medical research is only justified if there is a reasonable likelihood that the populations in which the research is carried out stand to benefit from the results of the research.

20. The subjects must be volunteers and informed participants in the research project.

21. The right of research subjects to safeguard their integrity must always be respected. Every precaution should be taken to respect the privacy of the subject, the confidentiality of the patient's information and to minimize the impact of the study on the subject's physical and mental integrity and on the personality of the subject.

22. In any research on human beings, each potential subject must be adequately informed of the aims, methods, sources of funding, any possible conflicts of interest, institutional affiliations of the researcher, the anticipated benefits and potential risks of the study and the discomfort it may entail. The subject should be informed of the right to abstain from participation in the study or to withdraw consent to participate at any time without reprisal. After ensuring that the subject has understood the information, the physician should then obtain the subject's freely-given informed consent, preferably in writing. If the consent cannot be obtained in writing, the non-written consent must be formally documented and witnessed.

23. When obtaining informed consent for the research project the physician should be particularly cautious if the subject is in a dependent relationship with the physician or may consent under duress. In that case the informed consent should be obtained by a well-informed physician who is not engaged in the investigation and who is completely independent of this relationship.

24. For a research subject who is legally incompetent, physically or mentally incapable of giving consent or is a legally incompetent minor, the investigator must obtain informed consent from the legally authorized representative in accordance with applicable law. These groups should not be included in research unless the research is necessary to promote the health of the population represented and this research cannot instead be performed on legally competent persons.

25. When a subject deemed legally incompetent, such as a minor child, is able to give assent to decisions about participation in research, the investigator must obtain that assent in addition to the consent of the legally authorized representative.

26. Research on individuals from whom it is not possible to obtain consent, including proxy or advance consent, should be done only if the physical/mental condition that prevents obtaining informed consent is a necessary characteristic of the research population. The specific reasons for involving research subjects with a condition that renders them unable to give informed consent should be stated in the experimental protocol for consideration and approval of the review committee. The protocol should state that consent to remain in the research should be obtained as soon as possible from the individual or a legally authorized surrogate.

27. Both authors and publishers have ethical obligations. In publication of the results of research, the investigators are obliged to preserve the accuracy of the results. Negative as well as positive results should be published or otherwise publicly available. Sources of funding, institutional affiliations and any possible conflicts of interest should be declared in the publication. Reports of experimentation not in accordance with the principles laid down in this Declaration should not be accepted for publication.

■ C. ADDITIONAL PRINCIPLES FOR MEDICAL RESEARCH COMBINED WITH MEDICAL CARE

28. The physician may combine medical research with medical care, only to the extent that the research is justified by its potential prophylactic, diagnostic or therapeutic value. When medical research is combined with medical care, additional standards apply to protect the patients who are research subjects.

29. The benefits, risks, burdens and effectiveness of a new method should be tested against those of the best current prophylactic, diagnostic, and therapeutic methods. This does not exclude the use of placebo, or no treatment, in studies where no proven prophylactic, diagnostic or therapeutic method exists.

    To further clarify the WMA position on the use of placebo controlled trials, the WMA Council issued, during October 2001, a note of clarification on article 29, which is available on this page.

30. At the conclusion of the study, every patient entered into the study should be assured of access to the best proven prophylactic, diagnostic and therapeutic methods identified by the study.

31. The physician should fully inform the patient which aspects of the care are related to the research. The refusal of a patient to participate in a study must never interfere with the patient-physician relationship.

32. In the treatment of a patient, where proven prophylactic, diagnostic and therapeutic methods do not exist or have been ineffective, the physician, with informed consent from the patient, must be free to use unproven or new prophylactic, diagnostic and therapeutic measures, if in the physician's judgment it offers hope of saving life, re-establishing health or alleviating suffering. Where possible, these measures should be made the object of research, designed to evaluate their safety and efficacy. In all cases, new information should be recorded and, where appropriate, published. The other relevant guidelines of this Declaration should be followed.

■ NOTE OF CLARIFICATION ON PARAGRAPH 29 of the WMA DECLARATION OF HELSINKI

The WMA is concerned that paragraph 29 of the revised Declaration of Helsinki (October 2000) has led to diverse interpretations and possible confusion. It hereby reaffirms its position that extreme care must be taken in making use of a placebo-controlled trial and that in general this methodology should only be used in the absence of existing proven therapy. However, a placebo-controlled trial may be ethically acceptable, even if proven therapy is available, under the following circumstances:

- Where for compelling and scientifically sound methodological reasons its use is necessary to determine the efficacy or safety of a prophylactic, diagnostic or therapeutic method; or
- Where a prophylactic, diagnostic or therapeutic method is being investigated for a minor condition and the patients who receive placebo will not be subject to any additional risk of serious or irreversible harm.

All other provisions of the Declaration of Helsinki must be adhered to, especially the need for appropriate ethical and scientific review.

From: World Medical Organization. (1996). Declaration of Helsinki. *British Medical Journal, 313,* 1448–1449.

Examples of Research That Might Be Eligible for Exempt Status and the Process for Requesting Exemption

Request for Exemption (Submit ONLY if your proposal qualifies for exemption status.)

Federal and State policy allow the Institutional Review Board to exempt certain projects from review. The description of exempt research is given below. It is taken from the Code of Federal Regulations Title 45, Part 46. If you think the Review Board might decide your project is exempt from review, please complete this form and attach it to your protocol form.

46.101(b)

Research activities in which the only involvement of human participants will be in one or more of the following categories are exempt from this policy (i.e., review by a human participants committee):

46.101(b)(1)

Research conducted in established or commonly accepted education settings, involving normal educational practices, such as:

(i) research on regular and special education strategies, or

(ii) research on the effectiveness of or the comparison among instructional techniques, curricula, or classroom management methods.

46.101(b)(2)

Research involving the use of educational tests (cognitive, diagnostic, aptitude, achievement), survey procedures, interview procedures or observation of public behavior, unless:

(i) information obtained is recorded in such a manner that human partic- ipants can be identified, directly or though identifiers linked to the par- ticipants **and**

(ii) any disclosure of the human participants' responses outside the research could reasonably place the participants at risk of criminal or civil liability or be damaging to the participants' financial standing, employability, or reputation.

4 6.101(b)(4)

Research involving the collection or study of existing data, documents, records, pathological specimens, or diagnostic specimens, if these sources are publicly available or if the information is recorded by the investigator in such a manner that participants cannot be identified, directly or through identifiers linked to the participants.

Action: If you believe your research may be exempt from Board review, please complete this form and attach it to your Protocol Form. **Only the Board is permitted to make the decision that a study is exempt from review.**

If you believe that your research is exempt from review, which of the paragraphs above justify the exemption?

____ 46.101(b)(1)

____ 46.101(b)(2)

____ 46.101(b)(4)

Project Title: _____

Principal Investigator: _____

Source: www.virginia.edu/researchandpublicservice/irbsbs

Sample Template for Medical Research Consent Form

Participant's Name_____ Medical Record # _____

■ CONSENT TO PARTICIPATE IN A RESEARCH STUDY

What is an Informed Consent?

You are being asked to take part in a clinical research study. Before you can make an informed decision whether to participate, you should understand the possible risks and benefits associated with this study. This process is known as informed consent. This consent form will provide you with the information about this study and your rights so that you can make an informed decision. No guarantees or assurances can be made regarding the results of this study.

This consent form may contain words or information you do not understand. Dr. _____ or the research study coordinator who is familiar with the study will explain anything that you do not clearly understand. Please ask as many questions as you need to make sure that you understand this study and why you are being asked to participate.

Be aware that your relationship with the study doctor bears certain differences from your relationship with your personal physician. Your personal physician individualizes the treatment of your specific problem with the expectation of a benefit to you. The research physician treats all subjects under a specific protocol to obtain general knowledge and with the understanding that you may or may not benefit from your participation in the study. Be sure to ask questions of the study physician if you want further clarification of this relationship.

It is essential that you are completely truthful regarding your health history and any symptoms or reactions you may experience during the study. If you are not truthful, you may harm yourself by participating.

Introduction

We invite you to participate in a study of... *{If this is a drug trial: (Enter name of drug)* an experimental drug that may *(summarize experience to date with the drug).}*

The purpose of this study is…

A total of _____participants will be enrolled in this study.

You are being asked to participate in this study because …

This study is being sponsored by …

[If there is an outside sponsor including a grant from NIH/DHHS or other private foundation enter the following sentence] The University of Virginia is receiving compensation from the sponsor to perform this study.

[Enter any information regarding potential conflict of interest here.]

[If the protocol involves a patent owned by UVA, insert the following: *As the owner of the patent of* (insert drug or device name) *the University of Virginia may profit if this study has positive results.]*

Investigational Procedures

If you choose to participate in this study, you will …

{This must be a clear, specific narrative of everything that will be done to the participant, beginning with the first visit/admission, etc., and proceeding through the final visit/discharge.

REMEMBER TO DEFINE ALL TERMS IN SIMPLE LAY LANGUAGE! Use terms such as investigational medications/procedures instead of therapy or treatment. Therapy or treatment may give the participant the wrong impression that the investigational medications/ procedures are proven to be effective. This should match what is listed in the research protocol.}

- *If material such as blood or spinal fluid is to be withdrawn, translate the total volume into teaspoons, tablespoons or ounces.*
- *State how many times you'll do each procedure and at what point each will be done.*
- *Specify the setting (GCRC, office visit, etc.),*
- *Give an approximation of the time involved in each phase and the time required for the entire study. Walk the participant through everything you'll be doing.*
- *{Do not use the term "sugar pill" to describe a placebo since patients with diabetes might confuse this with their diabetes medication.}*
- *ALL PROCEDURES THAT ARE EXPERIMENTAL INTERVENTIONS (invasive measurement, blood, tissue or data collection) PERFORMED SOLELY TO ANSWER THE RESEARCH QUESTION MUST BE IDENTIFIED AS SUCH, especially if the research procedures are "added on" to what is appropriate medical care for the participant.*
- *If randomization of treatment is involved, list the probability of receiving each treatment.*
- *If you're going to draw more than 300 mL of blood per month, the following screening criteria must be used:*

Hematocrit

- *> 41% for males*
- *> 38% for females*

- *For children, no more than 5% of the total estimated blood volume may be withdrawn; total blood volume is calculated at 70 cc/kg*
- *No one with body weight < 110 lbs. will be admitted to the study;*

If blood or tissue is to be taken, insert the following statement: The following tests will be done on the *blood/tissue* collected. When these tests are done any remaining *blood/tissue* will be thrown away.

The tests or examinations performed as part of this study should not be used as a substitute for your normal medical care. You should know that this study is not designed to detect any disease or abnormal condition. If you wonder whether you may have a disease or abnormal condition, please consult your doctor. Participating in this research study will not help you to know whether you have a disease or abnormal condition.

Exclusions

You should not participate in this study if....

Risks

Research studies often involve some risks. The risks of this study are ...

{Include any and all reasonably foreseeable risks; you may cite results from former studies. Be sure to include potential risks of withholding or delaying customary treatment, if this is pertinent. These need to match those listed in the research protocol and/or the investigator's brochure.}

{If you are drawing blood, insert the following:

The problems associated with blood drawing include discomfort from insertion of the needle (common), fainting at or about the time of blood drawing (infrequent), bruising at the site of blood drawing (infrequent), and infection at the same site (rare).}*

{If an intravenous catheter is placed for blood drawing, insert the following:

To allow safe and adequate collection of blood samples needed in the course of this study, you may occasionally need to have the first intravenous catheter replaced or have a blood sample taken from another vein.}*

{If you're drawing > 100 mL of blood in any 4-week period, insert the following:

If blood were to be drawn for any other purpose, such as a donation at the Blood Bank or in another laboratory, this could result in an excessive amount of blood being donated during the study period. Therefore, if asked to donate blood, you should inform such persons of this study and refuse further donation until *(insert time frame).}*

{If this study involves the use of ionizing radiation from a chest x-ray, bone mineral densities studies, bone age x-rays, knee x-rays, hip x-rays, sinus films, CT scans, or mammography, insert the appropriate language from the document titled "Uses of Ionizing Radiation That Do Not Need to be Reviewed by the

Radiation Safety Committee." If you use the exact wording as listed, the protocol and consent form will not need to be reviewed by the Radiation Safety Committee. You must however, send them a copy of the protocol and consent forms after the study is approved by the HIC. If this study involves the use of ionizing radiation other than those listed above, the Radiation Safety Committee must approve the wording.}

In addition, it is possible in any experiment that side effects that are not now known, could occur. Precautions will be taken to prevent harmful side effects. You should contact your study doctor or research coordinator if you think you are having side effects related to the study.

{If appropriate to the study add:

If you are pregnant, we want you to tell us and we will not include you in the experiment, because to do so might be harmful to your unborn baby. We also want you to avoid getting pregnant during this study and expect you to use an effective method of birth control. If you should become pregnant despite taking precautions, please immediately contact the investigator whose phone number is listed on this form and he/she will provide you with information and/or resources for your consideration.}

OR

If you are a male, it is advisable that you do not father a baby while participating in this study *or for* ____*months following the completion of this study.* To do so might be harmful to your unborn baby.

Benefits

If you participate in this study, you may experience...

{If the participant can reasonably expect any benefits, describe them. You may also include a statement that the research may benefit future patients or society in general. This must match what is stated in the research protocol. Also include the following statement: We do not guarantee or promise, however, that you will receive any of these benefits.}

{If there is no direct benefit to the participant, insert:

There is no direct benefit to you for participating in this study.}

Alternatives to Participating in This Study

Often, the treatment for your condition would be...

However, in order to *{insert explanation}*...we must necessarily *{withhold}{delay}* customary treatment, which would be...

Other alternatives to participating in this study include *{State appropriate alternative procedures or courses of treatment if any that might be advantageous to the participant. Often approved drugs/devices that are being studied are available to an individual without the need to participate in the study and these should be indicted by name if appropriate. }*

Another alternative is not to participate in this study.

{IF participants are normal volunteers, insert: The only alternative is not to participate.}

Privacy of Records

In addition to the members of the health care staff who usually have access to your medical records, your medical records and the consent form you sign may be inspected by the investigator of this study, his/her research staff, the sponsor *(list name, if applicable)*; federal agencies having oversight over this research, for example, the Food and Drug Administration (FDA); and the University of Virginia Human Investigation Committee (HIC) members or designates. The HIC is a special committee at the University of Virginia that reviews all medical research studies involving human participants. *{If appropriate add:* Your records may also be shared with governmental agencies in other countries where the study *drug/device* may be considered for approval.} Because of the need to release information to these parties, absolute confidentiality cannot be guaranteed; however, we will take every precaution to protect your privacy. The results of this research may be presented at meetings or in publications; however, your identity will not be disclosed. If you sign this form, you have given us permission to release information to these other people.

A copy of this consent form may be placed in your medical record. This means that everyone who is authorized to see your records will be able to find out that you are in this study. This is done so that if you have other health problems or need other treatment during the study, the doctors caring for you will be able to obtain sufficient information about what drugs or procedures you are receiving in the study and can treat you appropriately.

In the event anyone involved with this study is exposed to your blood or body fluids in a manner that might transmit an infectious disease to them, your blood may be tested for evidence of hepatitis, HIV (human immunodeficiency virus) or other infections without your further consent. You and the person exposed would be informed of the results of the test; however, the person exposed would not be informed of your identity. If your test result is positive, counseling will be offered.

Payment

You will receive $_____ for participating in and completing this study. *{If the payment will be prorated for incomplete participation, please make this clear.} {Or}* You will receive no payment for participating in this study. You should expect to receive your payment approximately *(insert time frame)* after the completion of the study *{or}* approximately *(insert time frame)* after each visit.

{If the payment will be prorated for incomplete participation, please make this clear. You will receive the payment (*insert specifics: e.g. in one lump payment approximately 2 to 4 weeks following the completion of the study.*)-*OR*-You will receive no payment for participating in this study.}

Financial Costs of the Research

{Be sure to indicate at this point whether the cost of the study or study related tests are covered all or in part by the sponsor. If all costs are not covered, explain which costs are covered and which are not. If not covered, indicate that should an insurance company refuse responsibility for the costs incurred, the participant will be held responsible, and what this includes. If any of the charges will be submitted to an insurance company please add the following: You may wish to check with your insurance company before the study starts to determine which of these charges they will cover.}

Compensation in Case of Injury

In the event you suffer physical injury directly resulting from the research procedures, no financial compensation for lost wages, disability, or discomfort is available. Medical treatment for physical injury directly resulting from the research procedure that is not covered by the sponsor or your insurance will be provided free of charge at the University of Virginia. If you have any questions concerning financial compensation for injuries caused by the experiment, you should talk to *{insert name of responsible investigator}* at *{telephone number}*.

You do not waive any liability rights for personal injury by signing this form.

{If the sponsors require their own indemnification statement, it may be added here.}

Right to Refuse to Participate or to Withdraw Early From the Study

Your care at this hospital will not be hurt if you decide not to participate in this study or if you decide now to enter but wish at a later time to stop the study. Of course, we will tell you anything we learn during the study that may help you decide whether to continue participating, or that is important to your overall health. *{For placebo-controlled trials:* We will not be able to tell you whether you received (*the name of the test medication*) or a placebo (an inactive substance) until the research is completed. Methods are in place to determine which medication you are receiving if there is an emergency and the doctor needs to know which medication you are taking.} *{If applicable enter the following statement.}* If you do decide to withdraw from the study the following procedures will need to be completed. *{Insert required procedures for study withdrawal}*

You may be withdrawn from the study without your permission at any time by the investigator or the sponsor conducting this study. Some situations in which this might occur is if you do not follow the instructions given to you or if the investigator feels your safety is at risk if you continue in the study.

Contact Information

If you have any questions about this study, please ask *{insert name of responsible investigator}* at *{telephone number}*.

If you have any questions regarding research participants' rights, please contact [insert name] at [insert telephone number]

Conclusion

I HAVE READ, OR HAD READ TO ME, THE ABOVE INFORMATION BEFORE SIGNING THIS CONSENT FORM. I HAVE BEEN OFFERED AN OPPORTUNITY TO ASK QUESTIONS AND HAVE RECEIVED ANSWERS THAT FULLY SATISFY THOSE QUESTIONS. I HEREBY VOLUNTEER TO TAKE PART IN THIS RESEARCH STUDY.

You will receive a *signed copy* of this form to keep.

Please check one of the following

_____ I agree to be contacted after the completion of this study for follow-up information.

_____ I do not agree to be contacted after the completion of this study for follow-up information.

PARTICIPANT (SIGNATURE)	PARTICIPANT (PRINT)	DATE	TIME

PERSON OBTAINING CONSENT (SIGNATURE)	PERSON OBTAINING CONSENT (PRINT)

DATE

Source: Retrieved 12/20/04: http://www.irb.virginia.edu

Sample Template for Behavioral Science Research Consent Form

■ Model Informed Consent Agreement

Page X of Y

Project Title: _____

Please read this consent agreement carefully before you decide to participate in the study.

Purpose of the research study:
The purpose of the study is…

What you will do in the study:
(Be specific.)

Time required:
You will spend about ___ hours in each session. The total experiment will require about ___ hours.

Risks:

Benefits: There are no direct benefits to you for participating in this research study. The study may help us understand… *(Limit to one brief statement.)*

Confidentiality: *(Only use the language below if it is appropriate for your study.)*

The information that you give in the study will be handled confidentially. Your information will be assigned a code number. The list connecting your name to this code will be kept in a locked file. When the study is completed and the data have been analyzed, this list will be destroyed. Your name will not be used in any report. *(Place audio/video tape erasure statement here if applicable.)*

Voluntary participation:
Your participation in the study is completely voluntary.

Right to withdraw from the study:
You have the right to withdraw from the study at any time without penalty. *(If payment or course credit is being offered, include the following phrase.)* You will still receive full payment *(or credit)* for the study. *(Place audio/video tape erasure statement here if applicable.)*

How to withdraw from the study:

If you want to withdraw from the study, tell the experimenter and quietly leave the room. There is no penalty for withdrawing. You will still receive full credit for the experiment. *(If deception is included in the study, let the participants know that they will be debriefed if they withdraw from the study and that their data will be destroyed.)*

Payment:

You will receive no payment for participating in the study. *(If payment or credit is being offered, describe it here.)*

Who to contact if you have questions about the study:

Researcher's Name *(If multiple PIs, list contact information for each person.)*

Department, Address

University of

Telephone:

Faculty Advisor's Name *(Include this information for student or staff research projects.)*

Department, Address

University of

Telephone:

Page X of Y

Project Title: _____

Who to contact about your rights in the study:

Include name and address.

Telephone:

Agreement:

I agree to participate in the research study described above.

Signature:_____ **Date:** _____

You will receive a copy of this form for your records.

Source: Adapted from http://www.virginia.edu/researchandpublicservice/irbsbs

Sample Template for Obtaining Consent from a Minor

Minors Consent Form (without tissue banking/genetic testing)
Template Revision Date: 01-01-02
PLEASE NOTE: If this study will involve the banking of tissue after this study is completed or involves any genetic testing, please use the Protocol and Consent Form Templates for Tissue Banking/Genetic Testing.
Participant's Name_____ Medical Record # _____

■ CONSENT FOR A MINOR TO PARTICIPATE IN A RESEARCH STUDY

What is an Informed Consent?

You or your child are being asked to take part in a clinical research study. Before you can make an informed decision whether to participate, you should understand the possible risks and benefits associated with this study. This process is known as informed consent. This consent form will provide you with the information about this study and your/your child's rights so that you can make an informed decision. No guarantees or assurances can be made regarding the results of this study.

This consent form may contain words or information you or your child do not understand. Dr. _____ or the research study coordinator who is familiar with the study will explain anything that you or your child do not clearly understand. Please ask as many questions as you need to make sure that you and your child understand this study and why your child is being asked to participate.

Be aware that your relationship with the study doctor bears certain differences from your relationship with your/your child's personal physician. Your personal physician individualizes the treatment of your/your child's specific problem with the expectation of a benefit to you/your child. The research physician treats all subjects under a specific protocol to obtain general knowledge and on the understanding that you/your child may or may not benefit from participation in the study. Be sure to ask questions of the study physician if you want further clarification of this relationship.

379

It is essential that you are completely truthful regarding your child's health history and any symptoms or reactions you/he/she may experience during the study. If you are not truthful, you may harm yourself/your child by participating.

Introduction

We invite your child _____ to participate in a study of…

The purpose of this study is… *{If you are doing a drug trial insert: (Insert name of drug)* an experimental drug which may *(summarize experience to date with the drug).*

A total of ____ participants will be enrolled in this study.

Your child is being asked to participate in this study because …

This study is being sponsored by …

{If there is an outside sponsor or through a grant from NIH/DHHS or other private foundation, enter the following sentence} The University of Virginia is receiving compensation from the sponsor to perform this study.

{Enter any information regarding potential conflict of interest here.}

{If the protocol involves a patent owned by UVA insert the following: As the owner of the patent of *(insert drug or device name)* the University of Virginia may profit if this study has positive results.

Investigational Procedures

If you and your child agree to participate in this study, your child will …

{This must be a clear, specific narrative of everything that will be done to the participant, beginning with the first visit/admission, etc., and proceeding through the final visit/discharge. REMEMBER TO DEFINE ALL TERMS IN *SIMPLE* LAY LANGUAGE! This must match what is listed in the research protocol.}

- *If material such as blood or spinal fluid is to be withdrawn, translate the total volume into teaspoons, tablespoons, or ounces.*
- *State how many times you'll do each procedure and at what point each will be done.*
- *Specify the setting (GCRC, office visit, etc.),*
- *Give an approximate idea of the time involved in each phase and the time required for the entire study. Walk the participant through everything you'll be doing.*
- *ALL PROCEDURES THAT ARE EXPERIMENTAL INTERVENTIONS (invasive measurement, blood, tissue or data collection) PERFORMED SOLELY TO ANSWER THE RESEARCH QUESTION MUST BE IDEN-TIFIED AS SUCH, especially if the research procedures are "added on" to what is appropriate medical care for the participant.*
- *Do not use the term "sugar pill" to describe a placebo since patients with diabetes might confuse this with their diabetes medication.*

- *If randomization of treatment is involved list the probability of receiving each treatment.*

{No more than 5% of the total estimated blood volume may be withdrawn.}
[Total blood volume is calculated at 70 cc/kg.]

{Use terms such as investigational medications/procedures instead of therapy or treatment. Therapy or treatment may give the participant the wrong impression that the investigational medications/ procedures are proven to be effective.}

If blood or tissue is to be taken insert the following statement: The following tests will be done on the *blood/tissue* collected. When these tests are done any remaining *blood/tissue* will be thrown away.

The tests or exams performed as part of this study should not be used as a substitute for your child's normal medical care. You should know that this study is not designed to detect any disease or abnormal condition. If you wonder whether your child may have a disease or abnormal condition, please consult his/her doctor. Participating in this research study will not help you to know whether your child has a disease or abnormal condition.

Exclusions

Your child should not participate in this study if....

Risks

Research studies often involve some risks. The risks of this study are …

{Include any and all reasonably foreseeable risks; you may cite results from former studies. Be sure to include potential risks of withholding or delaying customary treatment, if this is pertinent. These risks must match those listed in the research protocol and/or the investigator's brochure.}

{If an intravenous catheter is placed for blood drawing insert the following statement:

To allow safe and adequate collection of blood samples needed in the course of this study, your child may occasionally need to have the first intravenous catheter replaced or have a blood sample taken from another vein.}

{If you are drawing blood insert: The problems associated with blood drawing include discomfort from insertion of the needle (common), fainting at or about the time of blood drawing (infrequent), bruising at the site of blood drawing (infrequent), and infection at the same site (rare).}

{If this study involves the use of ionizing radiation from a chest x-ray, bone mineral densities studies, bone age x-rays, knee x-rays, hip x-rays, sinus films, CT scans, or mammography, insert the appropriate language from the document titled "Uses of Ionizing Radiation That Do Not Need to be Reviewed by the Radiation Safety Committee." If you use the exact wording as listed, the protocol and consent form will not need to be

reviewed by the Radiation Safety Committee. You must, however, send them a copy of the documents after the study is approved by the HIC.

If this study involves the use of ionizing radiation other than those listed above *Radiation Safety Committee must approve the wording.}*

In addition, it is possible in any experiment that side effects that are not now known could occur. Precautions will be taken to prevent harmful side effects. You should contact your study doctor or research coordinator if you think you are having side effects related to the study.

{If age appropriate, add: If your child is pregnant, we want you to tell us and we will not include her in the experiment, because to do so might be harmful to her unborn baby. We also want her to avoid getting pregnant during this study and expect her to use an effective method of birth control. If she should become pregnant despite taking precautions, please immediately contact the investigator whose phone number is listed on this form.
 OR

If your child is a male, it is advisable that he does not father a baby while on this study *or for* ____ *months following the completion of this study.* To do so might be harmful to his unborn baby. *}*

Benefits

If your child participates in this study, he/she may experience…

{If the participant can reasonably expect any benefits, describe them. You may also include a statement that the research may benefit future patients or society in general. These benefits must match those listed in the research protocol.}

We do not guarantee or promise, however, that he/she will receive any of these benefits.

{If there is no direct benefit to the participant, insert:
There is no direct benefit to your child for participating in this study.*}*

Alternatives to Participating in This Study

Often, the treatment for your child's condition would be…

However, in order to… *(insert explanation)*

we must necessarily *{withhold}{delay}* customary treatment which would be…

Other alternatives to participating in this study include *{State appropriate alternative procedures or courses of treatment if any that might be advantageous to the participant. Often approved drugs/devices that are being studied are available to an individual without the need to participate in the study and these should be indicted by name if appropriate}.*

Another alternative is not to participate in this study.

{IF participants are normal volunteers only, insert: *The only alternative is not to participate.}*

Privacy of Records

In addition to the members of the health care staff who usually have access to your child's medical records, your child's records and the consent form you sign may be inspected by the investigator of this study, his/her research staff, the sponsor (*list name, if applicable*); federal agencies having oversight over this research, for example, the Food and Drug Administration (FDA); and the University of Virginia Human Investigation Committee (HIC) members or designates. The HIC is a special committee at the University of Virginia that reviews all medical research involving human participants. *{When appropriate insert:* Your child's records may also be shared with governmental agencies in other countries where the study drug/device may be considered for approval.} Because of the need to release information to these parties, absolute confidentiality cannot be guaranteed; however, we will take every precaution to protect your child's privacy. The results of this research may be presented at meetings or in publications; however, your child's identity will not be disclosed. If you sign this form, you have given us permission to release your child's information to these other people.

A copy of this consent form may be placed in your child's medical record. This means that everyone who is authorized to see your child's records will be able to find out that your child is in this study. This is done so that if your child has other health problems or needs other treatment during the study, the doctors caring for your child will be able to obtain sufficient information about what drugs or procedures your child is receiving in the study and can treat your child appropriately.

In the event anyone involved with this study is exposed to your child's blood or body fluids in a manner that might transmit an infectious disease to them, your child's blood may be tested for evidence of hepatitis, HIV (human immunodeficiency virus) or other infections without your further consent. You and the person exposed would be informed of the results of the test, however, the person exposed would not be informed of your child's identity. If your child's test result is positive, counseling will be offered.

Payment

Your child will receive $_____ for participating in and completing this study. *{The payment should be in the form of age appropriate gift certificates and not in cash.} {Or}* Your child will receive no payment for participating in this study. You should expect to receive the payment approximately (*insert time frame*) after the completion of the study *{or}* approximately (*insert time frame*) after each visit.

{If the payment will be prorated for incomplete participation, please make this clear. You will receive the payment (*insert specifics: e.g. in one lump payment approximately 2 to 4 weeks following the completion of the study.*)-**OR**- You will receive no payment for participating in this study.}

Financial Costs of the Research

{Be sure to indicate at this point whether the cost of the study or study related tests are covered all or in part by the sponsor. If covered in part, specify which costs will be covered and which will not be covered. If not covered, indicate that should an insurance company refuse responsibility for the costs incurred, the participant will be held responsible, and what this includes.}

If any of the charges will be submitted to an insurance company, please add the following: You may wish to check with your insurance company before the study starts to determine which of these charges they will cover.

Compensation in Case of Injury

In the event your child suffers physical injury directly resulting from the research procedures, no financial compensation for such things as lost wages, disability, or discomfort is available. Medical treatment for physical injury directly resulting from the research procedure that is not covered by the sponsor or your insurance will be provided free of charge at the University of Virginia. If you have any questions concerning financial compensation for injuries caused by the experiment, you should talk *{insert name of responsible investigator}* at *{telephone number}*.

You do not waive any liability rights for personal injury by signing this form.

{If the sponsors require their own indemnification statement it may be added here.}

Right to Refuse to Participate or to Withdraw Early From the Study

The decision by you and your child not to participate in this study will not hurt your child's care at this hospital. If you decide to allow your child to participate, you may stop and withdraw your child at any time without hurting your child's care. Of course, we will tell you anything we learn during the study that may help you decide whether your child should continue participating, or that is important to your child's overall health. *{For placebo-controlled trials insert:* We will not be able to tell you whether your child received *(the name of the test medication)* or a placebo (a dummy medication) until after this research is completed. Methods are in place to determine which medication your child received if there is an emergency and the doctor needs to know.} *{If applicable enter the following statement.}* If you/your child decides to withdraw from the study the following procedures will need to be completed. *{Insert required procedures for study withdrawal}*

Your child may be withdrawn from the study without your permission at any time by the investigator or the sponsor conducting this study. Some situations in which this might occur is if you/your child does not follow the instructions given to you/your child or if the investigator feels your/your child's safety is at risk if you/your child continues in the study.

You and your child are making a decision whether or not he/she will participate in this study. If you sign this form, you are agreeing that your child will participate based on your reading and understanding this form. If you or your child have any questions about this study, please ask {insert name of responsible investigator} at {telephone number}.

If you have any questions regarding research participants' rights, please contact [insert name] and [insert address and telephone].

Conclusion

I HAVE READ, OR HAD READ TO ME, THE ABOVE INFORMATION BEFORE SIGNING THIS CONSENT FORM. I HAVE BEEN OFFERED AN OPPORTUNITY TO ASK QUESTIONS AND HAVE RECEIVED ANSWERS THAT FULLY SATISFY THOSE QUESTIONS. I HEREBY VOLUNTEER MY CHILD TO TAKE PART IN THIS RESEARCH STUDY. I CONFIRM BY SIGNING THIS FORM THAT I HAVE THE LEGAL AUTHORITY TO SIGN FOR THIS MINOR.

Please check one of the following

_____ I agree to be contacted after the completion of this study for follow-up information.

_____ I do not agree to be contacted after the completion of this study for follow-up information.

You will receive a *signed copy* of this form to keep.

MINOR PARTICIPANT (SIGNATURE) (If >15 and < 18 years of age)	MINOR PARTICIPANT (PRINT)	DATE	TIME
PARENT OR GUARDIAN(SIGNATURE)	PARENT OR GUARDIAN (PRINT)	DATE	TIME

{Insert the second parent signature line if the study has more than minimal risk and no benefit to the subject.}

PARENT OR GUARDIAN(SIGNATURE)	PARENT OR GUARDIAN (PRINT)	DATE	TIME
PERSON OBTAINING CONSENT (SIGNATURE)	PERSON OBTAINING CONSENT (PRINT)	DATE	TIME

Source: Adapted from http://www.irb.virginia.edu

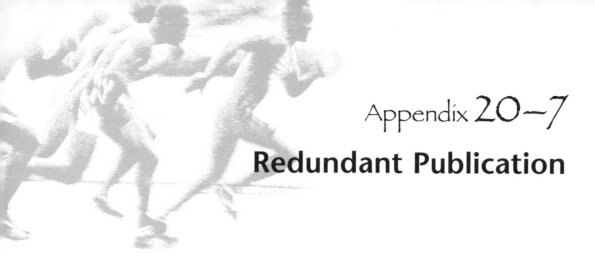

Appendix 20–7

Redundant Publication

■ The Editorial Policy Committee of the Council of Science Editors

Summary

The Committee on Editorial Policy has considered the matter of redundant (or duplicate or repetitive) publication and recommends that each journal have a clear policy regarding sole submission and the definition of redundant publication. Procedures should be developed to evaluate potential violations of such a policy; actions should be prescribed for cases in which a violation has been established. All of this information should be incorporated into the journal's instructions for authors.

Introduction

Journals that view their purpose as including the reporting of original work generally insist that papers be submitted to them solely, not having been published before or not under consideration by another journal. Violating this requirement by reporting substantially the same work more than once, without attribution of the original source(s), has been variously called duplicate, repetitive, or redundant publication. Of these terms, duplicate and, to a lesser extent, repetitive, connote identicality, and 2 papers need not be identical to be substantially the same. Thus, "redundant publication" is probably the favored term to describe this prac-

tice, and the term applies whether or not publication has actually occurred (that is, it includes submission in hopes of redundant publication).

Redundant publication is a matter of great concern to journal editors and editorial boards, mainly because it wastes a journal's most precious resources—its editorial pages and the time and talents of its reviewers and staff. And it displaces other meritorious reports. It can also distort the importance of an observation or treatment by artificially inflating its frequency, confound subsequent tabulations such as meta-analyses, subvert an academic reward system based on publication of scholarly work, and violate copyright laws.

Recognition

A working definition of redundant publication might be "publishing or attempting to publish substantially the same work more than once," but this raises the issue of how to recognize when 2 (or more) written reports are substantially the same. An all-inclusive, legalistic definition is probably not possible, although certain aspects or characteristics are usually evident on careful examination. At least 1 of the authors must be common to all reports (if there are no common authors, it is more likely plagiarism than redundant publication). The subject or study populations are often the same or similar, the methodology is typically identical or nearly so, and the results and their interpretation generally vary little, if at all. The papers may differ in form but not in substance; a useful general test is to ask if the reader of 1 paper would gain any new insights or perspectives from reading the other, at least with respect to those elements common to both papers. If the answer to this question is "Probably not," there is a strong likelihood that redundant publication exists. Nevertheless, the ultimate decision about whether 2 specific papers represent redundant publication has to be made on an individual basis, typically as a judgment by the editor(s) but guided by a journal policy established previously, and reached as fairly and objectively as possible.

A common circumstance in which concern about redundant publication should be raised is the one in which 1 of the papers clearly reports a subset of the other. The more comprehensive report may have been published first and the more focused later, or vice versa. In such instances, the components common to each publication should be examined and compared, first to verify their commonality, and then to make a judgment as to how much of the totality of the work they represent. If the common elements are clearly minor and secondary to the major "message" of the comprehensive report, it is probably not redundant publication (although the value of the secondary paper may be so low as to preclude acceptance). However, if the common elements represent the essence of the work, then redundant publication may well exist. No hard-and-fast rules govern the determination of what is "essence" or "major part," and judgment can only be based on a case-by-case determination. Again, it is often helpful to ask, "Would the reader of 1 gain anything from reading the other?"

Implicit in any definition is the caveat that any possibility of redundant publication is undeclared, in that there is no indication, in the letter or other materials accompanying a submission of the existence of other related manuscripts. Most journals state in their instructions that any potential overlap with other manuscripts, published, submitted, or in preparation, should be identified specifically to the editor and a copy of any relevant paper(s) provided. This provides the opportunity to use the peer-review process to define "substantially the same work" in a specific case. Failure to give this information strongly suggests some intent to deceive, although it may simply reflect the failure of authors to read the instructions of journals to which they submit their work. However, failure to mention, in the text of a paper, one's own work that is, at the very least, closely related is more worrisome and, given authors' penchant to self-citation, omitting it from the bibliography is probably prima facie evidence of redundant publication.

There are circumstances that might appear initially to fit the definition of redundant publication, but which clearly do not constitute the practice. A journal might want to publish, in part or even word-for-word, something that has appeared previously or will appear nearly simultaneously, because it is judged so important, or it possesses historic interest, or because the journal wants to be certain it is available to its readers. There is no redundant publication in this case as long as 1) the editors of both journals approve, preferably in writing, 2) the secondary version is printed with a clear statement of previous publication including the primary reference, and 3) appropriate permissions and copyright releases are secured. A similar circumstance is that in which there is a desire to publish something in a language other than that in which it appeared originally. Again, as long as all concerned are fully informed, give consent, and the steps listed above are followed, redundant publication is not at issue.

Other situations that are not usually considered to constitute redundant publication include publication of an abstract and presentation at a scientific meeting. However, a journal would be well advised to define the maximum length (for example, 300 words) that can appear in print, without being considered redundant. Problems can arise with news media, both the lay or popular media, and " controlled circulation" publications. If a journal wishes to prevent dissemination of major or essential portions of an article by these means, it should caution its authors specifically against making available full text, tables, and figures, before publication in the journal.

Electronic dissemination of a manuscript is a relatively new phenomenon, and firm guidelines have not been developed. Sending a paper to a small number of selected colleagues, for information or advice, is probably permissible. However, widespread dissemination in advance of publication would probably be regarded by most journals as violation of a "sole submission" requirement and therefore would constitute redundant publication.

Determination

Questions of redundant publication may be raised at any of several points: 1) both papers may have already appeared in print; 2) 1 paper may have been published and the other (the one of specific interest) may be under consideration or in press; 3) both papers may be under consideration at the same time. The last situation arises fairly frequently, because 1 expert reviewer may have been asked to evaluate both.

When such a question is raised, the editor needs to obtain a copy of the "other" paper and, by some process, compare it with the "index" paper so as to make a determination regarding redundant publication. When the "other" paper has already been published, there is no problem. However, when it is under consideration, the reviewer who called the editor's attention to possible redundant publication should not provide his or her review copy because that would violate the privileged nature of the peer review process. What can be done, however, is that the editor can ask the author to provide copies of all manuscripts related in any way to the "index" paper.

With copies of the 2 (or more) manuscripts in hand, the editor can institute a process to determine whether redundant publication exists. It is preferable for this process to include others who have not participated directly in the evaluation of the specific manuscript; other editors or members of an editorial or advisory board would be good candidates to constitute such a panel, along with perhaps an outside expert in the field. If feasible, identification of authors and institutions should be removed from the manuscripts examined by a review panel, which can give its judgment by either discussion to reach consensus or vote of individual members.

What should be communicated to the author(s) during the time a potential redundant publication is being evaluated? There are no clear guidelines in this regard, but the authors should be informed at some point in the evaluation process and permitted the opportunity to submit a written statement of their position, to be considered by the editor and/or the review panel. Whatever procedure is followed, it needs to be guided by the goal of maintaining the journal's integrity, but at the same time acknowledging the author's rights to due process.

Sanctions and Penalties

What should a journal do when it finds an author or authors in violation of its policies on redundant publication? If it involves a manuscript under consideration, at the very least the paper should be rejected. If it involves a report that has already appeared in print, then the journal should consider publishing a "notice of redundant publication" so that readers will be informed of the situation. If such a notice is listed in the journal's table of contents, appears on a numbered page of the journal, and is signed by the editor, it will be entered into the database of the National Library of Medicine and incorporated into its database, making the information available in literature searches. Additionally, some journals invoke specific sanctions against authors found in violation of redundant publication policies by refusing to accept any submissions from them for a specified length of time. In a few instances, groups of journals of a particular specialty or subspecialty have agreed to share information about cases of redundant publication. The journal may wish to notify the department or institution if an author is found guilty of redundant publication.

Recommendations

1. Journals that publish original work should develop policies, using their particular policy-making mechanisms, regarding requirements of sole submission. Abstracts or longer articles representing presentations at scientific meetings and electronic publications should be specified as part of such policies.
2. Once a journal has a policy about redundant publication, it should develop procedures to evaluate potential violations at any point at which they may come to light. Such procedures should be as fair as possible to all concerned, involving blinded review and an author's right to respond or explain.
3. Once a journal has a policy about redundant publication, it should identify action(s) to be taken when a violation of the policy is determined to have taken place.
4. All of the above policies and procedures should be announced prominently in the journal and should be incorporated into the journal's instructions to authors.

Index

Page numbers followed by "d," "f," and "t," indicate displays, figures, and tables, respectively.